Color Atlas of
Cytology of the Dog and Cat

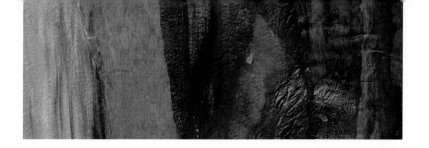

Color Atlas of Cytology of the Dog and Cat

Rebecca Baker, DVM, DVSc, Dipl ACVP,
Rockcliffe Park, Ontario, Canada

John H. Lumsden, DVM, MSc, Dipl ACVP,
Department of Pathology,
University of Guelph,
Guelph, Ontario, Canada

with 723 full-color illustrations

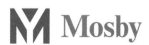 Mosby

St. Louis Baltimore Boston Carlsbad Chicago Minneapolis New York Philadelphia Portland
London Milan Sydney Tokyo Toronto

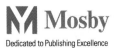

Publisher: John A. Schrefer
Executive Editor: Linda L. Duncan
Senior Developmental Editor: Teri Merchant
Project Manager: Carol Sullivan Weis
Senior Production Editor: Rick Dudley
Designer: Judi Lang

On the cover:

Images clockwise from left: Canine, fine needle, skin, basal cell tumor; canine, fine needle, skin mass, melanoma; canine, fine needle, axillary mass, liposarcoma; canine, fine needle, prostatic carcinoma.

Mosby, Inc.
A Harcourt Health Sciences Company
11830 Westline Industrial Drive
St. Louis, Missouri 63146

Printed in the United States of America

Library of Congress Cataloging in Publication Data

Baker, Rebecca, D.V.M.
    Color atlas of cytology of the dog and cat / Rebecca Baker, John
H. Lumsden.
        p.   cm.
    Includes bibliographical references.
    ISBN 0-8151-0402-2
    1. Dogs—Diseases Atlases.   2. Cats—Diseases Atlases.
    3. Veterinary cytology Atlases.   I. Lumsden, John, H.   II. Title.
    SF991.B26   1999
    636.77'0896—dc21   99-37111
                                                                              CIP

99 00 01 02 03 GW/KPT 9 8 7 6 5 4 3 2 1

To our families

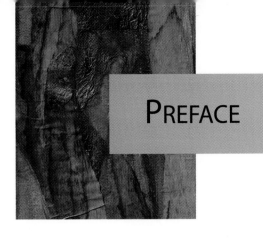

PREFACE

Color Atlas of Cytology of the Dog and Cat is a comprehensive treatment of diagnostic cytology for companion animals including illustrations of cells from common inflammatory, hyperplastic, and neoplastic lesions. A unique feature of this atlas is the addition of photographs of cells from normal tissues.

Diagnostic cytology is used by clinicians to investigate lesions that are visible, palpable, or identified using imaging techniques. As with any diagnostic test, when, where, and how the procedure is used greatly affect the reliability of the interpretation.

This atlas provides color photographs illustrating pertinent features of lesions observed in dogs and cats. Photographs were made from cytological samples harvested from confirmed lesions. This requirement limited our selection of representative lesions to those with sometimes less than ideal cytological features but also mimics the experience encountered daily by cytopathologists. Cytological features are illustrated using photographs of air-dried Wright's-stained cells. The marked influence of alternative fixatives and stains on the cellular cytoplasmic and nuclear features are illustrated using representative examples in Chapter 2. Awareness of these features assists understanding of the differences in appearance and thus descriptive terminology used in veterinary and human diagnostic cytology.

The photographs of representative cells from healthy young dogs and cats are included within organ systems. Cytological preparations were made immediately after euthanasia. Although artifactual changes must be considered when comparisons are made with cells obtained from live individuals, reference to these photographs is expected to be of value, especially to early students of cytopathology.

Reliable cytological interpretation requires examination of adequate, well-preserved, representative cells. The sampling procedures including the slide preparation techniques are frequently the major limitation to slide quality and interpretation and thus value to the clinician and patient. General sampling techniques are described in Chapter 2. Additional details and references are included for many sections.

Another feature of this atlas is the brief summary of lesions common to each organ system, with pertinent references, prevalence, and the reported strength or limitations for cytological diagnoses. To date there are too few studies documenting the diagnostic utility of cytopathology in veterinary medicine for various types of neoplasia, especially studies confirming the ability to provide prognostic information or showing correlation with histopathology. Reminding readers of this lack of documentation may stimulate prospective studies confirming the utility of cytopathology biopsies to identify neoplastic lesions and to predict their biological progression with, or without, the influence of therapy.

We are confident that this atlas will be a useful reference for clinicians and students of veterinary cytopathology. Review of sampling techniques and access to illustrations of cells from normal tissues and common lesions will improve the clinician's ability to assess sample quality. Resampling can be done immediately if required. The clinician may interpret common lesions or confidently refer quality slides to a cytopathologist. Together this will reduce clinician's time and costs to owner, as well as providing faster diagnosis and improving quality of patient care.

Rebecca Baker
John H. Lumsden

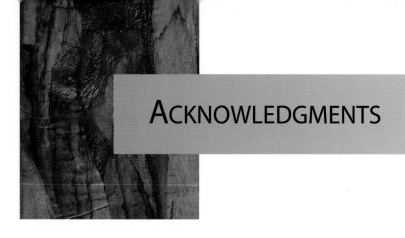

ACKNOWLEDGMENTS

Many individuals have contributed to the current state of development in veterinary diagnostic cytopathology. We have been directly influenced by several medical cytologists, especially Professors N. Soderstrom, J. Zajicek, and J. Frost, and veterinary cytologists, including Professors V. Perman, J. Rossel, and V. Valli. Each made specific contributions for which we are grateful. We specifically wish to thank Dr. Judy Taylor for her expertise and willingness to write and prepare photographs for Chapters 5 and 16. We wish to thank each faculty person, graduate student, and clinician contributing to the Ontario Veterinary College clinical pathology teaching files, including anatomic pathologists providing verification of diagnoses. We wish to thank Dr. T. French, Dr. K. Prasse, Dr. R. Duncan, Dr. R. Jacobs, Dr. W. Vernau, Dr. D. Borjesson, Dr. J. Zinkle, and colleagues, and each contributor to ASVCP study sets used to obtain photographs of case material. Also, we wish to thank Dr. Jeff McCartney for drafting legend descriptions for some of the photographs. Each added significantly to the range of case material and interpretation. We would like to express our gratitude to Linda Duncan of Mosby, whose persistent belief in the project kept us motivated and brought the project to completion.

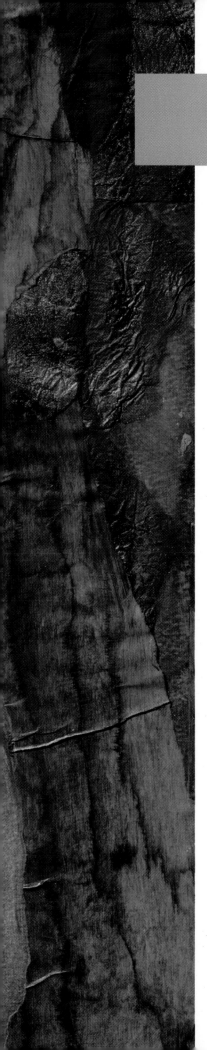

CONTENTS

Color Atlas of
Cytology of the Dog and Cat

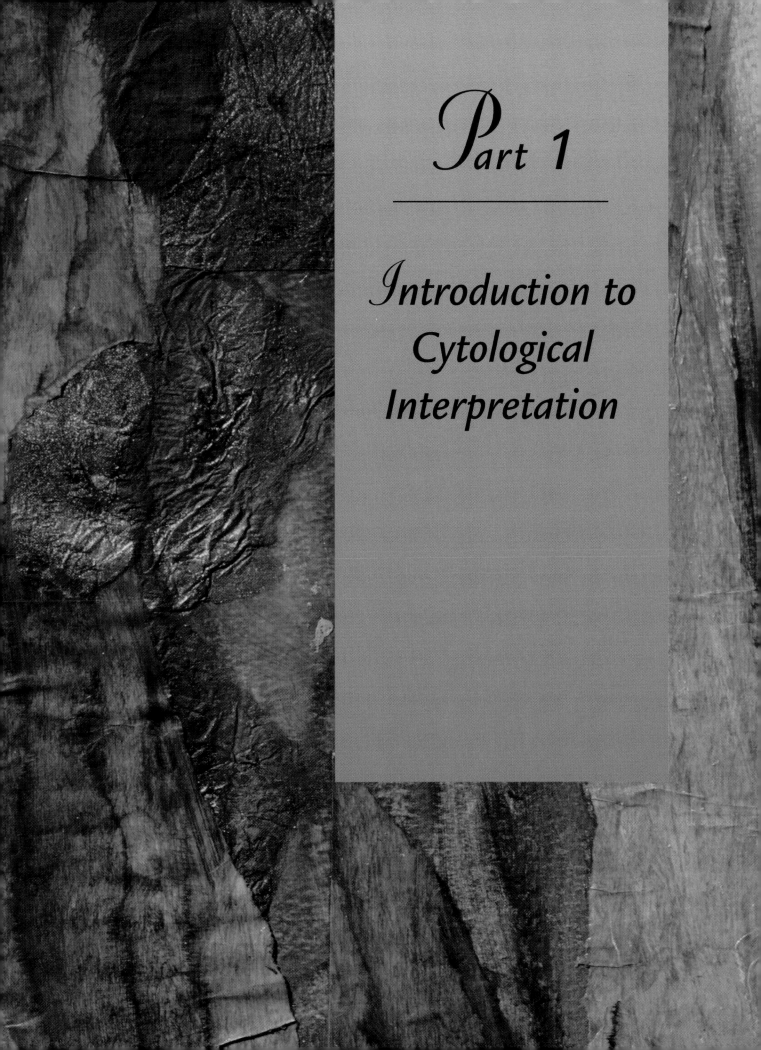

$\mathcal{P}$art 1

$\mathcal{I}$ntroduction to Cytological Interpretation

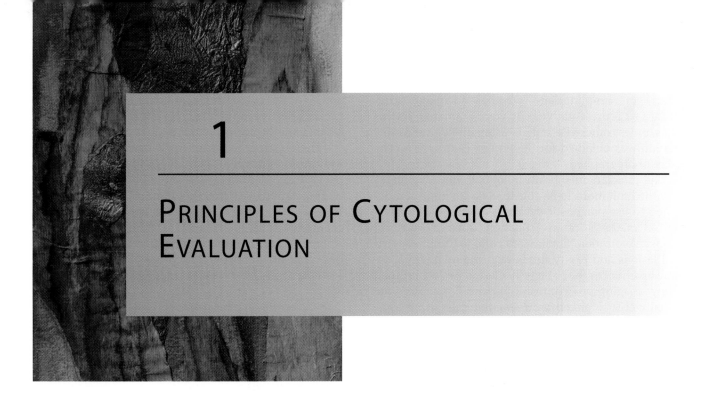

1

PRINCIPLES OF CYTOLOGICAL EVALUATION

ytopathology, or diagnostic cytology, is the microscopic examination of cells for investigation of clinical disorders. Cytopathology includes the procedures used to obtain and stain cells for microscopic examination, description of the cells, and collation of the morphological information with the clinical data, creating an interpretation or diagnosis benefiting the clinician and patient. Exfoliative or aspiration biopsy techniques are used to collect and examine cells for the investigation of inflammatory, infectious, and neoplastic lesions or disorders. *Exfoliative* cytology techniques are used to obtain cells from surface lesions and cavities. *Aspiration biopsy* techniques are used to obtain cells from lesions that are visible, palpable, or can be delineated using imaging techniques. Fine-needle aspiration biopsy (FN, FNA, FNAB) and aspiration biopsy cytology (ABC) are similar procedures used to biopsy cells. FNA biopsies should not be confused with the small-core biopsies used to obtain a small core of tissue for histological examination. Impression smears can be made from small-core biopsies for cytological examination.

Many biopsy and staining procedures are described in human (Bibbo, 1997; Cardozo, 1973; DeMay, 1996; Linsk, 1989; Orell, 1992; Söderström, 1966) and veterinary (Cowell, 1999; Duncan, 1994; Fournel-Fleury, 1994; Perman, 1979; Rebar, 1980) diagnostic cytology textbooks and handbooks. Most of the variation relates to the discipline training of the individuals who promoted the use of diagnostic cytology and the rapid introduction and acceptance for clinical use. Although cell fixation and staining procedures markedly alter the appearance of cells, various fixation and staining protocols have been used successfully. The microscopist must be familiar with the appearance of nor-

mal and abnormal cells, tissues, and lesions and apply basic principles for interpretation. Because each technique has strengths and weaknesses, use of more than one method of fixation and staining can be advantageous for challenging lesions.

EXPECTATIONS OF CYTOPATHOLOGY

Diagnostic cytology is used to screen for potential disease and to differentiate and identify a variety of lesions. Diagnostic cytology can be used independently or in conjunction with a surgical biopsy to obtain a definitive diagnosis or, at least, to obtain preliminary information that assists making clinical decisions regarding prognosis, treatment, or the need for further investigation. Cytological details are used to differentiate the type and the state of activity of cells. Inflammatory cells, bacteria, and fungi are visible when using Romanowsky's stains. For inflammatory lesions resulting from infectious agents, the organisms are often detected. These preliminary observations provide direction for sample handling and culture procedures, as well as an initial approach to therapy. If a lesion is noninflammatory, benign and neoplastic lesions can often be differentiated.

The diagnostic accuracy of cytological examinations is usually assessed against histopathology classifications. Although traditional, this comparison is not always valid. Controlled prospective studies are required to confirm the ability of histological and cytological classifications to predict biological behavior of neoplastic lesions. Many classification schemes have a limited ability to predict biological behavior, including response to therapy, and require further study. When correlations are made between cytological and histological diagnoses, it is necessary to consider the effects of sampling and whether adequate, well-preserved representative cells were examined. In this atlas, unless otherwise stated, histopathological confirmation was obtained for the lesions from which cells were photographed.

The clinician must be aware of both the advantages and the limitations to be able to make an informed decision to use diagnostic cytology, as opposed to alternative methods of investigation, such as surgical biopsy. Aspiration biopsies are obtained from superficial lesions and cavity fluids with minimal effort, expense, or risk to the patient. If a lesion can be outlined using imaging procedures, experienced operators are usually able to obtain representative cells using aspiration techniques. The effort, risk, and expense increase with deeper lesions but are usually low relative to surgical biopsy.

Biopsy samples must contain adequate, representative, and well-preserved cells. The clinician may interpret the cytology biopsy immediately in-clinic or may submit slides and cavity fluids to a laboratory for further processing and interpretation by a consulting cytopathologist. If truly interested, clinicians can develop skill in interpreting many lesions. Even if the slides are sent to a cytopathologist for interpretation, it is highly recommended that the clinician stain and examine one or more slides to confirm the presence of adequate numbers of intact and likely representative cells. This preliminary examination by the clinician ensures continuing improvement in the sampling and slide preparation techniques used, as well as the quality of biopsies submitted for consultation. Comparison of the interpretations between the clinician and the consulting cytopathologists, or reports from surgical biopsies, will result in increasing ability and confidence for interpretation of routine lesions and an increasing awareness of the strengths and limitations of diagnostic cytology.

The pathologist should be provided with the clinical history and the results from physical examination and related laboratory tests before a cytological diagnosis is attempted. Without such descriptive information, simple decisions, such as whether the cell harvest appears to be adequate or representative, are subjective. The clinical data provides considerable compensation for loss of tissue architecture when interpreting cytological biopsies. Although an experienced cytologist may be able to provide a useful clinical diagnosis for many lesions when the sample is less than adequate or when clinical data is not provided, the risk for incorrect interpretations increases dramatically if done routinely. The cytologist should know when to report an inadequate biopsy and when to delay interpretation until the clinical data is provided. The frequency of incorrect diagnoses resulting from inadequate samples and lack of clinical data versus the experience and interpretive ability of the cytopathologist is not known. Each factor is additive and must be considered when assessing the utility of cytopathology diagnoses.

When reporting results, the cytopathologist should indicate the degree of confidence in the diagnosis. If positive and definitive, this should be clear. If degrees of uncertainty exist, this should be stated. If additional investigation is required, this opinion should be reported.

In summary, the more important links in the chain of events leading to successful use of clinical cytology include:

- Selection of appropriate clinical cases for cytological examination, that is, can a cytological examination be expected to answer the clinical question?
- Successful biopsy of representative well-preserved cells
- Familiarity with the fixation and staining methods used
- Access to the pertinent clinical data, including the clinical questions to be answered, that is, some indication of the differential diagnoses
- The training, experience, and knowledge of the microscopist or cytopathologist

This atlas provides photographs of cells from normal tissues and from lesions with confirmed diagnoses. References are used to support statements relating to the prevalence of neoplasia in various organ systems and the diagnostic utility of cytological examinations.

References

Bibbo, M. *Comprehensive Cytopathology.* ed 2. WB Saunders, Philadelphia, 1997.

Cardozo, P.L. *Atlas of Clinical Cytology.* Targa b.v.'s-Hertogenbosch, The Netherlands, 1973.

Cowell, R.L., Tyler, R.D., and Meinkoth, J.H.: *Diagnostic Cytology and Hematology of the Dog and Cat.* ed 2. St Louis, 1999, Mosby.

DeMay, R.M. *The Art and Science of Cytopathology, volumes I and II, Aspiration Cytology.* ASCP Press, Chicago, 1996.

Duncan, J.R., Prasse, K.W., and Mahaffey, E.A. Cytology. In *Veterinary Laboratory Medicine Clinical Pathology.* ed 3. J.R. Duncan, K.W. Prasse, and E.A. Mahaffey (eds). Iowa State University Press, Ames, Iowa, 1994.

Fournel-Fleury, C., Magnol, J-P., and Guelfi, J-F. *Color Atlas of Cancer Cytology of the Dog and Cat.* C. Fournel-Fleury, J-P. Magnol, and J-F. Guelfi (eds). Conference Nationale des Veterinaires Specialises en Petits Animaux, Paris, 1994.

Linsk, J.A. and Franzen, S. *Clinical Aspiration Cytology.* JB Lippincott, Philadelphia, 1989.

Orell, S.R., Sterrett, G.F., Walters, M.N-I., et al. *Manual and Atlas of Fine Needle Aspiration Cytology.* Churchill Livingstone, New York, 1992.

Perman, V., Alsaker, R.D., and Riis, R.C. *Cytology of the Dog and Cat.* American Animal Hospital Association, South Bend, Ind, 1979.

Rebar, A.H. *Handbook of Veterinary Cytology.* Ralston Purina Company, St Louis, 1980.

Söderström, N. *Fine-Needle Aspiration Biopsy.* Grune & Stratton, New York, 1966.

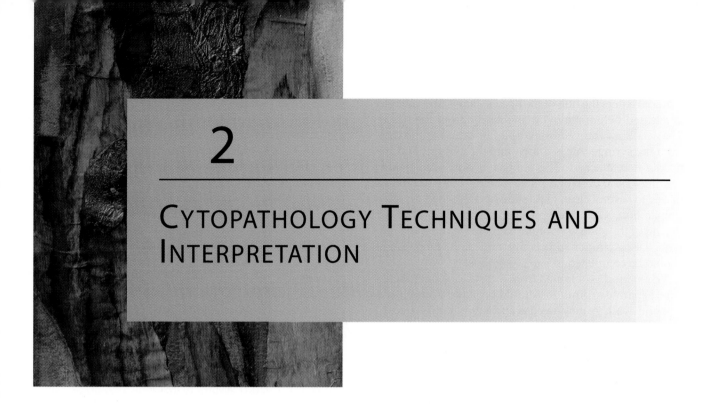

2

CYTOPATHOLOGY TECHNIQUES AND INTERPRETATION

SAMPLING TECHNIQUES

Fine-Needle Aspiration Biopsy

PRINCIPLES

FNA biopsies are used to biopsy cells from any palpable lesion.* Internal lesions are successfully aspirated using image-guided biopsies, but experience is required for consistent success (DeMay, 1996). Aseptic techniques must be used if there is a risk for infection. Sedation or anesthesia is used as required to reduce unnecessary pain and risk. Fine-needle aspirations are commonly obtained from superficial locations without the use of local anesthetics because the discomfort to the patient may be no greater than the injection of anesthetic solutions.

Cells are drawn into the barrel of the needle, transferred, and distributed onto a glass slide. The cells are immediately fixed and later stained. Although the basic techniques are simple, cell harvest and preservation are frequently less than adequate in submissions to consulting cytopathologists (Orell, 1992). Each individual should learn the principles and practice the basic techniques of aspiration biopsies before using on clinical cases. Repeated use is required to maintain the skill (Orell, 1992). Subtle adaptations are required for consistent success, especially when used for a variety of lesions and locations.

New 22-gauge needles and 10- to 12-ml plastic syringes are recommended. The needle must be long enough to penetrate the tissue area of interest. Smaller- and larger-bore needles, 25- to 20-gauge, and smaller

syringes can be used. Because differences in needle gauge and syringe diameter can significantly affect harvest, arrangement, and morphology of cells from some tissues, a similar needle gauge and syringe size should be used for routine sampling.

TECHNIQUE

The needle is attached to a syringe with the plunger depressed. After the needle is inserted into the tissue to be sampled, the plunger is withdrawn and held to maintain constant vacuum during the biopsy process, that is, to the 5- to 6-ml mark. Greater vacuum is required to harvest cells from fibrotic lesions. For vascular lesions, less vacuum may reduce the amount of blood aspirated. The quality of the aspiration biopsy depends on many factors, but four require special consideration, namely: amplitude, frequency, direction, and duration (DeMay, 1996). Long insertions (high amplitude), for example, 1.5 cm, increase yield compared with short insertions (low amplitude) of the needle tip. The intent is to keep the needle tip within the lesion or tissue of interest during sampling. Three insertions per second results in good cell yields. Changing the needle direction to mimic the shape of a fan or a cone will increase cell yield and the volume of lesion sampled. The direction of insertion should be changed only when the needle is most withdrawn. If the direction of the needle tip is changed when advanced, unnecessary laceration of tissues and increased aspiration of blood occur. This results in dilution of the primary cells of interest and increased risk for clotting. If clotting is initiated, sample quality, spreading of cells, and cell preservation may be seriously compromised.

---

*Cardozo, 1973; Cowell, 1999; DeMay, 1996; Fournel-Fleury, 1994; Jacobs, 1988; Linsk, 1989; Orell, 1992; Perman, 1979; Söderström, 1966.

Aspiration is stopped before or as soon as aspirate material enters the hub of the needle, that is, the vacuum is released before removing the needle from the tissue. The needle is removed from the lesion or tissue and then from the syringe. Air is drawn into the syringe, and the needle is reattached. The plunger is advanced gently, ejecting a *small* drop of aspirate material onto the surface of one to several clean glass slides as described for slide preparation. Cells are spread immediately. Rapid air drying of the slide is essential to preserve cell morphology. The aspiration procedure and slide preparation should be completed in 5 to 10 seconds.

When fluid is obtained from a cystic or a necrotic lesion, separate aspirations should be made from the peripheral wall. A new needle and syringe are used to separate origin of the cells.

If a syringe holder is available, one hand becomes free for palpating and outlining the lesion boundaries and thus helping direct the movement of the needle tip. Syringe holders are not required but are advantageous when aspirating most lesions.

Needle biopsies, also called *nonaspiration fine-needle biopsies,* are preferred by some cytopathologists, especially for vascular lesions (Cowell, 1999; DeMay, 1996; Orell, 1992). The needle, without an attached syringe, is inserted into the tissue of interest. Repeated short, dartlike movements are made advancing and withdrawing the needle several times. The needle tip is retained within the lesion, but the direction is changed to increase the area of the lesion investigated. A syringe is attached to the needle to eject cells from the needle lumen onto glass slides. Although cell harvest may be low, the reduced dilution with blood can result in greater visibility of the representative cells.

Common Problems Associated with Aspiration Biopsies

Rough movements cause excessive laceration of the tissues, especially when the needle tip is in the advance position (DeMay, 1996; Linsk, 1989; Orell, 1992). This is a common sampling error. The increased bleeding and release of thromboplastin activates clotting and proteolytic enzymes, leading to loss of intracellular details.

A constant vacuum should be maintained when aspirating cells. A pumping action *should not* be used. The confusion appears to relate to bone marrow biopsies, in which a pumping action is used to dislodge marrow granules (Jain, 1986).

Aspirated cells that enter the syringe are often lost for examination because they are not readily transferred to the glass slide. Excess blood can be removed from a slide by tipping against an absorbent material, such as tissue paper. Cell aggregates may become visible. The tip of a clean glass slide or coverslip is used to "pull off" the cells, which are spread over another glass slide or coverslip (Cowell, 1999; DeMay, 1996; Orell, 1992). Speed is essential. The aspiration procedure and the preparation of slides should be completed as quickly as possible.

FNA biopsies are used increasingly in conjunction with imaging techniques, including ultrasound and fluoroscopy. Each has advantages and disadvantages (DeMay, 1996; Orell, 1992). Directed biopsies can be obtained from deep lesions otherwise only accessible by surgical exposure. Additional time is usually required when using imaging techniques to guide aspiration biopsies. Needles may be rinsed with heparin (DeMay, 1996; Orell, 1992) or ethylenediaminetetraacetic acid (EDTA) solutions to retard clotting. Heparin alters cell morphology. The anticoagulant effects on morphology are kept to a minimum if the excess heparin solution is expelled, using a syringe to force air through the interior of the needle, before using for aspiration biopsy. With experience, very small lesions can be aspirated (DeMay, 1996; Orell, 1992).

Participation of the cytopathologist during the sampling procedure is recommended but not always practical (DeMay, 1996; Linsk, 1989; Orell, 1992). The radiologist, clinician, and cytopathologist must communicate and work as a team. Each should understand the potential influences of biopsy procedures on cell harvest and morphological details and thus the resulting cytological interpretation.

Exfoliative Cytology

IMPRESSION SMEARS

Impression smears are made from the surface of lesions or tissues (Cowell, 1999; Perman, 1979). Lesions of epithelial surfaces support bacterial growth with resultant chemotaxis of inflammatory cells that may obscure cells of primary interest. More commonly, impression smears are made from the cut surface of surgical biopsy or postmortem tissues. A fresh surface is created using a scalpel blade. Fluid is adsorbed using tissues or paper towels. The surface of a clean glass slide is brought to touch the tissue surface, removed, and the cells are rapidly air-dried. Variations in technique are described that enhance cell harvest and reduce the physical stress and shearing forces that increase cell rupture. For small pieces of tissue, such as a lymph node, the tissue is held in forceps and the glass slide is lightly "rolled" over the freshly dried cut surface without allowing any "sliding" action. When the glass slide is applied to the tissue surface and lifted perpendicularly, the suction created may reduce cell harvest.

Swabs, Scrapings, or Brushings

Cells are harvested and transferred to glass slides using various aids, such as cotton swabs, tongue depressors, and scalpel blades (Belford, 1998; Cowell, 1999; Perman, 1979). Cotton swabs can be used for collecting and transferring cells from vaginal and ear canals and from conjunctival and mucosal surfaces. A scalpel can be used to gently harvest a thin layer of cells from the surface of oral lesions or from postmortem and surgical biopsy tissues. A curved scalpel blade assists spreading of the cellular material in a very thin layer over the glass slide. The scalpel technique is especially useful when a high component of connective tissue cells are present within a tissue. Brush biopsies are very effective when used in conjunction with endoscopic techniques to harvest, transfer, and spread cells onto glass slides.

Fluids

Cytological examination of body cavity fluids usually includes determination of the protein concentration, nucleated cell count, and a morphological description of the cells. The percentage of major cell types may be estimated or counted. Direct smears may be adequate for cytological examination if the cell count is sufficiently high. The turbidity of the fluid is a useful indicator of cell concentration.

When cavity fluid cell counts are low, concentrated smear preparations are required for adequate examination. Cytocentrifuges are designed to concentrate cells from small aliquots of fluid directly onto glass slides. If not available, cells can be concentrated using any laboratory centrifuge. After centrifugation the supernatant fluid is removed, the cells are resuspended in a few drops of remaining supernatant, and small drops are transferred to glass slides and spread. Gravity sedimentation can also be used to concentrate cells. Gravity sedimentation is especially useful for cerebrospinal fluid (CSF) if a cytocentrifuge is not immediately available. The steps required for CSF slide preparation and fixation must be done carefully (see Chapter 6). Cells from fluids can be fixed in preservatives, but special filtration and staining procedures are required.

SLIDE PREPARATION

Noncytologists often do not appreciate the importance and the procedures required to make good smears (DeMay, 1996; Orell, 1992). The procedure is easier to demonstrate than to describe. For fine-needle aspirations the needle tip should touch the glass surface as the syringe plunger is advanced to *push* a small drop of aspirate material onto the glass surface. *Do not blow* the aspirate material from a distance onto the glass. Several slides can be prepared from the material within the barrel of a 1-inch needle. Each drop should not be much larger than the head of a pin. When the drop is too small, cells often rupture. When the drop is

too large (the more common problem), it is difficult to spread cells thinly and delicately over the glass surface.

Several techniques for smear preparation are described. The most commonly used is the *drawback and push away* method (Belford, 1998; Cowell, 1999; DeMay, 1996; Orell, 1992; Perman, 1979) as used for blood. A spreader slide is placed on the glass surface at about a 30- to 45-degree angle. The spreader slide is pulled back to the edge of the aspirate, allowing the cells and fluid to spread laterally by capillary action. As soon as the cells and fluid reach one half to two thirds the width of the slide, the spreader slide is advanced quickly and smoothly to distribute a thin layer of cells. The feather tip, which often contains the most significant cells, must remain within the working area of the slide. The distribution of cells on the slide can be adjusted by: (1) the angle of the spreader slide, (2) the length of time allowed for lateral movement, and (3) the volume of aspirate originally placed on the slide. Some cytologists recommend stopping the spreader slide so that a concentration of cells is deposited near the end of the smear (Cowell, 1999; Perman, 1979). This procedure has advantages and disadvantages. There is an increased concentration of cells, but the reduced rate of drying contributes to artifactual changes. Thick layers and clusters of cells often cannot be examined if only using Romanowsky's stains. If large aggregates of cells are visible at the feathered end, they may be spread immediately using the "squash" technique.

The "squash," or "pull-apart," technique is recommended if the texture of the aspirate prevents uniform distribution of the cells when using the drawback and push away method (Belford, 1998; Cowell, 1999; DeMay, 1996; Orell, 1992; Perman, 1979). The spreader glass slide is placed over the small drop of aspirate, and the two slides are separated using only horizontal force. If there is poor spreading of tissue fragments, *gentle* vertical pressure may be added while separating the slides. Unnecessary vertical pressure adds to the shearing forces, resulting in increased rupture of cells. The squash technique should be used when the aspirate contains excess mucin or small tissue particles and when the blood smear technique has not resulted in an expected distribution of cells. A needle bore greater than 21 gauge frequently results in small-core biopsies that spread poorly using the blood smear technique.

Optimal cell morphology may be expected when aspirates are spread between coverslips (Duncan, 1994; Orell, 1992). A small drop of aspirate is placed on a coverslip, another coverslip is placed at an angle over the aspirate, and the two cover slips are separated. Coverslip labeling and staining procedures require more technical input than do use of glass slides and automated staining procedures.

Fixation

AIR-DRYING

Air-drying is used routinely in veterinary cytopathology (Belford, 1998; Cowell, 1999; Perman, 1979). Air-drying must be accomplished quickly to attain optimal cytoplasmic and nuclear detail. Slow drying leads to many artifactual changes, particularly condensation, especially of the nucleus, with resulting loss of detail. Air-dried cells are usually stained with one of the Romanowsky's stains, but an aqueous stain, such as new methylene blue, can be used to advantage in some situations (Cowell, 1999; Perman, 1979).

In most medical cytopathology laboratories, at least in North America, ethyl alcohol is used to "wet-fix" cells before using bichrome or trichrome stains, such as hematoxylin and eosin (H&E) or Papanicolaou's stain (Pap stain) (Bibbo, 1997; DeMay, 1996; Orell, 1992). Because a monolayer of cells dries very quickly, each smear must be fixed *immediately* with a commercial alcohol-based spray fixative, preferably by an assistant, or by immersion into an alcohol-filled coplin jar (DeMay, 1996; Orell, 1992). When slides are prepared, cells are often allowed to dry before "wet" fixation. When this happens, cell morphology and tinctorial properties are poor and usually unsuitable for examination with either trichrome or Romanowsky's stains.

Although air-dried Wright's stained cells allow satisfactory interpretation of the majority of cytological biopsies, cytopathologists should be familiar with the advantages of alternative methods of fixation and staining. Because of the density of Romanowsky's stain uptake, especially within the nuclei, intracellular details are often obscured within tissue clusters or when there are multiple layers of cells. In contrast, cell relationships, borders, and nuclear details are still visible within dense cell clusters if cells are stained with bichrome or trichrome stains. Bichrome and trichrome stains require "wet" fixation to attain the morphological advantages offered by these stains.

In most clinical situations, immediate alcohol fixation is not practical or is not successful, based on the experience of the authors. After air-drying, cells can be rehydrated for 30 seconds in saline, immediately fixed in alcohol using dipping or a commercial spray fixative, and stained using a bichrome or trichrome stain (Chan, 1988; Jörundsson, 1999), as discussed in the following section on staining.

Staining (Figs. 2-1 to 2-11)

AIR-DRIED SMEARS

Romanowsky's Stains

In most laboratories the Romanowsky's stain used for hematology is used for routine cytology. Romanowsky's stains include Wright's stain, Giemsa stain, Wright's Giemsa stain, and May-Grünwald-Giemsa stain, as well as the "fast" stains developed for use in private clinics. These are alcohol-based stains for use on air-dried cells. If staining is to be delayed for more than a few days, cell preservation is enhanced if the air-dried cells are immersed for a few minutes in methyl alcohol. This procedure should not be confused with the rehydration and immediate fixation in alcohol procedures discussed for use with bichrome and trichrome stains. Tinctorial properties of cells can vary markedly when different Romanowsky's stains are used, especially between the fast Wright's type of stains. The microscopist must be familiar with the appearance of stain precipitate to prevent misinterpretation of infectious agents. Because Wright's stain is the predominant stain used by veterinary cytologists and for consistency, the majority of photographs included in this atlas are made from air-dried Wright's stained cells.

Aqueous Stains

New methylene blue (NMB) is an aqueous-based stain that allows immediate examination after application to air-dried cells. It was used extensively in veterinary cytology until the fast Wright's stains were marketed (Perman, 1979). NMB is still used to advantage when screening slides for cell harvest, inflammation, and some infectious agents. The nuclear chromatin aggregation more closely resembles the appearance expected with alcohol fixation and trichrome staining than for Romanowsky's stained cells. Nucleoli stain well. NMB is not good for cytoplasmic details, although fungal cell walls are often illustrated well because of negative staining. Because fungi and bacteria grow in aqueous but not in alcohol solutions, aqueous stains must be examined regularly for contamination.

Gram's Stain

Gram's stain is used to differentiate gram-negative and gram-positive bacteria. Bacterial presence, shape, and size are readily observed when using most Romanowsky's stains, but all bacteria are basophilic (Belford, 1998; Cowell, 1999; Perman, 1979).

Bichrome and Trichrome Stains

Trichrome stains, particularly Papanicolaou's stain, are used extensively in human medical laboratories. Trichrome stains are applied to cells that have been immediately wet-fixed. Sano's modified stain (Sano, 1949) is considered to be preferable to Papanicolaou's stain (Roszel, 1975).

H&E is used routinely for staining histological sections. Many histopathologists prefer using H&E stain for cytopathology interpretation because of their greater familiarity with cell tinctorial properties. Unfortunately, there is a marked loss of nuclear detail when air-dried cells are stained with H&E compared with the detail available when cells are rehydrated or immediately fixed with alcohol (see Figs. 2-5 and 2-6).

Routine and ultrafast trichrome and bichrome staining procedures can be used if air-dried cells are rehydrated and immediately wet-fixed (Chan, 1988). These procedures can be practical for use in a diagnostic referral laboratory. One or more unstained slides are kept in reserve, rehydrated, fixed, and stained when required to assist cell examination and interpretation. Although morphology is optimal when cells are rehydrated and fixed within a few hours of preparing the smear, morphology is still adequate for clinical use when rehydration is delayed 1 to 2 days (Jörundsson, 1999). Most of the advantages of bichrome or trichrome stains are attained, including excellent nuclear details and the ability to examine cells within tissue clumps. In addition, erythrocyte lysis increases the ability to examine the remaining cells.

Special Stains

Cytochemical and immunocytochemistry stains are used to assist the differentiation of the cell line or family origin, especially when cells are poorly differentiated (Bibbo, 1997; DeMay, 1996; Jain, 1988; Orell, 1992). Staining procedures must be validated for use with each cell type of interest within each species. An experienced stain technologist is required to attain repeatable and reliable staining results. Although of considerable academic interest, routine use of special staining techniques is the exception for most diagnostic laboratories. As well, when most required for classification of least-differentiated neoplastic cells, phenotypic expression may be unreliable.

Artifactual changes are created by each method used for fixation and staining. The changes affect cell diameter, nuclear-cytoplasmic ratio (N:C ratio), nuclear chromatin, nucleolar appearance, and tinctorial properties. The effects of fixation and staining differ with the cell type. In addition, the nuclear chromatin pattern effects may differ when hyperplasia and neoplasia are present. Sampling, fixation, and staining techniques must be applied consistently to allow differentiation of artifactual changes from biologically important changes in cell morphology.

The appearance of cells from a mast cell tumor, a poorly differentiated melanosarcoma, and a squamous cell carcinoma with secondary inflammation are included to illustrate the dramatic influence of fixation and staining techniques. Note the nuclear and cytoplasmic details, as well as the differences in tinctorial properties (Figs. 2-1 to 2-11).

SLIDE EXAMINATION (Figs. 2-12 to 2-22)

The slide is examined by holding it toward a source of light to determine size, location, and density of stained areas. The slide is scanned at a low magnification to identify the cellular areas within the slide and the cells requiring examination at higher magnification. The cells are examined for number, type, and state of preservation. In conjunction with the clinical data, the cells are also assessed as to whether they are likely representative of the lesion and whether they are present in sufficient number with adequate preservation for satisfactory cytological interpretation. Cells normally foreign to the source warrant particular attention. For example, squamous epithelial cells should not be present in a lymph node aspirate or a cavity fluid. If contamination from skin of the animal or operator is ruled out, further investigation is required to confirm or rule out the possibility of metastasis.

CYTOLOGICAL TERMINOLOGY

The terminology used when describing and interpreting cellular details for exfoliative and fine-needle cytology smears is similar to that used for histopathology sections, within limitations. Subtle to marked differences in definition have developed. When a full-thickness histological biopsy is examined, all cell layers and the depth and degree of changes within a lesion are visible. The cytoplasmic diameter and density often indicate the degree of cell differentiation. The nuclear appearance is assessed relative to the degree of cell maturation. Tissue architecture is used extensively in the histopathological classification. As well, local invasion, or metastasis, is relied on for differentiation between some benign and malignant tumors.

In contrast, when using exfoliative cytology to screen for epithelial lesions, differentiation between degrees of dysplasia and carcinoma in situ is based on the morphology of exfoliating superficial cells as indicators of changes occurring within cells from the deeper layers (DeMay, 1996; Frost, 1986; Orell, 1992). When cells are obtained using fine-needle aspirations, the original relationship between aspirated and surrounding cells or tissues is unknown. Interpretation becomes very dependent on awareness of the influence of the techniques used, as well as the location and description of the lesion.

In cytology, cytoplasmic criteria are used primarily to identify the cell family origin and the degree of maturation (DeMay, 1996; Frost, 1986; Orell, 1992). Nuclear details are relied on to identify the state of cell activity (Frost, 1986) and thus to differentiate benign from malignant transformation. Inflammation is a significant environmental factor that can alter cell morphology and confound interpretation (Frost, 1986).

Euplasia is a term that has been used to apply to the baseline "normal" state of activity expected in healthy cells (Frost, 1986). This activity varies with the cell type and the stage of differentiation. The morphology of euplastic cells is used as the basic frame of reference for each cell type. For example, the level of activity is very different for bone marrow cells compared with lipocytes and for parabasal cells compared with superficial squamous epithelial cells.

Retroplasia occurs when the general activity of cells is decreased (Frost, 1986). This may result from many processes, including aging, injury, degeneration, death, and necrosis. The duration can have significant influence on cell morphological changes. Differentiation of retroplasia from the artifactual changes induced during sample collection and handling is not always readily apparent when using Romanowsky's stains.

Proplasia includes those changes associated with an increase in cellular activity (Frost, 1986). Increased cellular activity is normal when associated with, for example, increased regeneration or increased secretion, but is likely abnormal when associated with atypical hyperplasia, dysplasia, or anaplasia. It is not uncommon for proplastic and retroplastic changes to coexist.

Dysplasia is the disordered or abnormal development of cells and tissues (Frost, 1986; Jones, 1996). In differentiated cells it is interpreted as a retrogressive change presenting as altered intercellular relationships, variation in size and shape of cells, nuclear hyperchromasia, increased N:C ratio, and increased mitotic activity (Frost, 1986; Jones, 1996). Dysplasia of *exfoliating* epithelial cells indicates altered development of all epithelial cell layers, if erosive lesions and sampling error are excluded. Dysplasia may indicate a response to inflammation if mild or early neoplastic change if severe (Bibbo, 1997; DeMay, 1996; Frost, 1986; Orell, 1992).

Metaplasia is the replacement of one type of fully differentiated cell with another, usually as part of an adaptive process involving alterations in stimuli to reserve cells (Frost, 1986; Jones, 1996).

Anaplasia is the reversion of cells to a less differentiated stage (Frost, 1986; Jones, 1996). Cell pleomorphism, nuclear hyperchromasia, and increased mitotic activities are features of anaplasia (Frost, 1986). Anaplasia may be reversible, as well as a precursor or a feature of neoplasia.

Hypertrophy applies to an increase in size of an organ (Jones, 1996). If the organ size increase is due to an increase in size of individual cells, it is called *cellular hypertrophy*, whereas an increase in the number of cells is called *hyperplasia*. Hyperplasia occurs in tissues containing cells that retain the ability for division. Hyperplasia is usually a response to hormonal influences or is a compensatory or an adaptive process. Multiple underlying stimuli may be involved. Hyperplasia may be a physiological or pathological response but denotes a benign change. Hematologists and cytologists sometimes use the terms *reactive* or *hyperplastic* when describing benign populations of lymphocytes or mesothelial cells with increased cytoplasmic basophilia, nuclear hyperchromasia and mitotic activity (Belford, 1998; Cowell, 1999; Jain, 1986). Some hyperplastic changes mimic those observed with neoplastic transformation. Differentiation is usually, but not always, accomplished if all available morphological and clinical data is considered.

Neoplasm refers to a new growth of cells that proliferate autonomously (Frost, 1986; Jones, 1996). The cells morphologically and functionally, to varying degrees, resemble normal cells from which they originate. There is loss of orderly patterns of growth. The new growth serves no useful function for its host and stems from a variety of causes (Jones, 1996).

Tumor refers to any neoplasm, whether benign or malignant (Jones, 1996). *Cancer* is a general term for malignant neoplasm.

Nuclear chromatin patterns are included within cytological descriptions (Bibbo, 1997; Cowell, 1999; DeMay, 1996; Orell, 1992). Chromatin patterns relate to the state of cell activity, especially the mitotic cycle. Terms used to describe nuclear chromatin include: amorphous, fine (smooth), reticular (lacy), and coarse. These terms are not used consistently among cytopathologists, partly because the method of fixation and staining markedly affects the artifactual creation of chromatin patterns. As developed for use in gynecology, nuclear criteria are very useful for differentiating malignant transformation of epithelial cells when the cells are fixed with alcohol and a trichrome stain applied (Bibbo, 1997; Frost, 1986). Distinctive chromatin patterns and chromatin density is used to assist differentiation between benign and malignant cells. When cells are air-dried and Romanowsky's stains applied, chromatin patterns are less apparent and much less distinctive (Cardozo, 1973; DeMay, 1996). Changes in nuclear chromatin patterns associated with malignancy are often described without acknowledging the association with the method of fixation and staining. This has led to some confusion regarding the significance of chromatin patterns for differentiating malignant transformation. Just as chromatin patterns differ as a result of the effects of fixation and staining, they also differ between cell type, degree of maturity, and state of activity.

CRITERIA AND REPORTING OF INFLAMMATORY LESIONS

The presence and type of inflammatory cells, including neutrophils, monocytes, macrophages, lymphocytes, plasma cells, and eosinophils, are determined during the initial examination of a slide. Algorithms may assist the thought process of beginners during the microscopic examination (Belford, 1998; Cowell, 1999) (Box 2-1). If inflammation is present, is there an obvious etiology? Are bacteria or fungi visible? Are they free or phagocytized? If agents are not immediately visible, do the neutrophil nuclear changes suggest the influence of toxins and indicate need for more detailed examination for bacteria and submission for culture? Do the numbers of mixed free and phagocytized pleomorphic bacteria in conjunction with marked chemo-

Box 2-1

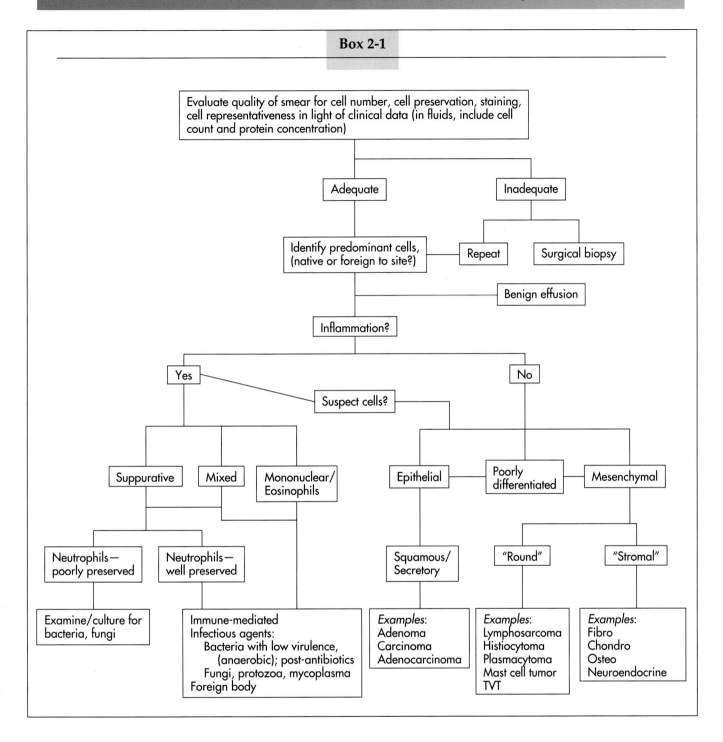

taxis of moderately preserved to well-preserved neutrophils indicate that the bacteria are possibly anaerobic agents and that special transport media and culture procedures should be considered? Diagnostic laboratories provide recommendations for sample collection and submission according to etiological agents suspected by the clinician (Cowell, 1999).

Acute, subacute, and *chronic* have been used by veterinary cytologists to classify types of inflammation (Rebar, 1980). Greater than 75% neutrophils is acute inflammation, and greater than 50% mononuclear cells is chronic inflammation. The ratio of neutrophils to

mononuclear cells does not predict duration. These definitions differ considerably from those used by histopathologists. Also, the definitions differ markedly between histopathologists and clinicians. In the experience of the authors, use of *acute, subacute,* and *chronic* as cytological descriptors of inflammation continues to create misunderstanding. Although alternative terminology has limitations, the advantages appear to outweigh the disadvantages.

The following are preferred descriptors of inflammation in cytological preparations. The inflammatory response is classified according to the predominant cell type(s) present. Additional descriptors may be added, including the mixture, or ratio, of cells.

> *Suppurative inflammation:* neutrophils predominate; "neutrophilic" and "purulent" are synonyms
>
> *Mixed inflammation:* monocytes or macrophages and neutrophils in various ratios
>
> *Mononuclear inflammation:* monocytes, macrophages, lymphocytes, plasma cells, or giant cells with few neutrophils

Because original architecture is unknown with cytological examinations, it is questionable whether pyogranulomatous or granulomatous inflammation should be used to classify a lesion, even if giant cells are present. Although additional knowledge of the lesion may support this biological response, the terminology is best restricted for use in histological classifications.

Neutrophil Morphological Changes

The presence or absence of "toxic" neutrophils is commonly reported for hematology and increasingly for cytology submissions. Unfortunately, there is lack of uniformity for the definition, use, and application of terminology.

In peripheral blood neutrophils, *cytoplasmic* granulation, vacuolation, basophilia, and the presence of Döhle's bodies are indications for "toxic" changes likely caused by toxins resulting from bacterial infections, severe inflammation, or extensive burns (Jain, 1986).

In contrast, for cytological examinations, neutrophil *nuclear* changes are examined to assess toxicity. The changes of interest are primarily the loss of filaments separating lobules, loss of normal chromatin clumping and density of chromocenters, and swelling of the nuclear lobules. Most of the morphological changes are due to chromatolysis or karyolysis. These nuclear changes are often called *lytic change, lysis,* or *toxicity* (Belford, 1998; Cowell, 1999). Although used routinely in veterinary cytopathology, such terminology is seldom used in human cytopathology. "Well-preserved" and "degenerated" neutrophils are briefly referred to as indicators of noninfectious and infectious etiology, respectively (DeMay, 1996).

Other nuclear changes observed in any aging population of neutrophils, especially when in cavity fluids, include karyopyknosis, karyorrhexis, and possibly apoptosis (Belford, 1998; Cowell, 1999). Cytoplasmic vacuolation of neutrophils within fluids and tissues, other than blood, is even less specific and usually is not reported (Perman, 1979). Nonspecific aging and degenerative changes often occur together. When neutrophil nuclear changes are marked in a purulent response, the microscopist should search diligently for infectious agents, that is, bacteria (Belford, 1998;

Cowell, 1999). If bacteria are not visible but nuclear swelling is apparent, and especially if supported by the patient signalment, recommendations should be made to the clinician to submit an aliquot for culture(s) (Belford, 1998; Cowell, 1999). The virulence and toxin production varies with the species and concentration of bacteria. Overall, certain aerobes traditionally produce more virulent toxins than do anaerobes. Thus, if there are many free and phagocytized pleomorphic bacteria visible, a suppurative or mixed inflammatory response, and neutrophils with minimal nuclear swelling, an aliquot should be submitted using specific transport media requesting culture for anaerobes (Belford, 1998; Cowell, 1999). Very swollen and degenerate neutrophils can be mistaken for macrophages. The microscopist should be informed if antibiotics have been administered.

The criteria used by cytopathologists and hematologists for classification of neutrophils as toxic in either cytology or blood samples should be defined and provided to the clinician. The currently recommended approach is to describe the specific changes observed, that is, within neutrophil nuclei for cytology samples and within neutrophil cytoplasm for blood samples.

Classification and Reporting of Neoplastic Lesions—Lumping versus Splitting

Detailed classification schemes are described for tumors involving most tissues and organs (Moulton, 1990). To be clinically relevant, classification schemes should be able to predict biological behavior, including expected response to surgical and radiation therapy or chemotherapy. For many types of tumors, criteria are still evolving. To date, histopathology is usually accepted as the gold standard for assessing accuracy of cytology diagnoses. Architecture, an important aspect of many histological classifications, cannot be determined from cytological examinations.

Cytological criteria for neoplasia rely heavily on nuclear changes (Bibbo, 1997; DeMay, 1996; Frost, 1986; Orell, 1992). The method of fixation and staining significantly affects the appearance and visibility of nuclear details. Some benign and malignant lesions can only be differentiated if there is histological evidence of local invasion or metastasis, especially when cells are well differentiated (DeMay, 1996). It is not surprising that there are differences in classification when comparing histopathology and cytopathology diagnoses. A more positive aspect is the degree of agreement between cytological and histological interpretations for most clinical cases.

Routine use of alternative methods of fixation and staining has not been adequately investigated in veterinary cytopathology for differentiating benign from well-differentiated malignant cells or for the classification of certain types of cells. Thus differentiation is usually limited to broad (lumping) versus detailed (splitting) classifications. The classifications applied should be limited to the current state of knowledge and the clinical objective. As part of the cytological interpretation, oncologists and owners expect to be informed whether there is any necessity or advantage to obtain a surgical biopsy. For some types of tumors the signalment, that is, breed, age, location, and cell type, may be the best predictor of expected biological progression. Within this atlas, broad classifications are used unless references are available to support the biological relevance of more definitive cytological classifications.

The following are simplistic guidelines used for differentiation and classification of tumors. If a palpable mass contains a monomorphic cell population, in the absence of inflammation, the diagnosis is most compatible with a tumor. The cell type, as determined primarily by the cytoplasmic features of the most differentiated cells, is used to categorize cells as epithelial or mesenchymal (Cowell, 1999; DeMay, 1996; Frost, 1986; Orell, 1992). Cytoplasmic shape, size, common borders, organelles, and secretory products (including extracellular matrix and cohesiveness) may lead to more specific classification of the cell line. Nuclear details are assessed and used to differentiate benign cells from malignant transformation. Nuclear details are interpreted in relationship to the type of cell, maturation, and expected activity.

Epithelial cells are round, cuboidal, or columnar depending on cell type and differentiation (Cowell, 1999; DeMay, 1996; Frost, 1986; Orell, 1992). The presence of common adjoining borders is a useful feature for epithelial cells. The cell type is further indicated by the presence of cilia, secretory activity, or, in the case of squamous epithelial cells, the appearance and tinctorial properties of the cytoplasm. As squamous epithelial cells mature, the N:C ratio decreases. Arrangement of cells may suggest acinar or papillary formation.

Mesenchymal cells include *spindle* and *round* cells (Belford, 1998; Cowell, 1999). Cytological details, such as shape, lysosomes, or the presence and type of extracellular matrix, may or may not allow further classification of spindle cells, especially when very anaplastic. Examples include hemangiopericytoma, fibrosarcoma, and chondrosarcoma. In contrast, several of the round, or *discrete*, cells, including hematopoietic cells, can be identified using a combination of cytoplasmic, nuclear, and tinctorial properties. Examples include lymphosarcoma, mast cell tumor, histiocytoma, plasmacytoma, and transmissible venereal tumor. Although melanosarcomas may consist of both round and spindle cells, even when poorly differentiated, some degree of cytoplasmic pigmentation is usually evident when using Romanowsky's stains (Belford, 1998; Cowell, 1999; Perman, 1979). It may not be possible to differentiate very anaplastic epithelial or

mesenchymal cells as to primary lineage. Just as there is overlap in nuclear criteria for proplasia (hyperplasia) and neoplasia (Frost, 1986), there is often overlap in the appearance of benign and well-differentiated malignant cells (Belford, 1998; Cowell, 1999; DeMay, 1996; Orell, 1992).

Cytochemical and immunocytochemical staining techniques can be used to differentiate the origin of certain specific cell lineages (Bibbo, 1997; DeMay, 1996; Orell, 1992). Unfortunately, phenotypic expression is less reliable in more anaplastic cells. A few cytochemical stains are practical for use in a diagnostic laboratory. Examples include stains for lipids (Sudan stain), specific carbohydrates (e.g., period acid–Schiff [PAS], Sudan black), and enzymes (e.g., esterase, alkaline phosphatase) (Jain, 1986). Sophisticated cytochemical and immunocytological stains are usually restricted to use in research laboratories. Each staining procedure must be validated for the species and cells of interest before being considered reliable for clinical diagnoses. This validation process should include correlation with histological diagnosis and biological progression.

Criteria of Malignancy

Criteria of malignancy are listed in most textbooks and atlases for cytology.* The fixation and staining methods must be considered when assessing nuclear morphological changes. The criteria of malignancy are based primarily on nuclear activity relative to the stage of differentiation (Frost, 1986). These criteria include hyperchromasia; anisokaryosis; high N:C ratio; multinucleation; increased and abnormal mitosis; and large, variably shaped single or multiple nucleoli and chromocenters. Chromatin patterns, nuclear molding, variation in nuclear membrane thickness, and angularity are readily visible when using alcohol fixation and trichrome staining but may be difficult to observe with air-dried Wright's stained cells. Variation in cell size (anisocytosis), cell shape (pleomorphism), and increased N:C ratio must be related to nuclear and cytoplasmic differentiation, as well as the state of cell activity. It is important to emphasize that many nuclear morphological changes of malignancy may be observed with hyperplasia, proplasia, and retroplasia and that all changes listed will not be seen in all neoplastic cells (Frost, 1986).

Both pleomorphism and monomorphism can be criteria of malignancy (Frost, 1986). Pleomorphism is a criterion in cell populations that are normally uniform in size and appearance, for example, epithelial cells. Conversely, monomorphism is of concern where pleomorphism is normally expected, for example, an aspi-

*Belford, 1998; Bibbo, 1997; Cowell, 1999; DeMay, 1996; Duncan, 1994; Frost, 1986; Linsk, 1989; Orell, 1992.

ration biopsy from a benign lymph node from which both follicular and medullary cells have been harvested. Very large cells and, for exfoliating epithelial cells, large aggregates of cells may be criteria of malignancy, although lack of normal cell adhesion is usually listed as a sign of malignancy (Cowell, 1999; DeMay, 1996; Orell, 1992). Changes in functional differentiation may be an indicator of malignancy, for example, if secretory or phagocytic activity is observed in cells not usually associated with such activity.

The cytopathologist must be familiar with cell biology, histology, histopathology, and oncology. As a cell matures, that is, becomes more differentiated, the cytoplasmic appearance usually becomes more distinctive, and for some types of cells, including hematopoietic and squamous cells, there are distinct changes in N:C ratio. The N:C ratio differs markedly for small and large lymphocytes. Erythrocytes and neutrophils are used to estimate cell and nuclear diameters, provided the effects of fixation and staining are considered.

In summary, cytoplasmic details are used to determine functional differentiation, that is, cell type and stage of differentiation. Cell activity, indicated by nuclear details relative to the cell type and stage of maturation, is used to differentiate proplasia and retroplasia from neoplasia (Frost, 1986). Many nuclear criteria of malignancy are also present in functionally active or proliferating benign cells, that is, proplastic change (Cowell, 1999; DeMay, 1996; Frost, 1986; Orell, 1992). Examples of proplasia include the appearance of mesenchymal cells within a healing bone fracture, mesothelial cells lining a fluid-filled cavity, and epithelial cells in association with chronic infectious diseases. When inflammation is present, proplasia or retroplasia may be expected, thus neoplasia must be interpreted very cautiously, if at all. Only intact well-preserved cells should be examined. Cell death, rupture of cytoplasmic or nuclear membranes, unusual or unfamiliar cell fixation, or staining methods contribute to morphological changes that can lead to misinterpretation. A population of uniform well-differentiated malignant cells may appear very similar to a benign population. The final cytological interpretation should incorporate patient clinical data, including growth rate, location, and size of tumor, as well as the expected biological behavior for the cell type and origin.

References

Belford, C. and Lumsden, J.H. Cytopathology. In *BSAVA Manual of Small Animal Clinical Pathology*. M.G. Davidson, R.W. Else, and J.H. Lumsden (eds). British Small Animal Veterinary Association, Cheltenham, UK, 1998.

Bibbo, M. *Comprehensive Cytopathology*. ed 3. WB Saunders, Philadelphia, 1997.

Cardozo, P.L. *Atlas of Clinical Cytology*. Targa b.v.'s-Hertogenbosch, The Netherlands, 1973.

Chan, J.K.C. and Kung, I.T.M. Rehydration of air-dried smears with normal saline: application in fine-needle aspiration cytologic examination. *Am J Clin Pathol* 89:30-34, 1988.

Cowell, R.L., Tyler, R.D., and Meinkoth, J.H. *Diagnostic Cytology and Hematology of the Dog and Cat*. ed 2. Mosby, St Louis, 1999.

DeMay, R.M. *The Art and Science of Cytopathology*, vol 2, Aspiration Cytology. ASCP Press, Chicago, 1996.

Duncan, J.R., Prasse, K.W., and Mahaffey, E.A. Cytology. In *Veterinary Laboratory Medicine Clinical Pathology*. ed 3. J.R. Duncan, K.W. Prasse, and E.A. Mahaffey (eds). Iowa State University Press, Ames, Iowa, 1994.

Fournel-Fleury, C., Magnol, J-P., and Guelfi, J.F. *Color Atlas of Cancer Cytology of the Dog and Cat*. C. Fournel-Fleury, J-P. Magnol, and J-F. Guelfi (eds). Conference Nationale des Veterinaires Specialises en Petits Animaux, Paris, 1994.

Frost, J.K. The cell in health and disease. An evaluation of cellular morphological expression of biological behavior. In *Monographs in Clinical Cytology*. ed 2. G.L. Wied (ed). Karger, New York, 1986.

Jacobs, R.M. Diagnostic cytology. In *Seminars in Veterinary Medicine and Surgery (Small Animal)*, vol 3, No 2, S.P. Arnoczky, P.R. Fox, and LP Tilley (eds). Grune & Stratton, New York, 1988.

Jain, N.C. *Schalm's Veterinary Hematology*. ed 4. Lea & Febiger, Philadelphia, 1986.

Jones, T.C., Hunt, R.D., and King, N.W. Disturbances of growth: aplasia to neoplasia. In *Veterinary Pathology*. ed 6. T.C. Jones, R.D. Hunt, and N.W. King (eds). Williams & Wilkins, Philadelphia, 1996.

Jörundsson, E., Lumsden, J.H., and Jacobs, R.M. Rapid staining techniques in cytopathology. *Vet Clin Pathol* 1999 (in press).

Linsk, J.A. and Franzen, S. *Clinical Aspiration Cytology*. JB Lippincott, New York, 1989.

Orell, S.R., Sterrett, G.F., Walters, M. N-I., et al. *Manual and Atlas of Fine Needle Aspiration Cytology*. Churchill Livingstone, New York, 1992.

Moulton, J.E. *Tumours in Domestic Animals*. ed 3. University of California Press, Berkeley, Calif, 1990.

Perman, V., Alsaker, R.D., and Riis, R.C. *Cytology of the Dog and Cat*. American Animal Hospital Association, South Bend, Ind, 1979.

Rebar, A.H. *Handbook of Veterinary Cytology*. Ralston Purina Company, St Louis, 1980.

Roszel, J.F. Genital cytology of the bitch. *Vet Scope* 19:2-15, 1975.

Sano, M.E. Trichrome stain for tissue section, culture or smear. *Am J Clin Pathol* 19:898- 899, 1949.

Söderström, N. *Fine-Needle Aspiration Biopsy*. Grune & Stratton, New York, 1966.

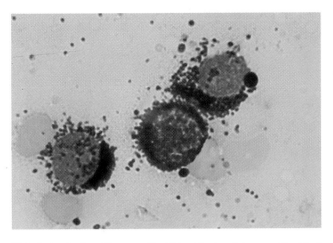

FIG. 2-1. Canine. Fine needle. Skin. Mast cell tumor. Air-dried, Wright's stain. Prominent metachromatic granules obscure nuclear details. (×630.)

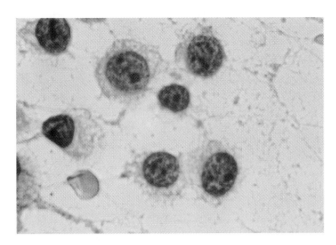

FIG. 2-2. Canine. Fine needle. Skin. Mast cell tumor. (Same case as Fig. 2-1.) Ethanol fixation, Papanicolaou's stain. Cytoplasmic granules are inapparent. Nuclear diameter is smaller. There is limited coarse nuclear chromatin clumping typical for alcohol fixation. (×630.)

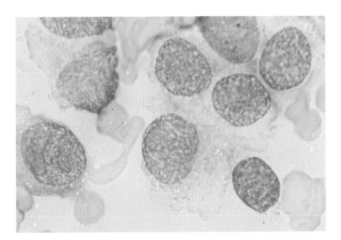

FIG. 2-3. Canine. Fine needle. Skin. (Figs. 2-4 to 2-9 are from same case.) Melanosarcoma poorly pigmented. Air-dried, Wright's stain. Cytoplasmic dimensions and borders are visible. Cytoplasm is pale blue and contains indistinct melanin "precursors." Nuclear chromatin pattern is prominent, and large nucleoli are indistinct but visible. (×630.)

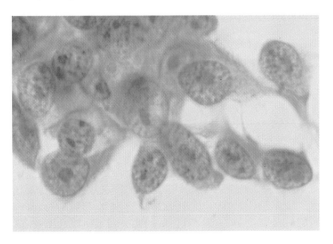

FIG. 2-4. Canine. Fine needle. Skin. Melanosarcoma poorly pigmented. Ethanol fixation, Papanicolaou's stain. Cytoplasmic detail is poor, although cell shapes and sizes are apparent. There is a fine nuclear chromatin pattern with prominent nucleoli and chromocenters. (×630.)

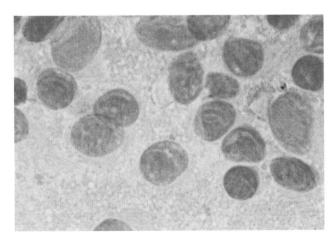

FIG. 2-5. Canine. Fine needle. Skin. Melanosarcoma poorly pigmented. Air-dried, hematoxylin and eosin stain. Cytoplasmic detail is inapparent. Nuclei are outlined, but internal details are poor. (×630.)

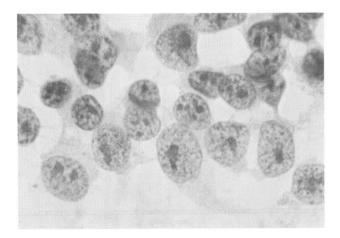

FIG. 2-6. Canine. Fine needle. Skin. Melanosarcoma poorly pigmented. Ethanol fixation, hematoxylin and eosin stain. Cytoplasmic borders and detail are poor. Nuclear membrane, heterochromatin pattern, chromocenters, and nucleoli are visible but have more uniform tinctorial properties than with trichrome staining in Fig. 2-4. (×630.)

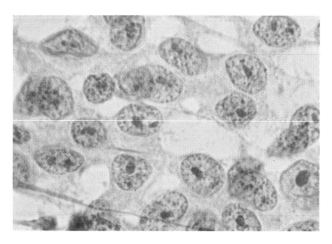

FIG. 2-7. Canine. Fine needle. Skin. Melanosarcoma poorly pigmented. Ethanol fixation, Sano's modified trichrome stain. Compare tinctorial and intracellular details with Fig. 2-4. Nucleoli are distinctive. (×630.)

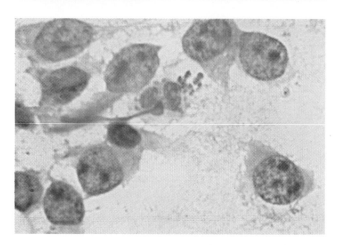

FIG. 2-8. Canine. Fine needle. Skin. Melanosarcoma poorly pigmented. Air-dried, Harleco stain. Cytoplasm and nuclear details are indistinct, although some blue granules are apparent within cytoplasm. (×630.)

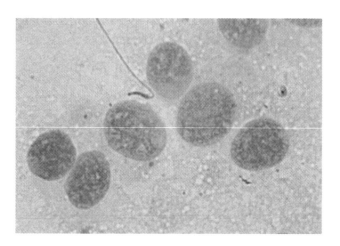

FIG. 2-9. Canine. Fine needle. Skin. Melanosarcoma poorly pigmented. Ethanol fixation, Harleco stain. Compare cytoplasmic and nuclear appearance, including diameter of cells and nuclei. (×630.)

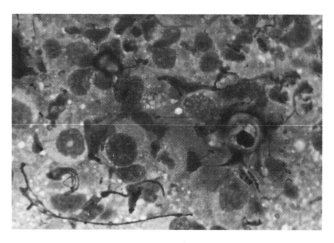

FIG. 2-10. Canine. Fine needle. Skin. Squamous cell carcinoma. Diff-Quick stain. Squamous epithelial cells are visible, but the cytoplasmic and nuclear details are indistinct because of necrosis and background inflammation. (×500.) (Courtesy E. Jörundsson.)

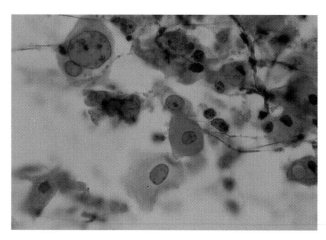

FIG. 2-11. Canine. Fine needle. Skin. Squamous cell carcinoma. Rehydration and ultrafast Papanicolaou's stain. Cytoplasmic details and tinctorial properties confirm squamous differentiation. Distinctive nuclear details, including chromatin patterns, support neoplastic transformation. (×500.) (Courtesy E. Jörundsson.)

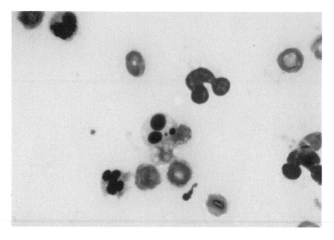

FIG. 2-12. Canine. Fine needle. Subcutaneous abscess. Karyorrhexis and karyopyknosis of neutrophil nuclei occur as a result of aging or toxins, that is, nonspecific, whereas loss of segmentation and karyolysis suggest the influence of toxins. No bacteria are present in this photograph. (×400.)

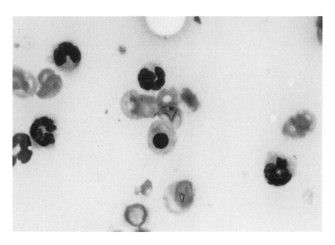

FIG. 2-13. Canine. Fine needle. Subcutaneous abscess. Neutrophil with pyknotic nucleus, in center of photograph, can be mistaken initially for a nucleated erythrocyte. (×400.)

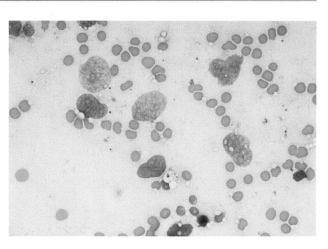

FIG. 2-14. Canine. Pleural fluid. Intact erythrocytes and many ruptured nuclei resulting from cell trauma during smear preparation. Prevalence of bare nuclei increases when poor collection and slide preparation techniques are used, especially when cells have increased fragility. (×100.)

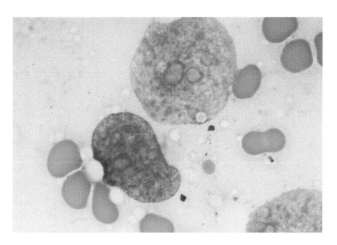

FIG. 2-15. Canine. Pleural fluid. Higher magnification illustrating loss of cytoplasm with dispersion of chromatin and resulting exposure of nucleoli. Only intact cells should be examined for nuclear and nucleolar morphology. (×500.)

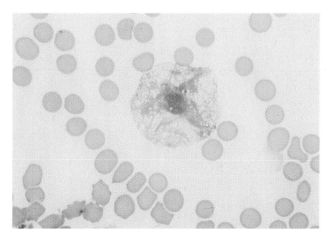

FIG. 2-16. Canine. Pleural fluid. Later stage of nuclear chromatin degeneration. Nuclear debris should not be confused with cellular elements. (×400.)

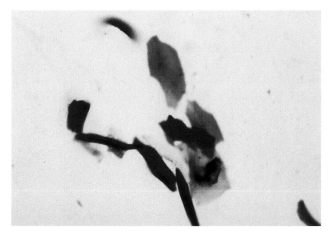

FIG. 2-17. Human finger imprint. Artifact. Superficial squamous epithelial cells exfoliating from operator's finger at time of sampling. (×100.)

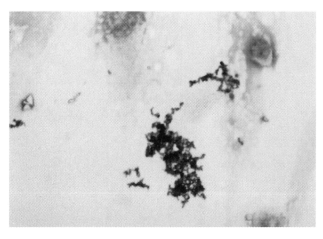

FIG. 2-18. Stain precipitate, often confused with bacteria. Morphology of stain precipitate is irregular and is usually out of focus with cellular elements. (×400.)

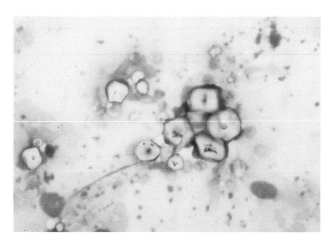

FIG. 2-19. Talc crystals. Contamination of sample from sterile gloves when using aseptic collection techniques. (×200.)

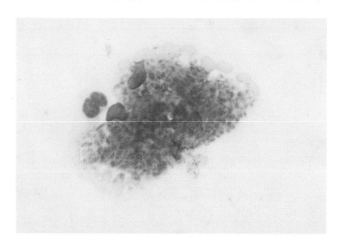

FIG. 2-20. Platelet clump. Bare nuclei are surrounded by a large platelet clump. Platelet clumps indicate aggregation during sampling. The clotting process is associated with release of proteolytic enzymes, which can greatly alter cellular morphology. (×250.)

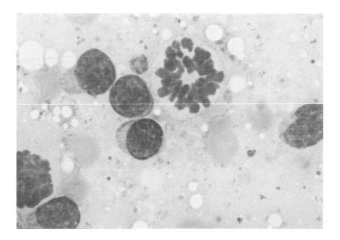

FIG. 2-21. Canine. Imprint. Skin. Normal mitotic figure. (×500.)

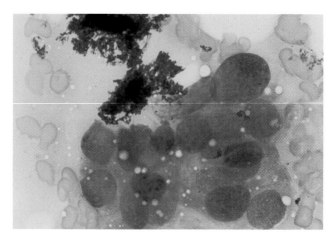

FIG. 2-22. Canine. Fine needle. Intestinal carcinoma. Ultrasound gel appearing as reddish-purple amorphous to fibrillar extracellular material not to be confused with a cell secretory product. (×500.)

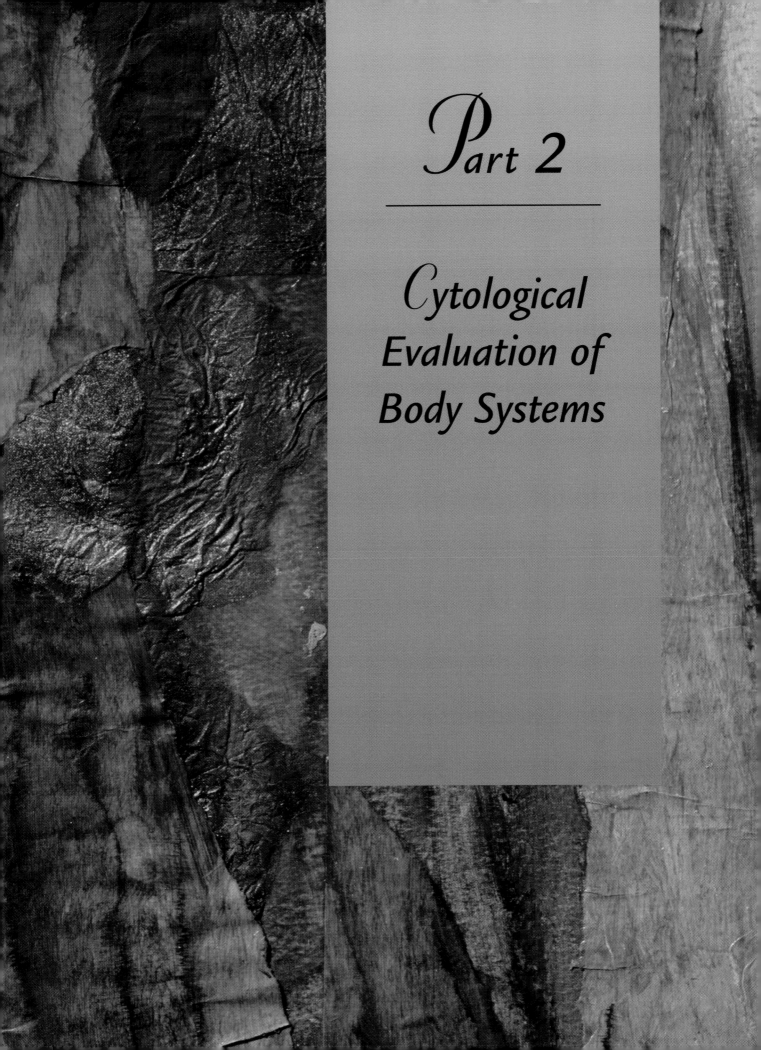

Part 2

Cytological Evaluation of Body Systems

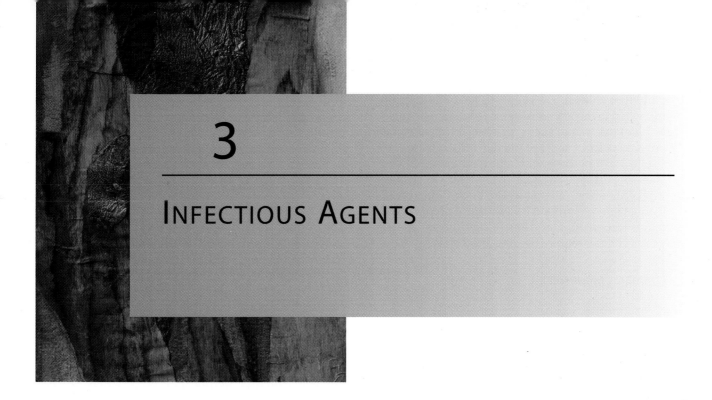

3

INFECTIOUS AGENTS

Many infectious agents are commonly observed and easily recognized using cytological examinations. The cytological appearance and the clinical presentation of common infectious agents are described.

TECHNIQUES

Infectious agents are responsible for initiating the inflammatory response observed in many tissues and fluids. The organisms are frequently observed during microscopic examination of Romanowsky's stained cytology preparations. Gram's stain and acid-fast stains are used for confirmation and characterization of bacteria. Aqueous stains, such as new methylene blue or trichome stains, enhance the visibility of negative-staining fungal cell walls. Fungal stains and many of the special stains used for histological sections can be used on cytology preparations to assist identification of specific infectious agents or to characterize host response.

Histoplasmosis (Figs. 3-1 to 3-4)

CLINICAL DIAGNOSIS

Histoplasma capsulatum is a dimorphic fungus that can infect many species. Dogs and cats younger than 4 years of age are more frequently infected (Clinkenbeard, 1987). Although diffuse reticuloendothelial system involvement can lead to disease in any organ, intestinal and pulmonary lesions are most common in dogs (Clinkenbeard, 1989), whereas anemia and lung disease are reported most frequently in cats (Clinkenbeard, 1987). In each of 11 cats biopsied, bone marrow aspirations were positive (Clinkenbeard, 1987).

CYTOLOGICAL DIAGNOSIS

Histoplasma capsulatum organisms are 2- to 4-µm, round to slightly oval bodies, that is, one quarter to one half the diameter of an erythrocyte (Tyler, 1999). With Romanowsky's stains the organisms are basophilic with a surrounding clear halo resulting from artifactual shrinking during fixation and staining (Wolf, 1995). Organisms are located within macrophages but may appear free. The host response observed during clinical disease is primarily mononuclear consisting predominantly of reactive macrophages.

Blastomycosis (Figs. 3-5 to 3-8)

CLINICAL DIAGNOSIS

Blastomyces dermatitidis is a dimorphic fungus that causes a typical pyogranulomatous infection in dogs and occasionally in cats (Breider, 1988; Miller, 1990). Inhalation of spores is the primary mode of infection. With pulmonary localization, clinical signs may be limited (Wolf, 1991). Systemic dissemination is common (Wolf, 1995), resulting in pulmonary, skin, ocular, or urogenital signs that initiate clinical examination. Primary cutaneous involvement is reported (Wolf, 1995; Yager, 1993).

CYTOLOGICAL DIAGNOSIS

Blastomyces dermatitidis organisms are approximately 8 to 25 µm in diameter and have a thick refractile outer wall. The single structure is more common, but broad-based budding forms, which are often stated to be characteristic, may be observed. The organisms are frequently intermixed with cellular debris and can often be observed while scanning the stained smear at low magnification. The organisms stain dark blue with

Romanowsky's stains, which may obscure internal details and the cell wall. The cell walls are outlined more clearly when using aqueous stains (such as new methylene blue), trichrome stains, or special fungal stains. There is usually a marked mixed inflammatory response to blastomycosis with a predominance of neutrophils. Neutrophil nuclear degenerative changes may be pronounced. Diagnosis can be confirmed readily if organisms are present in cytological preparations, although differentiation from *Cryptococcus* species may occasionally require use of special stains.

Coccidioides immitis (Figs. 3-9 and 3-10)

CLINICAL DIAGNOSIS

Coccidioides immitis is a geophilic dimorphic fungus endemic in semiarid areas. In North America, endemic areas include parts of California, Arizona, Nevada, Utah, New Mexico, and Texas. Infection occurs after inhalation of arthroconidia, leading to localized infection or, less frequently, disseminated coccidioidomycosis involving many organ systems, including bone and skin (Dungworth, 1993; Wolf, 1995). Cats are resistant to *Coccidioides* infection (Wolf, 1991).

CYTOLOGICAL DIAGNOSIS

Observation of *C. immitis* organisms is diagnostic, but the number present in tissues is low. The variable 10- to 70-µm spherules have a double-wall that is refractile in wet-mount preparations and blue-green with Romanowsky's stains. Small, globose, 2- to 5-µm endospores may be released from ruptured spherules. The host cellular response to *Coccidioides* infection is mixed and includes macrophages and neutrophils (Dungworth, 1993).

Cryptococcus neoformans (Figs. 3-11 to 3-14)

CLINICAL DIAGNOSIS

Cryptococcus neoformans is an encapsulated, yeastlike monomorphic organism. In the dog, the lung and central nervous system (CNS) are the most common sites of involvement (Wolf, 1989). In cats, *Cryptococcus* infection is the most frequently diagnosed systemic mycosis leading to nasal infections and single or multiple nodules involving the head and face (Dye, 1988; Wolf, 1989).

CYTOLOGICAL DIAGNOSIS

In cytological preparations the readily visible organisms frequently outnumber the inflammatory cells. At low magnification, large, clear areas of capsular material surround the smaller light-pink to gray organisms, which may appear creased or folded. The organisms are 1 to 7 µm with a 1- to 30-µm nonstaining capsule (Wolf, 1991). The cellular response often is minimal, presumably because of capsular shielding from the host's immune system. In our experience, macro-

phages tend to predominate. In one cat, cytological evaluation of bronchoalveolar fluid was predominantly eosinophilic (Hamilton, 1991). Nucleated cells included 29% macrophages, 14% neutrophils, 5% lymphocytes, and 52% eosinophils (Hamilton, 1991).

Sporothrix schenckii (Figs. 3-15 to 3-18)

CLINICAL DIAGNOSIS

The dimorphic fungus *Sporothrix schenckii* is a geophilic saprophyte with worldwide distribution. Infection usually occurs after a penetrating skin injury or wound contamination (Werner, 1993). The incubation period of 1 to 3 months leads to development of chronic granulomatous cutaneous, lymphocutaneous, or extracutaneous lesions that may ulcerate and discharge exudate. In dogs and cats the cutaneous and lymphocutaneous syndromes are most common. Subcutaneous nodules develop at the site of an injury. The nodules continue to develop as infection ascends along the lymphatic vessels. The skin lesions ulcerate and discharge and may cavitate, exposing muscle and bone (Dunstan, 1986). Disseminated sporotrichosis is reported rarely (Werner, 1993). Lesions are usually confined to the distal portion of the extremities, the head, or the base of the tail in cats (Dunstan, 1986) and the dorsal aspects of the head and trunk in dogs and cats (Wolf, 1995). Sporotrichosis should be suspected in any chronic nonhealing granulomatous skin lesion.

CYTOLOGICAL DIAGNOSIS

Impression or aspirate smears of exudate may contain low numbers (Wolf, 1995) of easily observed ovoid to elongate or cigar-shaped 3- to 10-µm organisms free or phagocytized by macrophages (Dunstan, 1986). With Romanowsky's stains, the pale blue organisms have a pink, slightly eccentric nucleus surrounded by a clear halo (Tyler, 1999). Although the pleomorphic appearance of the *Sporothrix* organisms in exudates is characteristic, it may be difficult on morphology alone to differentiate *Histoplasma* and *Cryptococcus* organisms (Dunstan, 1986). In the cat the profusion of organisms is the basis for serious public health concern. In dogs and humans, fewer organisms are observed than in cats (Yager, 1993). Cytology preparations must be examined carefully. Culture and histopathology may be required for confirmation. There is a mixed purulent to mononuclear host response.

Prototheca (Figs. 3-19 to 3-20)

CLINICAL DIAGNOSIS

Prototheca spp. are colorless algae closely related to *Chlorella* spp. *Prototheca* spp. cause rare opportunistic infections in dogs and cats. They are ubiquitous in sewage and water. In dogs, disseminated disease occurs within the gastrointestinal tract, eye, and CNS, which is the most commonly affected. Cutaneous nodules can occur. In cats, only cutaneous involvement is reported (Coloe, 1982).

CYTOLOGICAL DIAGNOSIS
Cytology smears of aspirates or scrapings contain low to moderate numbers of organisms intermixed with a mild mixed, but predominantly mononuclear, host response (Barker, 1993; Yager, 1993). An imprint of an affected colonic lymph node demonstrated lymphocytes, increased plasma cells, neutrophils, activated macrophages, and large numbers of *Prototheca* organisms (Bird, 1988).The organisms range from 5-μm spheres to 1- to 16-μm ovoids (Barker, 1993; Tyler, 1999) with a small, pink-staining nucleus and a clear cell wall. Two to 20 sporangiospores within a sporangium is characteristic. Most organisms are free, but some can be found within macrophages. They may be confused with cryptococcal or yeast organisms (Barker, 1993; Yager, 1993).

Leishmania donovani (Figs. 3-21 to 3-23)

CLINICAL DIAGNOSIS
Leishmania donovani is a protozoan parasite that infects dogs and rarely cats (Bravo, 1993). It is endemic in parts of Europe, Africa, and Asia and is transmitted by the sandfly. Leishmaniasis is a disease of the reticuloendothelial system and as such mimics histoplasmosis. In the dog, cutaneous and visceral forms are described. The cutaneous form develops at the site of the insect bite, leading to chronic ulcers. The more common visceral form results in chronically debilitated dogs that have oculonasal discharge, diarrhea, and lymphadenopathy.

CYTOLOGICAL DIAGNOSIS
In cytological preparations, the protozoan mammalian form (the amastigote) is round, is approximately 2 μm in diameter, and has a vesicular nucleus and small kinetoplast (Bravo, 1993; Yager, 1993). The host response is neutrophilic or macrophagic with lymphocytes and plasma cells (Tyler, 1999). Plasma cells are increased in bone marrow aspirates from chronically infected dogs. Hyperplastic lymph nodes contain increased lymphoblasts, plasma cells, and *Leishmania*-laden macrophages (Ferrer, 1992). The organisms are readily visible free or within macrophages from aspirates of bone marrow, spleen, or lymph nodes (Bravo, 1993).

Mycobacteria (Fig. 3-24)

CLINICAL DIAGNOSIS
Feline leprosy and skin diseases resulting from atypical mycobacteria should be considered as separate entities (White, 1982). "Cat leprosy" appears as single or multiple cutaneous, subcutaneous, or submucosal lesions anywhere over the body, usually in cats younger than 3 years. Ulceration may occur. The diagnosis is made on the basis of finding numerous intracellular, readily acid-fast staining organisms and a negative culture for *Mycobacterium bovis* and atypical mycobacteria.

Atypical mycobacteria are facultative opportunistic agents from the Mycobacteriaceae family found in soil and water. Atypical mycobacteria are associated with skin diseases in cats (White, 1982) and occasionally subcutaneous granulomas in dogs (Yager, 1993). The infection appears to enter through wound contamination and is observed in the dorsal lumbosacral and ventral abdomen of the cat and head and trunk of the dog (White, 1982; Yager, 1993). Subcutaneous nodules may ulcerate, releasing purulent exudate containing few to many free or phagocytized, variably acid-fast staining organisms.

CYTOLOGICAL DIAGNOSIS
Mycobacterial organisms in feline leprosy are outlined as numerous negative images within the cytoplasm of Romanowsky's stained macrophages or giant cells. The feline leprosy mycobacteria usually stain well with acid-fast stains, in contrast to the weak to poor staining of atypical mycobacteria. Special culture procedures are required for confirmation and differentiation (White, 1982; Yager, 1993). The host cellular response is primarily mononuclear, as demonstrated in the impression smears of a subcutaneous mass containing a pure population of macrophages with phagocytized negative-staining bacilli (Kramer, 1988).

Cytauxzoan (Fig. 3-25)

CLINICAL DIAGNOSIS
Cytauxzoonosis is a tickborne protozoal disease caused by the piroplasm *Cytauxzoon felis*. The disease is reported in cats from the mid-southern to southeastern United States. The bobcat is the natural host, with ticks being the apparent vector (Meinkoth, 1996). Infected cats become pyrexic, anorectic, dehydrated, icteric, depressed and invariably die (Hauck, 1982; Wagner, 1980).

CYTOLOGICAL DIAGNOSIS
As fever develops, *Cytauxzoon* organisms may be observed in a low percentage of erythrocytes. The 1- to 1.5-μm round to oval signet ring–shaped intraerythrocytic *C. felis* organisms must be differentiated from *Haemobartonella felis*, which are multiple, 0.1- to 0.8-μm cocci or 1.0- to 1.5-μm rods that locate on the periphery of the erythrocyte membrane. Impression smears of infected organs may demonstrate variable numbers of basophilic intracytoplasmic structures, schizonts, within mononuclear phagocytes of the bone marrow,

spleen, lung, or lymph node (Meinkoth, 1996). Large, swollen, infected macrophages (80 to 100 μ) may be seen (Meinkoth, 1996). The cytoplasm is usually extended by a single large schizont containing developing merozoites (Meinkoth, 1996).

Toxoplasmosis (Figs. 3-26 to 3-28)

Clinical diagnosis

Felidae are the definitive host for the protozoan *Toxoplasma gondii*. *T. gondii* can infect a wide range of species, leading to asymptomatic systemic infection (Barker, 1993; Wolf, 1991). Animals with overwhelming infection, often immunocompromised individuals, develop clinical signs related to the primary organ system involved. Often, toxoplasmosis in dogs and cats is diagnosed after death. General signs of fever, anorexia, and lethargy may be associated with respiratory distress, neurological signs, hepatitis, or paresis resulting from myositis (Barker, 1993; Peterson, 1991; Wolf, 1991). In dogs, toxoplasmosis is often associated with canine distemper (Barker, 1993).

Cytological diagnosis

In cytological preparations, such as lung aspirations or impressions of necropsy tissues, toxoplasmosis is diagnosed when tachyzoites are observed. The tachyzoites are 5-μm by 2-μm crescent-shaped bodies that stain pale blue to purple, often with a dark-staining eccentric nucleus. The organisms may be observed intracellularly and extracellularly in body fluids of dogs and cats during the 1- to 3-week acute phase of the disease (Dubey, 1986). Occasionally the organisms have been reported in blood and CSF (Dubey, 1986). Fifteen cats were experimentally infected with *Toxoplasma* (Hawkins, 1997). Tachyzoites were found, usually in low numbers, in 14 of 15 bronchoalveolar lavage samples (Hawkins, 1997).

Neospora caninum

Clinical diagnosis

Neospora caninum is a protozoan parasite recently recognized and previously confused with *Toxoplasma gondii* (Dubey, 1990a; Dubey, 1990b). It causes multifocal neurological disease, myositis, myocarditis, and dermatitis in puppies (Hay, 1990) and dogs (Dubey, 1992). Tissue tachyzoites of neospora appear similar to those of toxoplasma. Experimentally infected cats develop lesions that are morphologically similar to toxoplasmosis (Dubey, 1990b).

Cytological diagnosis

Cytological descriptions of this organism have not been reported and would require special techniques for differentiation from *Toxoplasma*. The organisms cannot be differentiated on morphology alone.

Pneumocystis carinii (Figs. 3-29 and 3-30)

Clinical diagnosis

Pneumocystis carinii is an opportunistic pulmonary pathogen observed in immunosuppressed dogs (Rakich, 1989). In humans the organisms are observed in bronchoalveolar lavage fluids, sputum, or FNAs of the lung (Chaudhary, 1977). In dogs it is often fatal (Sakura, 1996).

Cytological diagnosis

In a lung imprint, *Pneumocystis* cysts were described as 5 to 10 μm in diameter and containing 4 to 8 intracystic bodies 1 to 2 μm in diameter (Cowell, 1989). Transtracheal aspiration of four miniature dachshunds with respiratory difficulty and interstitial pneumonia revealed *P. carinii* organisms in all four dogs (Lobetti, 1996). The dogs had a mixed macrophage and neutrophil cellular infiltrate (Lobetti, 1996). Bronchoalveolar lavage from one dog included 73% neutrophils, 21% macrophages, and 6% lymphocytes (Sakura, 1996). Multinucleate bodies, approximately the size of a red blood cell, were seen and suspected to be *P. carinii* (Sakura, 1996). Each multinucleate cell contained up to eight small violet-red nuclei (Sakura, 1996). Eosinophilic empty structures were present extracellularly (Sakura, 1996). These two appearances were confirmed to be the cyst and trophozoite stages of *P. carinii* (Sakura, 1996).

Ehrlichia

The clinical and cytological description of *Ehrlichia* infection is described in Chapter 6.

Chlamydia (Figs. 3-31 to 3-33)

Clinical diagnosis

Chlamydia psittaci causes transient rhinitis and chronic conjunctivitis in cats.

Cytological diagnosis

The conjunctival inflammatory response to *Chlamydia* is primarily neutrophilic. The organisms appear as aggregates of coccoid basophilic 0.5- to 1-μm elementary bodies or as larger 3- to 5-μm basophilic particulate forms on squamous cells (Lavach, 1977; Prasse, 1989). Conjunctival scrapings are diagnostic when organisms are observed but often have disappeared by the time the cat is presented for examination (Prasse, 1989).

Nocardia and Actinomyces (Figs. 3-34 to 3-36)

Clinical diagnosis

Nocardia and *Actinomyces* are saprophytic bacteria that cause suppurative or granulomatous inflammatory reactions in dogs and cats. Infection may be confined to local skin abscessation or disseminate to other organs, primarily the lung or CNS (Marino, 1993). Empyema associated with *Nocardia* or *Actinomyces* is frequently described as "tomato soup"-like in consistency (Marino, 1993).

CYTOLOGICAL DIAGNOSIS

These organisms are branching, filamentous, gram-positive rods. With Romanowsky's stains the bacteria are light purple to blue with purple to pink dots along the filamentous structure. Pleomorphic populations of free and phagocytized rods, cocci, and filamentous structures may be observed in clinical cases. The bacteria induce marked chemotaxis of neutrophils and macrophages but less neutrophil nuclear degeneration than expected for most aerobes, presumably because of less potent cytotoxin production. Neutrophils have varying degrees of chromatolysis, karyopyknosis, and karyorrhexis. Large bacterial colonies may be present. The characteristic cytological appearance of numerous pleomorphic bacteria alerts the clinician to the need for both anaerobic and aerobic culture techniques, as well as directing clinical treatment until confirmed.

Neorickettsia helminthoeca (Figs. 3-37 and 3-38)

CLINICAL AND CYTOLOGICAL DIAGNOSES

The disease known as salmon fluke poisoning in dogs is caused by ingestion of a rickettsial agent, *Neorickettsia helminthoeca*, found in fish containing the trematode metacercariae *Nanophyetus salmincola*. It is limited geographically to the west coast of the United States and Canada (Breitschwerdt, 1995). The clinical disease is characterized by fever, depression, vomiting, and diarrhea (Breitschwerdt, 1995). With Wright's stain, intracytoplasmic bodies can be seen in macrophages of lymph node imprints.

Mycoplasma Infection (Figs. 3-39 and 3-40)

See Chapter 12.

FUNGAL INFECTIONS THAT FORM HYPHAE IN TISSUES

Several categories of hyphal-forming fungal infections exist. Most cause a pyogranulomatous cellular response with a mixture of neutrophils, macrophages, lymphocytes, giant cells, and occasionally plasma cells. In cytological preparations the fungal hyphae may or may not be easily seen depending on the number and type present and the stain used. Differentiation requires use of histological and culture criteria.

Zygomycosis

CLINICAL DIAGNOSIS

Zygomycosis is the term used to describe granulomatous skin reactions caused by several fungal species, such as *Mucor*, *Absidia*, *Rhizopus*, and *Mortierella* (Bentinck-Smith, 1989). The current term replaces the term *phycomycosis* (Bentinck-Smith, 1989). Infections of the digestive tract are most common, but any tissue may be involved (Miller, 1985).

CYTOLOGICAL DIAGNOSIS

Many zygomycetes do not stain with Romanowsky's stains and appear as negative fungal images intermixed with the mixed cellular response of neutrophils, macrophages, and giant cells. Most of these fungi form poorly septate hyphae.

Phaeohyphomycosis

CLINICAL DIAGNOSIS

Phaeohyphomycosis is an infection in which pigmented fungi cause single or multiple subcutaneous nodules, rarely in dogs and sporadically in cats (Yager, 1993). In the cat, lesions tend to occur on the face and distal extremities (Yager, 1993).

CYTOLOGICAL DIAGNOSIS

Aspirates of microabscesses or impressions of draining sinuses may contain evidence of pyogranulomatous inflammation and negative-staining hyphal organisms. The septate hyphae vary in width, length, and branching pattern with possible dilated segments up to 25 μm resembling chlamydospores (Yager, 1993). Special fungal stains may be required for confirmation. Unstained sections allow confirmation that fungi are pigmented.

Aspergillosis (Fig. 3-41)

CLINICAL DIAGNOSIS

Aspergillus fumigatus is most commonly associated with nasal disease in the dog and cat causing severe destruction of the nasal turbinates. The term *aspergillosis* is applied to other *Aspergillus* and *Penicillium* spp., which appear similar cytologically (Sharp, 1989). Specific identification requires fungal culture. Aspergillosis is rare in the cat (Sharp, 1989). Aspergillus is best detected using nasal flushes (Rakich, 1989).

CYTOLOGICAL DIAGNOSIS

The cellular response to aspergillus is primarily neutrophilic. Large numbers of moderately lytic neutrophils can be seen intermixed with macrophages and lymphocytes. Negatively staining large (4 to 6 μm wide) septate branching hyphae with parallel sides may be seen, or alternatively the hyphae may stain dark purple with Romanowsky's stain. Careful examination is required because the few hyphae may be obscured by cellular debris or may protrude from the edges of clusters of cells.

Pythium insidiosum

CLINICAL DIAGNOSIS

Pythium insidiosum is an aquatic organism associated primarily with gastrointestinal granulomas, but it may cause subcutaneous granulomas in the dog (Howerth, 1989; O'Neill, 1984). *P. insidiosum* is responsible for many of the reported gastrointestinal phycomycoses (Miller, 1985). Male, large-breed dogs less than 3 years of age are overrepresented in some studies (Taboada, 1995).

CYTOLOGICAL DIAGNOSIS

The 6- to 12-μm wide fungal hyphae have irregular branches and rare septae. Aspiration of a *Pythium*-positive abdominal mass contained neutrophils, macrophages, and eosinophils but no organisms (Bentinck-Smith, 1989). Organisms can be difficult to observe with regular staining procedures. Methenamine silver has been recommended (Yager, 1993). A scraping of a duodenal mass described a mixture of neutrophils, macrophages, epithelioid cells, lymphocytes, plasma cells, and multinucleated giant cells (Whitney, 1990).

References

Barker, I.K., Van Dreumel, A.A., and Palmer, N. The alimentary system. In *Pathology of Domestic Animals*. ed 4. K.V.F. Jubb, P.C. Kennedy, and N. Palmer (eds). Academic Press, San Diego, 1993.

Bentinck-Smith, J., Padhe, A.A., Maslin, W.R., et al. Canine pythiosis-isolation and identification of *Pythium insidiosum*. *J Vet Diagn Invest* 1:295-298, 1989.

Bird, K.E., Whitney, M.S., and Relford, R.L. *Case 14.* ASVCP Annual Slide Review Session, Kansas City, Mo, 1988.

Bravo, L., Frank, L.A., and Brenneman, K.A. Canine leishmaniasis in the United States. *Compend Cont Ed Pract* 15:699-708, 1993.

Breider, M.A., Walker, T.L., Legendre, A.M., et al. Blastomycosis in cats: five cases (1979-1986). *J Am Vet Med Assoc* 193:570-572, 1988.

Breitschwerdt, E.B. The rickettsiosis. In *Textbook of Veterinary Internal Medicine*. S.J. Ettinger and E.C. Feldman (eds).WB Saunders, Philadelphia, 1995.

Chaudhary, S., Hughes, W.T., Feldman, S., et al. Percutaneous transthoracic needle aspiration of the lung. Diagnosing *Pneumocystis carinii* pneumonitis. *Am J Dis Child* 131: 902-907, 1977.

Clinkenbeard, K.D., Cowell, R.L., and Tyler, R.D. Disseminated histoplasmosis in cats: 12 cases (1981-1986). *J Am Vet Med Assoc* 190:1445-1448, 1987.

Clinkenbeard, K.D., Wolf, A.M., Cowell, R.L., et al. Canine disseminated histoplasmosis. *Compend Cont Ed Pract* 11:1347-1358, 1989.

Coloe, P.J. and Allison, J.F. Prototothecosis in a cat. *J Am Vet Med Assoc* 180:78-79, 1982.

Cowell R.L. and Tyler, R.D. Figure 8. In *Diagnostic Cytology of the Dog and Cat*. R.L. Cowell and R.D. Tyler (eds). American Veterinary Publications, Goleta, Calif, 1989.

Dubey, J.P. Toxoplasmosis in cats. *Feline Practice* 16:12-27, 1986.

Dubey, J.P. Neosporum caninum infection. In *Current Veterinary Therapy XI, Small Animal Practice*. R.W. Kirk and J.D. Bonagura (eds). WB Saunders, Philadelphia, 1992.

Dubey, J.P., Koestner, A., and Piper, R.C. Repeated transplacental transmission of Neospora caninum in dogs. *J Am Vet Med Assoc* 197:857-860, 1990a.

Dubey, J.P., Lindsay, D.S., and Lipscomb, T.P. Neosporosis in cats. *Vet Pathol* 27:335-339, 1990b.

Dungworth, D.L. The respiratory system. In *Pathology of Domestic Animals*. ed 4. K.V.F. Jubb, P.C. Kennedy, and N. Palmer (eds). Academic Press, San Diego, 1993.

Dunstan, V., Reimann, K.A., and Langham, R.F. Feline sporotrichosis. *J Am Vet Med Assoc* 189:880-883, 1986.

Dye, J.A. and Campbell, K.L. Cutaneous and ocular cryptococcosis in a cat: case report and literature review. *Comp Anim Pract* 2:34-44, 1988.

Ferrer, L. Leishmaniasis. In *Current Veterinary Therapy XI, Small Animal Practice*. R.W. Kirk and J.D. Bonagura (eds). WB Saunders, Philadelphia, 1992.

Hamilton, T.A., Hawkins, E., and DeNicola, D.B. Bronchoalveolar lavage and tracheal wash to determine lung involvement in a cat with cryptococcosis. *J Am Vet Med Assoc* 198:655- 656,1991.

Hawkins, E.C., Davidson, M.G., Meuten, D.J., et al. Cytologic identification of *Toxoplasma gondii* in bronchoalveolar lavage fluid of experimentally infected cats. *J Am Vet Med Assoc* 210:648-650, 1997.

Hauck, W.N. and Snider, T.G. Cytauxzoonosis in a native Louisiana cat. *J Am Vet Med Assoc* 180:1472-1474, 1982.

Hay, W.H., Shell, L.G., Lindsay, D.S., et al. Diagnosis and treatment of *Neospora caninum* infection in a dog. *J Am Vet Med Assoc* 197:87-89, 1990.

Howerth, E.W., Brown, C.C., and Crowder, C. Subcutaneous pythiosis in a dog. *J Vet Diagn Invest* 1:81-83, 1989.

Kramer, J. and Brobst, D. *Case 11.* ASVCP Slide Review Session, Kansas City, Mo, 1988.

Lavach, J.D., Thrall, M.A., Benjamin, M.M., et al. Cytology of normal and inflamed conjunctivas in dogs and cats. *J Am Vet Med Assoc* 170:722-727, 1977.

Lobetti, R.G., Leisewitz, A.L., and Spencer, J.A. Pneumocystis carinii in the miniature dachshund: case report and literature review. *J Small Anim Pract* 37:280-285, 1996.

Marino, D.J. and Jaggy, A. Nocardiosis, a literature review with selected case reports in two dogs. *J Vet Intern Med* 7:4-11, 1993.

Meinkoth, J.H., Cowell, R.L., and Cowell, A.K. What is your diagnosis? *Vet Clin Pathol* 25:48, 59, 1996.

Miller, P.E. and Schoster, L.M. Feline blastomycosis: a report of three cases and literature review (1961 to 1988). *Am Anim Hosp Assoc* 26:417-423, 1990.

Miller, R.I. Gastrointestinal phycomycosis in 63 dogs. *J Am Vet Med Assoc* 186:473-478, 1985.

O'Neill, C.S., Short, B.G., Fadok, V.A., et al. A report of subcutaneous pythiosis in five dogs and a review of the etiologic agent *Pythium spp*. *Am Anim Hosp Assoc* 20:959-966, 1984.

Peterson, J.L., Willard, M.D., Lees, G.E., et al. Toxoplasmosis in two cats with inflammatory intestinal disease. *J Am Vet Med Assoc* 199:473-476, 1991.

Prasse, K.W. and Winston, S.M. The eyes and associated structures. In *Diagnostic Cytology and Hematology of the Dog and Cat*, ed 2. R.L. Cowell, R.D. Tyler, and J.H. Meinkoth (eds). Mosby, St Louis, 1999.

Rakich, P.M. and Latimer, K.S. Cytology of the respiratory tract. In *Vet Clin North Am Sm Animals, Clinical Pathology: Part II*, B.W. Parry (ed), 19:823-850. WB Saunders, Philadelphia, 1989.

Sakura, A., Saari, S., Jarvinen, A.K., et al. Pneumocystis carinii pneumonia in dogs: a diagnostic challenge. *Vet Diagn Invest* 8:124-130, 1996.

Sharp, N. Nasal aspergillosis. In *Current Veterinary Therapy X, Small Animal Practice*. R.W. Kirk (ed). WB Saunders, Philadelphia, 1989.

Taboada, J. and Merchant, S.R. Protozoal and miscellaneous infections. In *Textbook of Veterinary Internal Medicine*. S.J. Ettinger and E.C. Feldman (eds). WB Saunders, Philadelphia, 1995.

Tyler, R.D., Cowell, R.L., and Meinkoth, J.H. Cutaneous and subcutaneous lesions: masses, cysts, ulcers and fistulous tracts. In *Diagnostic Cytology and Hematology of the Dog and Cat*, ed 2. R.L. Cowell, R.D. Tyler, and J.H. Meinkoth (eds). Mosby, St. Louis, 1999.

Wagner, J.E., Ferris, D.H., Kier, A.B., et al. Experimentally induced cytauxzoonosis-like disease in domestic cats. *Vet Parasit* 6:305-311, 1980.

Werner, A.H. and Werner, B.E. Feline sporotrichosis. *Compend Cont Ed* 15:1189-1197, 1993.

White, S.D., Ihrke, P.J., Stannard, A.A., et al. Cutaneous atypical mycobacteriosis in cats. *J Am Vet Med Assoc* 182:1218-1222, 1982.

Whitney, M., Bird, K., and Gossett, R. *Case 6*. ASVCP Slide Review Session, Phoenix, 1990.

Wolf, A.M. Systemic mycosis. *J Am Vet Med Assoc* 194:1192-1196, 1989.

Wolf, A.M. Systemic mycotic and protozoal infections in cats. *Vet Int* 3:11-18, 1991.

Wolf, A.M. and Troy, G.C. Deep mycotic diseases. In *Textbook of Veterinary Internal Medicine*. S.J. Ettinger and E.C. Feldman (eds). WB Saunders, Philadelphia, 1995.

Yager, J.A., Scott, D.W., and Wilcock, B.P. The skin and appendages. In *Pathology of Domestic Animals*, ed 4. K.V.F. Jubb, P.C. Kennedy, and N. Palmer (eds). Academic Press, San Diego, 1993.

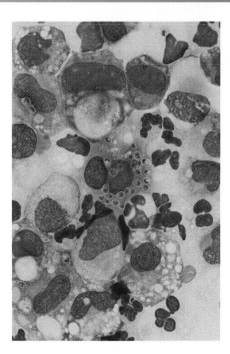

FIG. 3-1. Canine. Peritoneal fluid. Histoplasmosis. Mixed inflammatory response. Multiple small, round, clear, walled organisms are visible within the cytoplasm of the central mononuclear cell. The organisms are most compatible with *Histoplasma capsulatum.* (×400.)

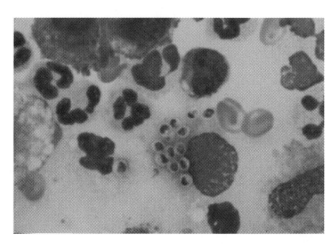

FIG. 3-2. Canine. Peritoneal fluid. Histoplasmosis. Mixed inflammatory response surrounding large central macrophage, which contains *Histoplasma* organisms. (×630.)

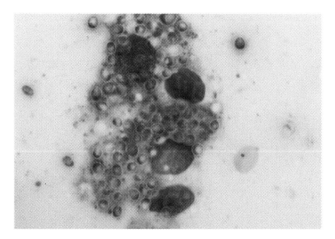

FIG. 3-3. Canine. Fine needle. Liver. Histoplasmosis. Numerous *Histoplasma capsulatum* organisms are visible extracellularly and within macrophages. (×400.)

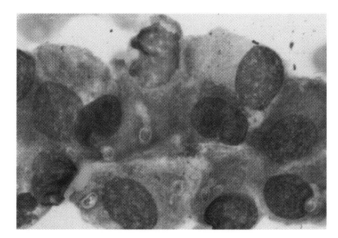

FIG. 3-4. Canine. Fine needle. Lung mass. Histoplasmosis. Large epithelioid macrophages contain 1- to 4-μ organisms typical of *Histoplasma capsulatum.* (×500.)

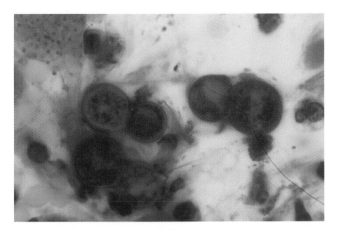

FIG. 3-5. Canine. Imprint. Skin. Blastomycosis. New methylene blue stain. The 8- to 25-μ round *Blastomyces dermatitides* organisms have a negative to basophilic staining cell wall. The cell wall and internal structures of the organism have greater visibility when using non-Romanowsky's stains, such as new methylene blue or Papanicolaou's stain. (×400.)

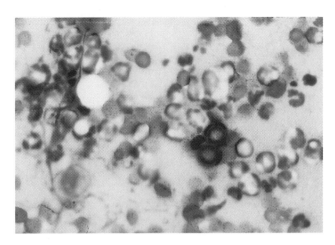

FIG. 3-6. Canine. Synovial fluid. Blastomycosis. Organisms are often first observed enmeshed in inflammatory cells while scanning at low magnification. The double-walled dark blue–staining structure of *Blastomyces* is prominent among the inflammatory components. (×250.)

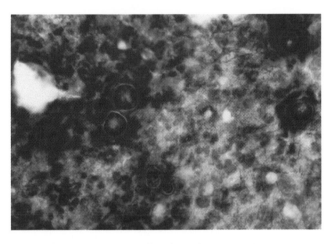

FIG. 3-7. Canine. Fine needle. Skin. Blastomycosis. Low-power view of *Blastomyces dermatitides*. Organisms are surrounded by a suppurative cellular response. (×250.)

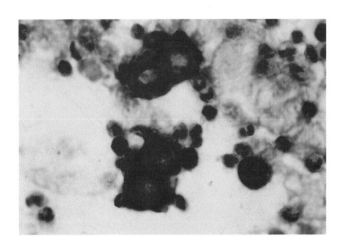

FIG. 3-8. Canine. Imprint. Skin. Blastomycosis. Typical appearance of *Blastomyces dermatitides* using Romanowsky's stains. (×400.)

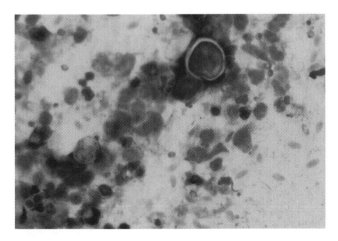

FIG. 3-9. Llama. Imprint. Lung. Coccidioidomycosis. Large, poorly staining round bodies are the spherules of coccidioidomycosis. These spherules can be 10 to 100 μ in diameter. (×400.)

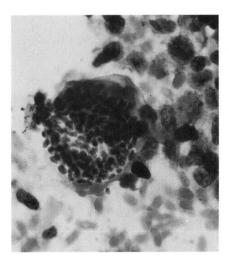

FIG. 3-10. Llama. Imprint. Lung. Coccidioidomycosis. Oval erythrocytes and mixed inflammatory response visible in background. The cluster of endospores are released as a result of rupture of the green refractile calyx-like wall. (×400.)

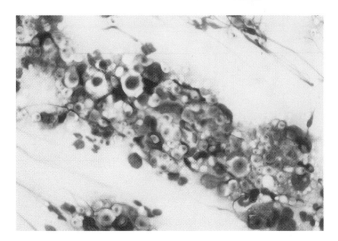

FIG. 3-11. Feline. Skin. Fine needle. Cryptococcosis. Numerous variably sized *Cryptococcus neoformans* organisms with light to dark purple center (1-7 μ) and thick negative-staining capsule (1-30 μ). (×200.)

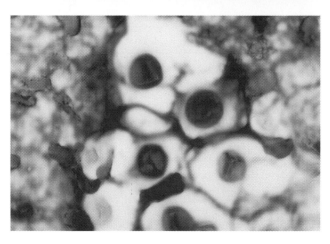

FIG. 3-12. Canine. Fine needle. Lymph node. Numerous *Cryptococcus neoformans* organisms. (×400.)

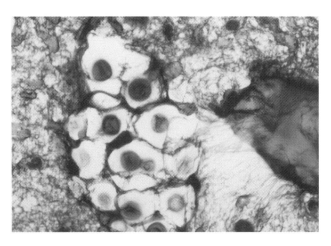

FIG. 3-13. Canine. Fine needle. Lymph node. Cryptococcosis. *Cryptococcus neoformans* organisms illustrating budding in the central organism and the typical lack of inflammatory response. (×250.)

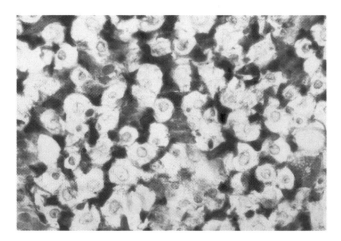

FIG. 3-14. Canine. Fine needle. Aqueous humor. Cryptococcosis. *Cryptococcus neoformans* organisms are visible within the aqueous fluid. (×100.)

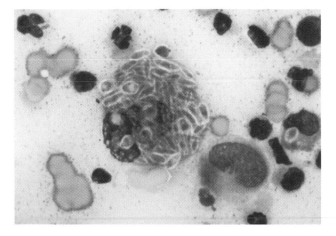

FIG. 3-15. Feline. Imprint. Skin of digit. Sporotrichosis. Large macrophage contains intracytoplasmic, oval to cigar-shaped *Sporothrix schenckii* organisms. The organisms are 2 to 4 μ, are lightly basophilic, and have a pink eccentric nucleus surrounded by a clear halo. (×400.) (Courtesy Cheryl Swenson, 1993.)

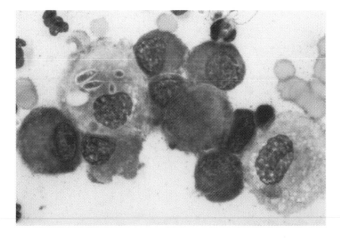

FIG. 3-16. Feline. Imprint. Skin of digit. Sporotrichosis. (Same case as Fig. 3-15.) Macrophage contains many intracellular *Sporothrix schenckii* organisms. The presence of the basophilic epithelioid macrophages suggests a granulomatous inflammatory response. (×400.) (Courtesy Cheryl Swenson, 1993.)

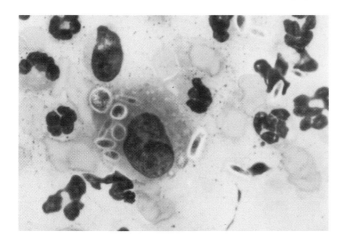

FIG. 3-17. Feline. Imprint. Skin of digit. Sporotrichosis. (Same case as Fig. 3-15.) A macrophage contains *Sporothrix schenckii* organisms. The organisms have a light-purple to eosinophilic internal structure and a negative-staining wall. If elongated organisms are not observed, differentiation from *Histoplasma* may be difficult using light microscopy. (×500.) (Courtesy Cheryl Swenson, 1993.)

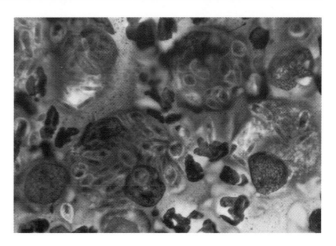

FIG. 3-18. Feline. Imprint. Skin of digit. Sporotrichosis. (Same case as Fig. 3-15.) *Sporothrix* organisms may be observed both intracellularly and extracellularly in cytological preparations. A mixed cellular response is expected. (×500.)

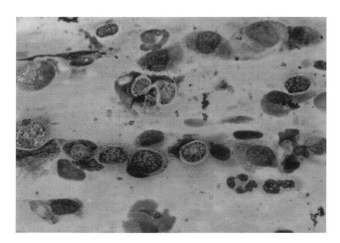

FIG. 3-19. Canine. Rectal scraping. Prototothecosis. Mixed cellularity including neutrophils and mononuclear cells. Mucosal epithelial cells and macrophages are present. The large oval bodies with thin negative-stained wall and stippled central region are compatible with *Prototheca* spp. (×400.)

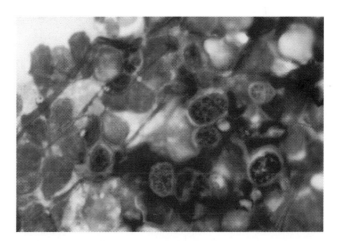

FIG. 3-20. Canine. Imprint. Colonic lymph node. *Prototheca*. Numerous pleomorphic round to oval organisms, 2 to 13 μ by 2 to 15 μ, with basophilic granular cytoplasm and thick hyaline negative-staining cell walls consistent with *Prototheca* spp. (×200.) (Courtesy Karyn Bird, 1988.)

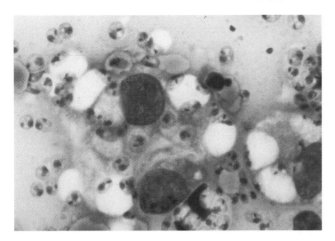

FIG. 3-21. Feline. Fine needle. Mass on ear pinnae. *Leishmania* infection. Numerous 0.5- to 2-μ round organisms consistent with *Leishmania* amastigotes are present free and within macrophages. The organisms have clear to pale basophilic cytoplasm, an oval basophilic nucleus, and a small dark kinetoplast on the margin of the organism opposite the nucleus. Diff-Quick stain. (×500.) (Courtesy R. Gossett, 1991.)

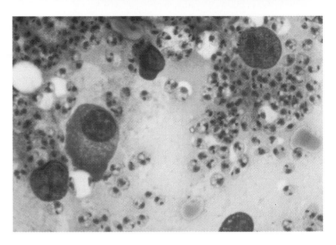

FIG. 3-22. Feline. Fine needle. Mass on ear pinnae. *Leishmania* infection. (Same case as Fig. 3-21.) There are many free and intracellular *Leishmania* spp. organisms. Plasma cells are part of the typical mononuclear inflammatory response. Diff-Quick stain. (×400.) (Courtesy R. Gossett, 1991.)

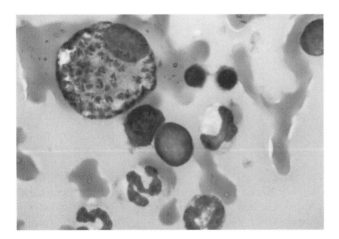

FIG. 3-23. Canine. Fine needle. Lung. *Leishmania* infection. The large macrophage contains many round to oval organisms consistent with *Leishmania* spp. There is a mixed inflammatory response. (×400.)

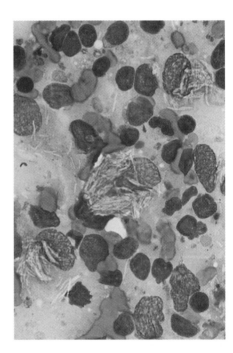

FIG. 3-24. Feline. Fine needle. Lymph node. Mycobacteriosis. Mixed population of moderately preserved mononuclear cells, including macrophages. Closely associated with the macrophages are many small, sharply tipped, long, narrow, negative-staining organisms compatible with mycobacteria. *Mycobacterium avium* was confirmed by culture and polymerase chain reaction (PCR) analysis. (×400.)

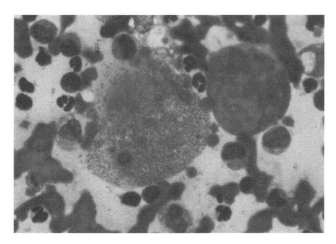

FIG. 3-25. Two huge mononuclear cells with abundant cytoplasm, eccentric nuclei, and prominent nucleoli. These cells contain many developing *Cytauxzoon merozoites,* which appear as either small, dark-staining bodies or larger irregularly defined clusters. (Wright's stain, original magnification ×250.) (Courtesy Dr. French, Cornell University. From Cowell, R.L., Tyler, R.D., and Meinkoth, J.H. *Diagnostic Cytology and Hematology of the Dog and Cat,* ed 2. Mosby, St Louis, 1999.)

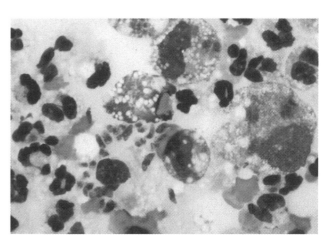

FIG. 3-26. Feline. Peritoneal fluid. Feline infectious peritonitis and toxoplasmosis. Free and phagocytized oval to lunate 5-μ by 2-μ crescent-shaped pale blue structures with a small, dark, eccentrically located nucleus consistent with *Toxoplasma gondii* tachyzoites. (×400.) (Courtesy T.W. French, 1993.)

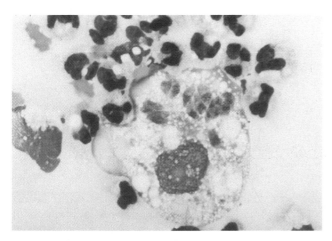

FIG. 3-27. Feline. Peritoneal fluid. *Toxoplasma* infection. (Same case as Fig. 3-26.) Several *Toxoplasma gondii* tachyzoites are visible within a large, foamy macrophage. A mixed inflammatory response is illustrated by the degenerating neutrophils surrounding the macrophage. (×400.) (Courtesy T.W. French, 1993.)

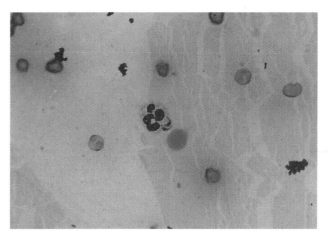

FIG. 3-28. Feline. Sediment smear. Respiratory fluid. Toxoplasmosis. Two small, elongated organisms are visible within the cytoplasm of the neutrophil. (×400.)

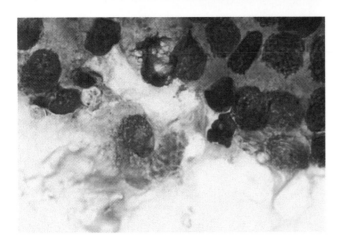

FIG. 3-29. Canine. Fine needle. Lung. *Pneumocystis.* A *Pneumocystis carinii* cyst is closely associated with a ruptured macrophage located on the periphery of the cluster of degenerate mononuclear cells. The 4- to 6-μ cysts contain four to eight intracystic bodies. (×630.)

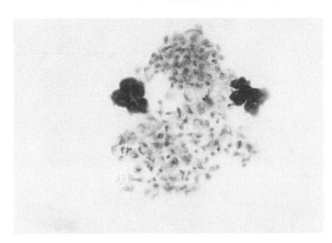

FIG. 3-30. Canine. Fine needle. Lung. *Pneumocystis* infection. Numerous 1- to 2-μ intracystic bodies are spread between two ruptured nuclei. (×630.)

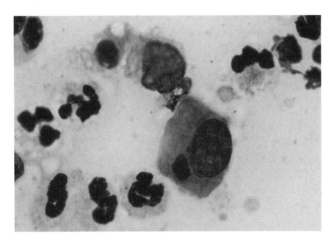

FIG. 3-31. Feline. Scraping. Conjunctiva. *Chlamydia.* Initial body within a conjunctival epithelial cell. (×630.)

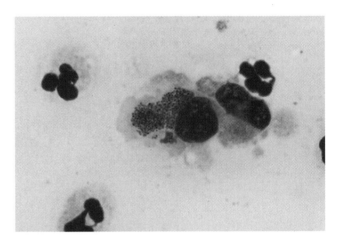

FIG. 3-32. Feline (7 weeks). Scraping. Conjunctiva. *Chlamydia.* Small, round basophilic elementary bodies of *Chlamydia psittaci* in the cytoplasm of a conjunctival epithelial cell. Organisms are diagnostic when observed but have often disappeared by the time animal is presented for examination. (×630.)

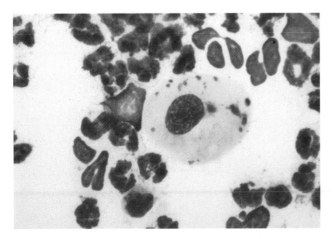

FIG. 3-33. Feline. Scraping. Conjunctiva. *Chlamydia.* Elementary bodies within conjunctival epithelial cells. (×400.)

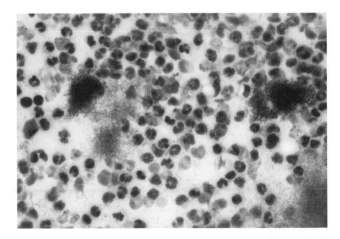

FIG. 3-34. Canine. Pleural fluid. Septic pleuritis. Large blue clusters of filamentous bacteria, likely *Actinomycetaceae* spp. Intermixed with large numbers of neutrophils. (×200.)

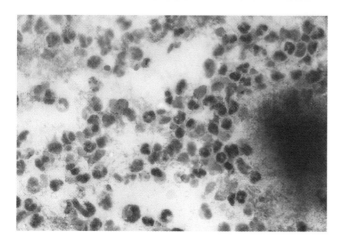

FIG. 3-35. Canine. Pleural fluid. Septic pleuritis. These large clusters of filamentous organisms are described grossly as "sulfur granules." (×200.)

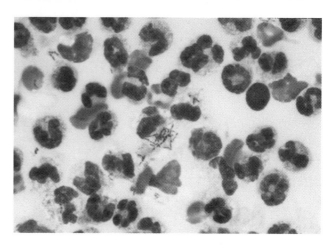

FIG. 3-36. Canine. Pleural fluid. Septic pleuritis. Suppurative inflammatory response is typical for the anaerobic *Actinomycetaceae* spp. Neutrophil cytoplasm must be carefully searched to identify these filamentous types of bacteria. (×400.)

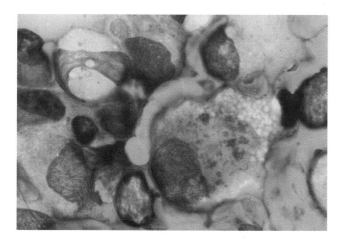

FIG. 3-37. Canine. Fine needle. Lymph node. *Neorickettsia helminthoeca.* Salmon fluke poisoning. The large macrophage contains the causative agent, *N. helminthoeca.* (×200.)

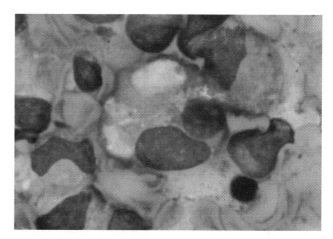

FIG. 3-38. Canine. Impression. Mesenteric lymph node. Salmon fluke poisoning. A large basophilic intracytoplasmic morula is prominently located adjacent to the nucleus of the central large mononuclear cell. (×500.)

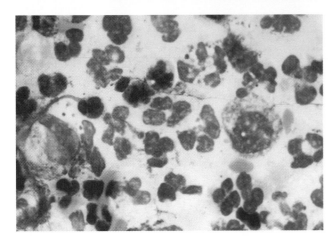

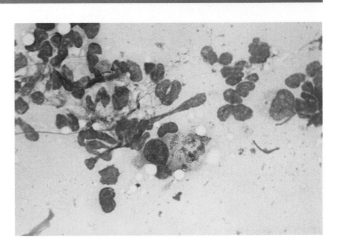

FIG. 3-39. Feline. Fine needle. Dermal abscess. *Mycoplasma.* Primarily degenerating neutrophils and two mononuclear phagocytic cells. Fine granularity in the cytoplasm of the mononuclear cell is compatible with mycoplasma. (×400.)

FIG. 3-40. Feline. Scraping. Conjunctiva. *Mycoplasma.* Fine to aggregated basophilic bodies are visible within the epithelial cell cytoplasm. There is a background of degenerating neutrophils. (×312.)

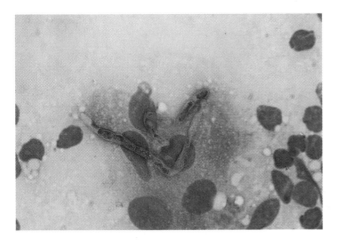

FIG. 3-41. Canine. Fine needle. Prescapular lymph node. Aspergillosis. The long, narrow, angular negative-stained organism with narrow stained central region is compatible with fungal etiology probably caused by *Aspergillus* spp. (×630.)

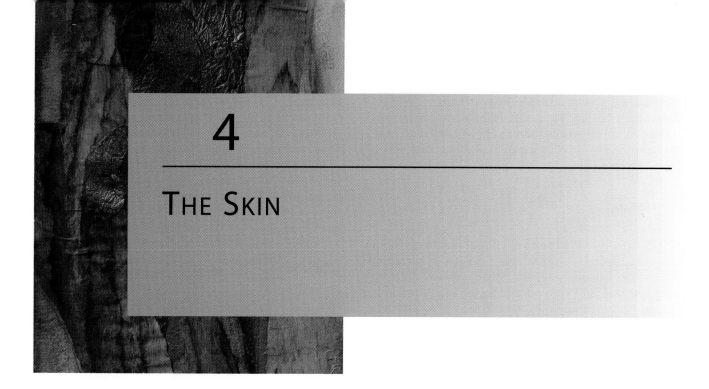

4

THE SKIN

One of the more effective and frequently used applications for diagnostic cytology is the examination and differentiation of cutaneous and subcutaneous lesions. A good aspiration, with cells spread into a thin layer and stained, will provide information adequate for the clinical diagnosis and prognosis of many lesions. At a minimum it will provide guidance for immediate treatment of infection or the need for further evaluation, including special culture techniques or histology. Absence of inflammation usually rules out an infectious cause.

Conversely, the limitations of the technique are dramatically illustrated by the range of appearance of skin "lumps" routinely presented to the clinical cytologist. Minimal differences separate hyperplasia, benign adenoma, and well-differentiated malignancy for many lesions. Differentiation may not be possible without the aid of tissue architecture and evidence of local invasion. However, with experience, most lesions can be categorized sufficiently to provide useful clinical guidance. Obscure anaplastic lesions often are as challenging for the histopathologist as for the cytopathologist. Diagnosis may require use of electron microscopy, special stains, and immunohistochemical characterization.

The outline and classification scheme of Yager and Wilcock (1994) is used in an attempt to unify classification of skin lesions. Description will be limited to skin-associated lesions or tumors for which cytological descriptions have been reported or for which the authors consider there are identifying features.

TECHNIQUES

The previously described techniques for aspiration biopsy, impression smears, and scrapings are applicable for lesions of the skin.

NORMAL TISSUE

Surface scrapings of normal superficial epidermis contain fully keratinized squamous epithelial cells. Deeper scrapings contain basilar epithelial cells, follicular elements, and erythrocytes.

NONNEOPLASTIC DISEASE

Granulation Tissue

CLINICAL AND CYTOLOGICAL DIAGNOSES

The histological diagnosis of granulation requires evidence of tissue architecture. Because architecture is not preserved in cytology preparations, this classification is not appropriate. Cytological diagnosis must be limited to the cellular inflammatory response observed. However, a mononuclear response with a predominance of macrophages and benign reactive stromal cells with an appropriate clinical description provides support for this interpretation. The sampling technique used will affect the harvest, distribution, and appearance of cells.

Hematoma/Seroma (Figs. 4-1 and 4-2)

CLINICAL DIAGNOSIS

Hematomas and seromas are common after trauma or surgery. Fine-needle aspirations are used for confirmation and to rule out infectious, inflammatory, or neoplastic causes.

CYTOLOGICAL DIAGNOSIS

Aspirate fluid may be clear to colored depending on the number and degenerative state of the erythrocytes. The erythrocyte preservation and macrophage response changes with the duration of the lesion. Platelets are absent unless there is fresh hemorrhage. There may be low to moderate numbers of macrophages with or without erythrocytophagy and evidence of hemoglobin breakdown products, including hemosiderin in older lesions.

Abscess (Figs. 4-3 to 4-7)

CLINICAL DIAGNOSIS
Skin abscesses are a common clinical diagnosis especially in the cat. Normal oral flora are a common source of bacterial agents, which enter via bite wounds. Soil- and water-borne bacteria and fungi often gain entry through wounds. There are reports implicating a wide range of etiological agents, including mycoplasma (see Chapter 3).

CYTOLOGICAL DIAGNOSIS
The stage of lesion development and the aspiration site (i.e., central or wall area) affects the cell harvest in pyogranulomatous lesions. Early neutrophil predominance may eventually be replaced by a mixed or mononuclear response. The infectious agents release toxins and induce cytokine activation, which initiate cell chemotaxis and varying degrees of cellular degenerative change. Neutrophil accumulation and nuclear morphology provide immediate evidence for local chemotaxis, as well as the presence and virulence of cytotoxins. Many anaerobic bacteria and mycoplasma initiate active neutrophil chemotaxis but minimal neutrophil nuclear degenerative change. In contrast, some aerobic bacteria and fungi induce marked neutrophil nuclear lysis. These degenerative or lytic changes are recognized as swelling and loss of filaments separating nuclear lobules. Nuclear chromatolysis is considered to be more specific for cytotoxins than karyorrhexis and karyopyknosis, which can be associated with normal "aging" of the cells. With marked nuclear degeneration, neutrophils may appear indistinguishable from macrophages. In a pyogranulomatous or mixed response, variable numbers of macrophages, lymphocytes, and plasma cells may be present.

Bacteria may be observed intracellularly and extracellularly. If bacteria are not readily observed where there is prominent neutrophil accumulation and nuclear degeneration, careful examination and culture are indicated. Where neutrophils predominate, but no bacteria are found, treatment with antibiotics before cytological evaluation should be suspected. Clinical history is critical. If pleomorphic bacteria are present in large numbers and there is less-than-expected neutrophil nuclear degeneration, the possibility of anaerobic bacteria should be considered and appropriate sample collection, transport, and culture initiated.

Most bacteria stain light blue to dark blue with Romanowsky's stains. Staphylococcal organisms typically appear in small grapelike clusters, whereas streptococci and peptococci usually appear in chains. Gram's, acid-fast, fungal, and other special stains may be required to demonstrate and differentiate characteristics of some agents originally observed using Romanowsky's stain. Chapter 3 contains further details describing specific infectious agents and host responses.

Granuloma

CLINICAL AND CYTOLOGICAL DIAGNOSES
Granuloma is a histological term for a cellular infiltrate consisting primarily of macrophages. Epithelial macrophages and/or giant cells are also a feature. These cellular characteristics are easily identified with aspirate preparations, and a diagnosis of mononuclear inflammation is given. Inciting causes include mycotic agents and foreign bodies.

NEOPLASTIC DISEASE

EPITHELIAL TUMORS

Cystic Epidermal Tumors, Epidermal Inclusion Cysts, Follicular Cysts, and Infundibular Cysts (Figs. 4-11 to 4-16)

CLINICAL DIAGNOSIS
Cystic epidermal tumors include the histologically differentiated epidermal cysts, follicular cysts (infundibular, matrical, isthmus), and intracutaneous cornifying epithelioma (Walder, 1992; Yager, 1994). On cytological examination, each of these lesions may appear similar and are classified as epidermal inclusion cysts.

Cystic epidermal tumors have an outer wall of squamous epithelium with a keratin-filled center. They account for 6% (Yager, 1994) of canine skin tumors but are less common in the cat. Cystic epidermal tumors are benign skin lesions that can be surgically removed and have no tendency to recur (Yager, 1994).

CYTOLOGICAL DIAGNOSIS
Fine-needle aspirations of cystic epidermal tumors contain keratinized epithelial cells with pyknotic nuclei distributed in a background of blue amorphous cellular debris. Nuclei are often pyknotic if present. Clear, notched, rectangular cholesterol crystals resulting from cell breakdown may be present. Cholesterol crystals are often dissolved by the alcohol in Romanowsky types of stains, leaving behind their negative image, cholesterol clefts. A typical cellular inflammatory reaction may be present within the blue background debris if the cysts have ruptured.

Basal Cell Tumors (Figs. 4-17 to 4-19)

CLINICAL DIAGNOSIS

Although basal cell tumors represent 22% of skin tumors in cats and 6% in the dog (Yager, 1994), they are seldom diagnosed cytologically in the referral cases submitted to the Ontario Veterinary Teaching Hospital. The term *basal cell tumor* can be used broadly to encompass any tumor arising from epithelium of epidermal or adnexal origin (Walder, 1992). Some authors believe the term should be restricted to the syndrome in cats in which no adnexal differentiation is seen (Walder, 1992). It is suggested that *trichoblastoma* is a more appropriate term for many of the more common basal tumors seen in dogs and cats (Walder, 1992). Thus many tumors diagnosed as basal cell tumors cytologically, which previously would have been similarly diagnosed histologically, are now being classified histologically as trichoblastomas. *Basal cell carcinoma* (basal cell epithelioma) is reserved for those tumors with a potentially aggressive nature (Tyler, 1999; Walder, 1992). Basal cell tumors, or trichoblastomas, may be large and can ulcerate, but metastasis is not reported (Yager, 1994).

CYTOLOGICAL DIAGNOSIS

Aspirates or impression smears of basal cell tumors and trichoblastomas contain uniform small cells with basophilic cytoplasm and a high N:C ratio (1:1 ratio). They occasionally occur in a row or ribbon of cells (Barton, 1987). Melanin pigment may be observed in both basal cells and melanocytes (Barton, 1987). Histological examination may be required for diagnosis because basal cells can be observed in epidermal inclusion cysts and other benign adnexal or follicular tumors.

Basal Cell Tumors with Follicular and/or Adnexal Differentiation, Including Trichoepithelioma, Pilomatrixoma, and Sebaceous Gland Adenoma or Carcinoma (Figs. 4-20 to 4-22)

CLINICAL DIAGNOSIS

Basal cell tumors with follicular (e.g., trichoepithelioma and pilomatrixoma) or adnexal (e.g., sebaceous gland hyperplasia, adenoma, and carcinoma) differentiation are common in dogs and, except for trichoblastomas, are uncommon to rare in cats (Yager, 1994). Basal cell tumors with follicular differentiation account for approximately 2% of skin tumors in the dog (Yager, 1994). Benign sebaceous tumors account for approximately 8% of all canine skin masses (Scott, 1990; Yager, 1994) but only 2% in cats (Yager, 1994). Sebaceous adenocarcinomas are rare (Yager, 1994).

CYTOLOGICAL DIAGNOSIS

Few reports describe the cytological appearance of these tumors. Cytological preparations from tumors with sebaceous differentiation contain moderate numbers of cells with abundant foamy cytoplasm and small central nuclei (Tyler, 1999). Cytological diagnoses should be restricted to benign epithelial or adnexal tumor with or without sebaceous differentiation because a cytological distinction cannot be made between a basal cell tumor with sebaceous differentiation and sebaceous gland hyperplasia or adenoma.

Cytologically, cystic epidermal tumors, basal cell tumors or trichoblastomas, and basal cell tumors with follicular or adnexal (sebaceous) differentiation may all contain basal cells with areas of keratinized debris. Cytological differentiation is not always possible. These tumors may represent different degrees of differentiation and cytologically classification may not be important because each has a benign clinical course. These tumors are often removed surgically because of their physical appearance.

The following guidelines are proposed, recognizing the limitations for cytological diagnosis of these tumors. Two approaches are possible. First, an epithelial inclusion cyst is diagnosed if only keratinized debris is seen. A basal cell tumor or trichoblastoma is diagnosed if basal cells predominate. A diagnosis of sebaceous gland hyperplasia or sebaceous adenoma is made if there is a pure population of sebaceous types of cells. Conversely, an umbrella cytological diagnosis can be made that includes all of these tumors, that is, benign epidermal or adnexal tumor with or without sebaceous differentiation. Hopefully, a consensus will ultimately be reached in this area. From a clinical viewpoint, either the umbrella diagnosis or the more specific diagnosis will rule out the more serious skin neoplasms.

Perianal Gland (Hepatoid) Tumor (Figs. 4-23 to 4-26)

CLINICAL DIAGNOSIS

The perianal tumor is an adnexal tumor with a specific cytological appearance. Perianal gland tumors are the third or fourth most common cutaneous neoplasm in the dog (Ross, 1991; Yager, 1994). Most of these perianal gland tumors are benign; however, it is difficult with histology and may be impossible cytologically to differentiate hyperplasia from adenoma.

CYTOLOGICAL DIAGNOSIS

The "hepatoid" cytological appearance of perianal cells is characteristic. On fine-needle biopsy these cells exfoliate readily and have a round central nucleus with a prominent nucleolus. Cells are often present in large sheets or clusters. The cytoplasm is finely granular and pink. Small flattened cells called *reserve cells* can occasionally be seen around the larger hepatoid cells.

Perianal Gland Carcinoma (Figs. 4-27 and 4-28)

CLINICAL DIAGNOSIS
Perianal gland carcinoma accounts for 3% to 17% of all perianal tumors (Vail, 1990). Between 5% and 15% of these tumors will metastasize locally late in the disease (Vail, 1990; Yager, 1994).

CYTOLOGICAL DIAGNOSIS
Perianal gland carcinoma can be difficult to distinguish from an adenoma both cytologically and histologically (Vail, 1990). Without the histological criteria of tumor invasiveness, cytologists must rely on the usual criteria of malignancy, including nuclear pleomorphism, hyperchromasia, and increased N:C ratio.

Tumors of Sweat Glands (Paratrichial) (Figs. 4-29 to 4-31)

CLINICAL DIAGNOSIS
Sweat gland tumors account for 2% of canine and feline skin tumors. Benign tumors are more common in the dog but rare in the cat (Yager, 1994). Sweat gland carcinomas and ceruminous gland tumors of the horizontal ear canal in the cat are very aggressive and frequently metastasize to distant sites (Legendre, 1981; Yager, 1994).

CYTOLOGICAL DIAGNOSIS
Cytological reports are absent, but the usual criteria of epithelial malignancy are to be expected.

Apocrine Gland Anal Sac Carcinoma

CLINICAL DIAGNOSIS
Adenocarcinoma of the anal sac is reported in dogs. This tumor develops most commonly in old female dogs (Hause, 1981; Ross, 1991). Adenocarcinoma of the anal sac is rare but carries a guarded prognosis because the tumor has often metastasized to regional lymph nodes at the time of diagnosis (Ross, 1991). Differentiation of apocrine carcinomas from perianal gland carcinoma is important because each has a very different prognosis. Based on immunohistochemical features, both anal glands and anal sac glands may be the site of origin for these carcinomas (Vos, 1993).

CYTOLOGICAL DIAGNOSIS
Cytological reports are rare, but it is assumed that the usual characteristics of malignancy should be applied.

Squamous Cell Carcinoma (Figs. 4-32 to 4-38)

CLINICAL DIAGNOSIS
In dogs, squamous cell carcinoma accounts for 2% (Yager, 1994) to 5% (Bostock, 1972) and in cats 15% of all cutaneous tumors (Miller, 1991; Yager, 1994). Although squamous cell carcinoma may develop at any site in the body, they are more frequently diagnosed in the skin, digits, oral cavity, and tonsil (Yager, 1994). In 112 dogs, 18% of squamous cell carcinomas involved the oral cavity with a high rate of involvement of the limbs, digits, scrotum, and lips (Strafuss, 1976). The nailbed has a predilection, especially in large black breeds (Madewell, 1982; O'Rourke, 1985; Paradis, 1989) in which the tumors may be multiple (Paradis, 1989). In dogs chronically exposed to sun, the nose and thinly haired flank areas are also predisposed (Madewell, 1982). Most canine cutaneous squamous cell carcinomas have a low rate of metastasis, and if surgical excision is complete, the prognosis is good (Yager, 1994). The exception is digital squamous carcinomas, which are reported to metastasize or invade locally in up to 20% of cases (Madewell, 1982; Paradis, 1989; Yager, 1994). In dogs with squamous cell carcinoma originating from subungual epithelium, 95% survived for at least 1 year, whereas only 60% were alive if the squamous cell carcinoma originated in other parts of the digit (Marino, 1995). Although squamous cell carcinomas are the second most common intraoral tumor in dogs, the tendency for late metastasis leads to a more favorable prognosis than with other intraoral neoplasms, such as melanoma (Oakes, 1993). In contrast, the prognosis with tonsillar squamous cell carcinoma is poor because metastasis to the local lymph nodes has usually occurred at the time of diagnosis (Oakes, 1993).

In cats, particularly if white, the preferred sites for squamous cell carcinoma are the thinly haired skin of ear tips, nasal planum, and lips. Over 80% of squamous cell carcinoma lesions in the cat are on the head (Ruslander, 1997). Squamous cell carcinomas are the most common intraoral tumor in the cat (Bostock, 1972). The prognosis is very poor for intraoral tumors because of local uncontrolled recurrence (Bostock, 1972; Cotter, 1981), whereas for skin tumors the prognosis depends on the degree of cellular anaplasia (Bostock, 1972). Although the skin tumors become locally invasive, they rarely metastasize (Lana, 1997). In a study including 61 cases of squamous cell carcinoma affecting the nasal planum and pinnae, affected cats were older and white, and none had evidence of metastasis (Lana, 1997). Some 58 of 61 cats were white or had white ear tips, supporting the probable influence of sunlight on the pathogenesis (Lana, 1997).

CYTOLOGICAL DIAGNOSIS
The cytological diagnosis of squamous cell carcinoma is frequently made with a high degree of confidence,

especially when collated with pertinent clinical information. Cellular atypia can vary from mild to extreme. In aspiration slides, cells may be single or arranged in obvious epithelial clusters. Intercellular bridges representing desmosomal junctions may be visible, especially if wet fixation and trichrome stains are used. Nuclei may be small and condensed, as expected in well-differentiated squamous epithelial cells, or they may be large with marked anisokaryosis and prominent nucleoli.

Asynchrony in nuclear and cytoplasmic differentiation is an important indicator of malignancy. As the normal squamous cell matures and keratinizes, the nucleus undergoes pyknosis and karyorrhexis and then disappears, leaving an anuclear squame. As the nuclear chromatin condenses, the cytoplasm becomes keratinized or blue-green in appearance. With malignant transformation, normal progressive differentiation disappears. Cells may have an open vesicular and even vacuolated nucleus despite advanced keratinization of the cytoplasm or a small pyknotic nucleus in a parabasilar or early intermediate squamous epithelial cell.

The cytoplasm may be vacuolated with increased concentration around the nucleus, forming a nuclear halo. The presence of "tadpole cells" with the cytoplasm blunted and displaced to one side have traditionally been associated with malignancy in humans. They are less frequently seen in squamous cell carcinoma cytological preparations from dogs and cats, possibly because of species differences or differences in fixation and staining.

ROUND CELL TUMORS (DISCRETE CELL TUMORS)

Histiocytic Diseases

Several histiocytic syndromes are recognized in dogs. These include cutaneous histiocytoma, cutaneous histiocytosis, systemic histiocytosis, malignant histiocytosis, and histiocytic sarcoma. New evidence suggests that the proliferation of histiocytes is common to all these diseases (Affloter, 1997). Both macrophages and dendritic cells can be classified as histiocytic because both originate from a common precursor cell in the bone marrow (Affloter, 1997). These histiocytic proliferative disorders (HPDs) result from a proliferation of the dendritic cell line (Affloter, 1997). Dendritic cells function in the presentation of antigen to T lymphocytes and thus in the production of an antigen-specific immune response (Affloter, 1997). Phenotypic evaluation of these cells classifies them further as Langerhans' cells (Affloter, 1997). Therefore canine histiocytic proliferative disorders are essentially Langerhans' cell histiocytosis (Affloter, 1997). Phenotypic differences between the various types of Langerhans' cells distinguishes the different syndromes (Affloter, 1997).

Cutaneous Histiocytoma (Figs. 4-40 and 4-41)

CLINICAL DIAGNOSIS

Cutaneous histiocytoma originates from epidermal Langerhans' cells (Affloter, 1997). It appears as a benign dermal nodule in the skin of dogs. The majority, 60% to 80%, occur in dogs less than 5 years of age (Yager, 1994). These tumors regress spontaneously on their own.

CYTOLOGICAL DIAGNOSIS

On FNA, cell harvest is low to moderate, containing a pleomorphic population of mononuclear cells 12 to 26 μ in diameter (Tyler, 1999). There is moderate anisocytosis. Nuclei are usually round but may be indented with only rare nucleoli. Nuclear chromatin is finely granular. As these tumors naturally regress, increased numbers of benign lymphocytes appear, often confusing the diagnosis. The stage of tumor regression must be considered whenever a diagnosis of histiocytoma is contemplated.

Cutaneous Histiocytosis

CLINICAL DIAGNOSIS

A syndrome known as cutaneous histiocytosis is described in dogs (Bender, 1989; Calderwood Mays, 1986). Multifocal cutaneous lesions develop that appear similar to cutaneous histiocytoma (Bender, 1989; Calderwood Mays, 1986). Phenotypically these dendritic cells display increased epidermal antigens (compared with cutaneous histiocytoma) consistent with activated epidermal Langerhans' cells (Affloter, 1997). The lesions can wax and wane over months to years.

CYTOLOGICAL DIAGNOSIS

Aspirates from three dogs contained cells with round to oval nuclei (Calderwood Mays, 1986). Nucleoli were not prominent. Cells usually had abundant foamy cytoplasm. The cells resembled those of the standard cutaneous histiocytoma. Some aspirates had neutrophils, and others had lymphocytes interspersed (Calderwood Mays, 1986).

Systemic Histiocytosis (Fig. 4-42)

CLINICAL DIAGNOSIS

Systemic histiocytosis is a disease of young adult (approximately 4 years) male Bernese mountain dogs that has also been reported in rottweilers, golden and Labrador retrievers, and several other breeds (Affloter, 1997; Paterson, 1995). Systemic histiocytosis and cutaneous histiocytosis are classified under the umbrella of "reactive histiocytosis." As with cutaneous histiocytosis, these cells are consistent with activated epidermal Langerhans' cells (Affloter, 1997). The skin is consistently affected, but regional lymph nodes, eyes, and nasal cavity may also be affected (Affloter, 1997; Paterson, 1995). Tissues become infiltrated with benign-appearing histiocytic cells. The disease is not usually fatal, but the protracted course of remissions and relapses usually leads to euthanasia of affected dogs.

CYTOLOGICAL DIAGNOSIS

Histiocytic infiltrates in systemic histiocytosis do not exhibit malignant criteria, unlike the pleomorphic cells of malignant histiocytosis (Paterson, 1995). Histologically the skin is infiltrated with large round cells that have open vesicular, possibly indented nuclei (Affloter, 1997). Lymphocytes and neutrophils may be intermixed (Affloter, 1997). Cytological reports are rare.

Malignant Histiocytosis (Figs. 4-43 to 4-50)

CLINICAL DIAGNOSIS

Malignant histiocytosis is a malignant disease initially described in older Bernese mountain dogs but also described in rottweilers and golden, Labrador, and flat-coated retrievers (Affloter, 1997; Hayden, 1993). The phenotypic origin of these cells is still unclear (Affloter, 1997). Clinically the dogs present with non-responsive generalized signs, including anorexia, lethargy, neurological signs, and weight loss (Peaston, 1993; Rosin, 1986). It is a multisystem infiltrate of a systemic progressive proliferation of histiocytes and carries a poor prognosis. The primary organs affected include the spleen, lymph nodes, lung, and bone marrow (Affloter, 1997). The skin is only rarely involved (Affloter, 1997). Malignant histiocytosis is characterized histologically by the presence of giant cells, atypical histiocytes, and abnormal mitosis.

CYTOLOGICAL DIAGNOSIS

One cytology report of malignant histiocytosis describes large cells with a low to moderate N:C ratio and moderate anisocytosis and anisokaryosis (Newlands, 1993). Cell borders were distinct, and cell shape was variable (Newlands, 1993). The cytoplasm was slightly basophilic with a variable amount of fine vacuolation and erythrocytophagy (Newlands, 1993). Occasional multinucleated cells were present (Newlands, 1993). Another report describes cells that varied markedly in size and had indistinct cell borders. N:C ratio was variable but often high. Nuclei had coarse hyperchromatic chromatin patterns with multiple prominent nucleoli (Moroff, 1990). An FNA from a chest mass was highly cellular with abundant vacuolated cytoplasm (Ramsey, 1996). Nuclei were large with irregular nuclei and coarse stippled nuclear chromatin and large numbers of mitosis (Ramsey, 1996). A liver imprint in an affected Bernese mountain dog showed a pleomorphic population of mononuclear cells (Peaston, 1993). Cells were

stellate, spindle, and round with marked anisokaryosis, and with a moderate N:C ratio. Binucleation and erythrocytophagy were occasionally seen (Peaston, 1993). Bone marrow aspirates contained large pleomorphic mononuclear cells with abundant vacuolated cytoplasm and hemosiderin pigment (Peaston, 1993). In seven affected dogs, cytology preparations revealed highly cellular samples containing pleomorphic large mononuclear cells with marked anisokaryosis (Brown, 1994). Nucleoli were prominent. Mitosis was present and often abnormal (Brown, 1994). In four of the cases, erythrophagocytosis, leukophagocytosis, and multinucleation were present (Brown, 1994).

Histiocytic Sarcoma

CLINICAL AND CYTOLOGICAL DIAGNOSES

Canine histiocytic sarcoma presents as a soft-tissue skin mass. Flat-coated retrievers are predisposed, but it is also seen in golden and Labrador retrievers and rottweilers (Affloter, 1997). These tumors are solitary and locally aggressive (Affloter, 1997). Histiocytic sarcomas are frequently located on extremities, near joints, but are also reported in spleen, stomach, liver, and tongue (Affloter, 1997). Histiocytic sarcomas that develop in or near joints may have been previously misdiagnosed as synovial sarcomas. Both histiocytic sarcoma and malignant histiocytosis represent the neoplastic aggressive forms of Langerhans' cell proliferation. Again the phenotypic origin of these cells is unclear (Affloter, 1997). Histologically these cells are large, pleomorphic, and round (Affloter, 1997). Nuclei are large, indented, or twisted (Affloter, 1997). Bizarre mitosis and multinucleate forms are common (Affloter, 1997). Similar changes are expected cytologically. As research into these canine histiocytic disorders continues, classification and distinctions between the various categories will likely improve.

Mast Cell Tumors (Figs. 4-51 to 4-56)

CLINICAL DIAGNOSIS

In the dog, mast cell tumors represent 15% to 20% of all skin tumors (Yager, 1994). There is a reported breed predilection for boxers, pugs, and Boston terriers. Mast cell tumors are usually solitary, but multiple cutaneous tumors (cutaneous mastocytosis) are reported rarely in dogs (Davis, 1992). The behavior of canine mast cell tumors is highly correlated to histological grading when cellular criteria of malignancy and the mitotic figures per high-power field are the primary criteria (Yager, 1994). In dogs, more than 80% with grade 1 tumors and 50% with grade 2 tumors will be alive after 4 years, whereas with grade 3 tumors less than 10% survive a year (Yager, 1994). Similar prognostic grading in the cat has not been shown to be of value (Buerger, 1987), although tumors with increased mitotic activity and marked anisocytosis were associated with recurrence or spread (Wilcock, 1986). Cytological grading of tumors has not been assessed and correlated with the histological system or biological prognosis. At present we are restricted to a cytological diagnosis of mast cell tumor.

In the cat, mast cell tumors account for 1% to 6% of all feline neoplasms, and 10.3% to 20% of the cutaneous masses (Miller, 1991; Wilcock, 1986). Mast cell tumors are the second most common feline skin tumor (Wilcock, 1986). Only 2% are malignant (Miller, 1991; Wilcock, 1986). Feline mast cell tumors may be single or multiple. Most feline mast cell tumors are composed of normal-appearing mast cells and are classified as mastocytoma, mast cell type (Wilcock, 1986). In 10% to 20% of feline mast cell tumors the predominant cell appears "histiocytic," leading to the classification of mastocytoma, histiocytic type (Wilcock, 1986). Cats with this histiocytic type are typically younger (Miller, 1991). Most of the described cases have been in Siamese cats (Chastain, 1988; Miller, 1991; Wilcock, 1986). The tumor masses are frequently multiple and usually regress spontaneously (Miller, 1991; Wilcock, 1986).

No cytology reports of these skin variants are available.

In the cat, cutaneous mast cell tumors are a separate entity from visceral mastocytosis. Approximately half of feline mast cell tumors occur in the skin and half in the viscera (Macy, 1986). The visceral tumors frequently involve the liver and spleen. Approximately half are leukemic at the time of diagnosis (Macy, 1986). Although visceral mast cell tumors appear similar to the cutaneous form on cytological examination, visceral mast cell tumors have a guarded prognosis (Macy, 1986).

CYTOLOGICAL DIAGNOSIS

Mast cell tumors are easily diagnosed using most cytology techniques and Romanowsky's stain. The staining technique used will affect the intensity and color of mast cell granules. Mast cell granules are not readily visible using routine H&E, Papanicolaou's stains, and some of the "fast" Wright's stains. Granules vary from 0.2 to 5 μ in diameter. Well-differentiated mast cells are round and 7 to 20 μ in diameter with an eccentric nucleus. Mast cell tumors exfoliate readily, but cells are fragile and often rupture during preparation of slides. The released granules are scattered throughout the background. Eosinophils may be present, especially in the dog. Intact cells are round and discrete with pale-staining nuclei and inconspicuous nucleoli. With Wright's stain, the nuclei may be obscured by the prominent purple-staining granules.

Anaplastic tumors are rarely reported cytologically. The cells are poorly granulated and have marked anisokaryosis and prominent nucleoli. Even in extremely anaplastic mast cell tumors a few small positive granules are usually present and can be identified using Wright's stain. This cytological observation may assist the histopathological differentiation of a round cell tumor of undetermined origin. It is suggested that these anaplastic tumors have a greater likelihood of metastasis or aggressive local recurrence, but no studies have been reported correlating cytological appearance to behavioral tendencies of the tumor.

Canine Extramedullary Plasmacytoma (Figs. 4-57 to 4-61)

CLINICAL DIAGNOSIS

Tumors of plasma cells that arise outside of bone are termed *extramedullary plasmacytomas* (Clark, 1992). They have been reported in the gastrointestinal tract, skin, oral cavity, gingiva, and tongue (Brunnert, 1992; Clark, 1992; Rakich, 1989). Plasmacytomas occur predominantly in older dogs (Rogers, 1991). The cutaneous form may account for up to 2% of canine skin tumors (Yager, 1994). Histological evidence suggests that these tumors have a benign clinical course despite many of the cytological criteria of malignancy. Surgical excision is curative in more than 90% of the cutaneous cases, and unlike myelomas, plasmacytomas do not appear to be associated with paraneoplastic diseases (Frazier, 1993).

CYTOLOGICAL DIAGNOSIS

Although cytological reports are rare (Rakich, 1989), plasmacytomas should be included in the list of possible round cell tumors. In five reported cases (Rakich, 1989) the cells were described as discrete, appearing "plasmacytoid" with prominent anisocytosis and anisokaryosis. Binucleation or multinucleation may be a feature. Mitoses were rare to abundant. Cytoplasm may be scant to abundant (Rakich, 1989). Differentiation from multiple myeloma depends greatly on the site (skin) and lack of evidence of bone lysis and/or gammopathy. It may be impossible using cytology to differentiate plasmacytoma from the rare myeloma metastatic to the skin.

Transmissible Venereal Tumor (Figs. 4-62 and 4-63)

CLINICAL DIAGNOSIS

Transmissible venereal tumor is an uncommon transplantable tumor of dogs. Transmission occurs at the time of mating. Typical cutaneous nodules are produced in the genital and oronasal area. The tumors usually remain localized but may disseminate widely, either through multiple implantations at sites of injury and abrasion or by true metastasis. Many tumors regress spontaneously (Yager, 1994). Surgical excision combined with chemotherapy is usually curative (Rogers, 1991).

CYTOLOGICAL DIAGNOSIS

The cytological appearance of the cells in transmissible venereal tumors is characteristic. Aspiration or impression slides are highly cellular. The cells are discrete and round. Nuclei are round with a distinctive clumped, coarse granular chromatin and one or two prominent nucleoli (Richardson, 1981). Most cells are large (16 to 24 µ) compared with neutrophils (10 µ). Cytoplasmic vacuolation may be present. There may be low numbers of intermixed lymphocytes and plasma cells. Mitotic figures may be numerous (Rogers, 1991).

SPINDLE CELL TUMORS

Spindle cell tumors arise from mesodermal tissue and consequently may be found in any anatomic location. In general they are locally invasive with poorly defined tumor margins. Hemangiosarcoma may be the exception, having a higher metastatic rate (Graham, 1993). Soft-tissue sarcomas account for 14% to 17% of all malignancies in dogs and 7% to 9% in cats (Graham, 1993). Aggressive surgical resection is the treatment of choice in most cases regardless of tumor type or origin.

Spindle Cell Tumors of Canine Soft Tissue (Hemangiopericytoma, Schwannoma) (Figs. 4-64 to 4-67)

CLINICAL DIAGNOSIS

It is often impossible to differentiate hemangiopericytoma and schwannoma using histology at the light microscope level. Consequently, they are classified together as spindle cell tumors of canine soft tissue (Yager, 1994). Hemangiopericytoma is a tumor of pericytes that line the blood vessels. Schwannoma is a tumor of the nerve sheath or Schwann cell. Although these tumors usually do not metastasize, they are locally invasive. The rate of recurrence at the site of previous excision can lead to euthanasia (Pstotino, 1988). These tumors account for 4% (Bostock, 1986) to 7% (Yager, 1994) of canine skin tumors and are rare in cats.

CYTOLOGICAL DIAGNOSIS

For cytological classification, it is logical to include all spindle cell tumors of soft-tissue origin within one group. FNA of these tumors yields a moderate number of spindle-shaped cells arranged singly or occasionally in clusters, suggesting a whorling pattern. Nuclei are round to elongate with one or two inconspicuous to prominent nucleoli. Cytoplasm is gray-blue and "veillike" (Barton, 1987). Differentiation from other spindle cell tumors may at times be impossible. Evidence of cytological atypia (hyperchromasia and anisokaryosis) is suggestive of fibrosarcoma.

Malignant Fibrous Histiocytoma (or Giant Cell Tumor of Soft Parts) (Figs. 4-68 to 4-72)

CLINICAL DIAGNOSIS

Malignant fibrous histiocytoma is an infiltrative spindle cell sarcoma found most commonly in the skin, especially of the distal extremities (Yager, 1994). Malignant fibrous histiocytoma has been reported in dogs but more frequently in cats (Allen, 1988; Garma-Avina, 1987; Pace, 1994). Local recurrence is common, whereas distant metastasis is rare, as with other spindle cell sarcomas (Yager, 1994). The finding of malignant fibrous histiocytoma in the spleen of the dog warrants a poor prognosis (Hendrick, 1991).

CYTOLOGICAL DIAGNOSIS

On cytological examination the predominant cells are neoplastic, appearing as fibroblasts, histiocyte-like cells, and giant cells. The primary tumor cells are pleomorphic, varying in appearance from fusiform to round, large, and "plump." Large giant cells are routinely present and may resemble osteoclasts (Gibson, 1989). Multinucleation with dyskaryosis may be present. Often nucleoli are prominent and irregular (Desnoyers, 1994). Extracellular amorphous eosinophilic material may be prominent and likely represents collagen production by the tumor. The exact identification of this tumor may be difficult because other spindle cell sarcomas may exhibit multinucleation and extracellular eosinophilic material, which is common to spindle cell origin neoplasms (Pace, 1994). Because spindle cell tumors presumably arise from a common primitive mesenchymal cell, and because local invasion and recurrence, as opposed to metastasis, is a common biological behavior, cytological or histological differentiation has limited clinical significance unless further evidence for correlation with biological behavior or response to treatment is demonstrated.

Fibroma, Collagen Nevus, and Fibroadnexal Dysplasia

CLINICAL AND CYTOLOGICAL DIAGNOSES

Fibroma, collagen nevus, and fibroadnexal dysplasia require a histological diagnosis. These are all benign skin lesions. Aspiration reveals low numbers of normal-appearing stromal cells with low N:C ratio, abundant cytoplasm, and inconspicuous nucleoli. Differentiation from granulation tissue may be impossible.

Vaccine Reaction (Figs. 4-73 and 4-74)

CLINICAL AND CYTOLOGICAL DIAGNOSES

A vaccine-induced cellular reaction that develops into a subcutaneous nodule, may be evaluated cytologically. In the cat it is important to distinguish these reactions from the vaccine-induced fibrosarcomas

(Coyne, 1997). Nucleated cells vary depending on the time from vaccination and the area sampled. Cells include a combination of lymphocytes, mononuclear cells, and macrophages. A characteristic pink amorphous intracellular and extracellular substance may be present (Tyler, 1999) and is presumed to be adjuvant. Reactive stromal cells may be present, and differentiation from neoplasia may require histological biopsy.

Fibrosarcoma (Figs. 4-75 to 4-80)

CLINICAL DIAGNOSIS

In dogs, fibrosarcomas account for 2% (Yager, 1994) to 7% (Bostock, 1972) of cutaneous tumors and 9% of skeletal neoplasms (Ablin, 1991). In cats, fibrosarcomas are the second or third most common skin tumor, representing 11% (Yager, 1994) to 25% (Bostock, 1972) of all cutaneous masses and are the second most common intraoral neoplasm (Cotter, 1981). Feline sarcoma virus is responsible for multiple fibrosarcomas in young cats (Kass, 1993). As well, cats can develop sarcomas at sites of previous vaccination (Coyne, 1997; Kass, 1993). Aluminum hydroxide and aluminum phosphate used as adjuvants in feline vaccines may induce proliferation of mesenchymal cells that undergo neoplastic transformation (Kass, 1993). The postvaccinal sarcomas reported include fibrosarcoma, malignant fibrous histiocytomas, osteosarcoma, rhabdomyosarcoma, and chondrosarcoma (Hendrick, 1994). In both dogs and cats with fibrosarcomas the best treatment is complete surgical removal. The clinical prognosis is poorer when complete removal is impossible.

CYTOLOGICAL DIAGNOSIS

On cytological examination the primary cells can vary from classical well-differentiated stromal cells to bizarre anaplastic cells with little or no differentiating characteristics. Typically the cells are single and have round to elongated nuclei, mild to marked anisokaryosis, frequently large bizarre nucleoli, and round to bipolar basophilic cytoplasm. Fine pink cytoplasmic granulation may be present.

Differentiation between granulation tissue, fibroma, and well-differentiated fibrosarcoma may be difficult to impossible in some cases. The nuclear features of neoplasia, such as anisokaryosis and large prominent nucleoli, are often present in marked hyperplasia. The extent of cell exfoliation may be a useful guide in this differentiation. Cell exfoliation is poor from benign stromal tumors and is somewhat higher from fibrosarcomas, especially if less differentiated. Exfoliation is also high with benign stromal hyperplasia, but greater cell heterogeneity is expected.

In cats after injection with rabies vaccine, aspirate cellularity increased for 21 days and consisted of macrophages and lymphocytes (Schultze, 1997). A blue amorphous substance was seen in the macrophages of some cats injected with rabies virus vaccine (Schultze, 1997). Feline rhinotracheitis, calicivirus, and panleukopenia virus vaccine and feline leukemia virus vaccine sites had moderate cellularity at week 1, which slowly decreased with time (Schultze, 1997).

Lipoma (Figs. 4-81 to 4-83)

CLINICAL DIAGNOSIS

Lipomas are benign mesenchymal tumors of normal-appearing adipocytes. Lipomas are very common in dogs. Aggressive tissue invasion by otherwise normal-appearing adipocytes is diagnosed as infiltrating lipoma (Yager, 1994). On histological examination, differentiation is determined solely on the basis of tissue invasion. Cytological distinction may be impossible (Yager, 1994). Infiltrative lipomas do not metastasize but are very invasive locally, making complete surgical removal difficult (Kramek, 1985; McChesney, 1980).

CYTOLOGICAL DIAGNOSIS

When aspirate material from a lipoma is placed on a glass slide, it appears clear unless mixed with blood cells and remains in a globular shape. The material appears to spread well initially but quickly becomes irregular as it coalesces and aggregates as expected for a drop of oil. The aspirate material dries poorly. These physical characteristics are useful indicators of lipomatous origin. The microscopic appearance of Wright's stained aspirates of lipomas and infiltrating lipomas is of normal-appearing fat cells, single or more often in large clusters, mixed with erythrocytes and occasional small blood vessels. The cells are large and show a thin membrane delineating an area of abundant clear cytoplasm. Nuclei are located at the edge of the cell and are small and often appear pyknotic. If cells rupture, only bare nuclei or a few erythrocytes may be visible. Fat stains can confirm lipid content but are seldom required for routine interpretation. Accidental aspiration of normal fatty tissue instead of the lesion of concern should always be considered when fat cells are aspirated.

Liposarcoma (Figs. 4-84 to 4-86)

CLINICAL DIAGNOSIS

Liposarcoma is rarely diagnosed in dogs and cats. Metastasis to distant sites and local aggressiveness are reported in affected dogs and cats (Doster, 1986; Tanimoto, 1987).

CYTOLOGICAL DIAGNOSIS

In cytological preparations from a canine liposarcoma, pleomorphic adipocytes were described that varied from normal size with low N:C ratio and abundant cytoplasm to smaller cells with a high N:C ratio, some basophilia of the cytoplasm, and one to multiple lipid droplets (Messick, 1989). Some cells were multinucleated (Messick, 1989) and had peripheralization of the nucleus by lipid contents (Messick, 1989). Similar cells without lipid droplets were interpreted as primitive mesenchymal cells (Messick, 1989).

Myxoma and Myxosarcoma (Figs. 4-87 to 4-91)

CLINICAL DIAGNOSIS

Myxomatous tumors are rare in the dog and cat, with the skin being the usual focus in the dog (Grindhem, 1990). These tumors probably arise from multipotential mesenchymal cells (Grindhem, 1990).

CYTOLOGICAL DIAGNOSIS

A cytological report in one dog describes a population of large mononuclear cells with eccentric nuclei and low to high N:C ratio (Grindhem, 1990). The cytoplasm was pale and vacuolated and occasionally had an eosinophilic fringe. The background was stippled eosinophilic, suggestive of mucin. Similar cells were observed in a local lymph node (Grindhem, 1990).

Hemangioma

CLINICAL DIAGNOSIS

In the dog, 2% (Bostock, 1972) to 5% (Yager, 1994) of all cutaneous tumors are hemangiomas. In dogs the skin is the most common site, with the spleen being second (Srebernik, 1991). Hemangioma accounts for 1% (Miller, 1992) to 2% (Yager, 1994) of skin tumors in the cat.

CYTOLOGICAL DIAGNOSIS

Typical benign stromal cells predominate in hemangioma. Differentiation of benign endothelium, hemangioma, or well-differentiated hemangiosarcoma is not reliable using cytological examination.

Hemangiosarcoma (Figs. 4-92 to 4-98)

CLINICAL DIAGNOSIS

Hemangiosarcoma is a malignant neoplasm of endothelial cells, which may be cutaneous or visceral. In the dog the most frequently reported visceral location is the spleen, followed by the heart and liver (Srebernik, 1991). The prognosis is poor (Brown, 1985).

Cutaneous hemangiosarcoma has been associated with solar radiation in the dog (Hargis, 1992) and cat (Miller, 1992) and accounts for 1% of skin tumors in the dog and 2% to 3% in the cat (Yager, 1994). Cutaneous hemangiosarcoma is reported to lead to death in 30% of affected dogs (Culbertson, 1982; Hargis, 1992). It is often difficult to determine whether cutaneous hemangiosarcoma is primary or metastatic from internal tumors. In the cat the incidences of cutaneous and visceral forms are about equal (Scavelli, 1985). The cutaneous form has a high rate of local recurrence in the cat, frequently leading to euthanasia (Esplin, 1986; Miller, 1992).

CYTOLOGICAL DIAGNOSIS

The histological appearance of hemangiosarcoma varies from well-differentiated tumors containing benign-appearing endothelial cells to severely anaplastic stromal cells typical of sarcomas. This is also true cytologically. Sarcomas of well-differentiated endothelial cells may be impossible to differentiate from hemangiomas. Typically, hemangiosarcomas contain large, plump, fleshy, stromal cells. Nuclei are frequently 5 to 6 erythrocytes in diameter, and anisokaryosis may be dramatic. Nucleoli are multiple, irregular, and prominent. N:C ratio may be high. There may be erythrocytophagy and/or cytoplasmic hemosiderin. Red blood cells are usually present in the background. Cellularity is usually low but may be moderate, especially in the more anaplastic tumors. Hemangiosarcoma cells frequently demonstrate some of the most bizarre cellular atypia seen cytologically.

Melanoma (Figs. 4-99 to 4-105)

CLINICAL DIAGNOSIS

Melanomas arise from melanosomes, the pigment-producing cells of the skin. In dogs, benign melanomas account for 4% and malignant melanomas 1.6% (Yager, 1994) of cutaneous tumors. Melanomas are the most common neoplasm of the canine oral cavity and eye (Bolon, 1990). Location of the melanoma is important in determining prognosis. Only 5% to 15% of cutaneous melanomas are behaviorally malignant (Yager, 1994), with the exception of tumors involving the digits, in which 50% are associated with malignant behavior (Aronsohn, 1990; Marino, 1995). Melanomas of the oral cavity routinely metastasize and carry an extremely poor prognosis regardless of histological appearance (Bolon, 1990). Melanomas of the mucocutaneous lip junction are also associated with a poor prognosis (Aronsohn, 1990; Bolon, 1990; Yager, 1994).

In the cat, benign and malignant melanomas accounted for 3% of all skin tumors (Yager, 1994). In one study of 29 cats with melanomas, 19 were ocular, 5 were oral, and 5 were dermal tumors (Patnaik, 1988). Metastasis occurred in 63% of intraocular tumors and all palpebral tumors (Patnaik, 1988). In cats, as in dogs, oral melanomas have a high rate of metastasis (Patnaik, 1988). In a study of 57 cutaneous melanomas in cats, mean survival time after surgical removal was 4.5 months. All 16 cats available for postmortem had peripheral metastasis (vander Linde-Sipman, 1997).

CYTOLOGICAL DIAGNOSIS

On cytological examination, melanomas vary from mesenchymal to epithelial in appearance, even within the same aspirate, as a result of the neuroectodermal origin. The cytoplasm is light blue to dark blue and may contain distinct green-brown round to elongated granules as seen in samples from eye tissue, brown to black distinct granules, or fine gray-blue dustlike particles in the cytoplasm. In highly pigmented tumors the background of the slide may be black and cell details may be obscured. Even in tumors containing otherwise poorly differentiated cells, with Romanowsky's stains the cytoplasmic appearance of melanin and melanin precursors allows identification of melanoma origin. Completely amelanotic melanomas are rare and with careful searching some melanin can usually be found. Extreme anaplastic changes are observed in poorly differentiated melanomas. Cells may contain very large nuclei, three to four red blood cells in diameter, multiple prominent irregular nucleoli, and multiple aberrant mitosis. In well-differentiated melanomas in which few characteristics of malignancy are present, differentiation between benign or malignant tumors requires histological examination.

References

Ablin, L.W., Berg, J., and Schelling, S.H. Fibrosarcoma of the canine appendicular skeleton. *Am Anim Hosp Assoc* 27:303-309, 1991.

Affloter, V.K. and Moore, P.F. Histiocytosis. In *Proceedings of the 14th Annual Congress ESVD-ECVD*, Pisa, Italy, Sept 5-7, 1997.

Allen, S.W. and Duncan, J.R. Malignant fibrous histiocytoma in a cat. *J Am Vet Med Assoc* 192:90-91, 1988.

Aronsohn, M.G. Distal extremity melanocytic nevi and malignant melanomas in dogs. *J Am Anim Hosp Assoc* 26:605-612, 1990.

Barton, C.L. Cytologic diagnosis of cutaneous neoplasia: an algorithmic approach. *Compend Cont Ed Pract* 9:20-33, 1987.

Bender, W.M. and Muller, G.H. Multiple resolving cutaneous histiocytoma in a dog. *J Am Vet Med Assoc* 194:535-537, 1989.

Bolon, B., Calderwood-Mays, M.B., and Hall, B.J. Characteristics of canine melanomas and comparison of histology and DNA ploidy to their biologic behavior. *Vet Pathol* 27:96-102, 1990.

Bostock, D.E. The prognosis in cats bearing squamous cell carcinoma. *J Small Anim Pract* 13:119-125, 1972.

Brown, C.A. and Chalmers, S.A. Diffuse cutaneous mastocytosis in a cat. *Vet Pathol* 27:366-369, 1990.

Brown, D.E., Thrall, M.A., Getzy, D.M., et al. Cytology of canine malignant histiocytosis. *Vet Clin Pathol* 23:118-122, 1994.

Brown, N.O., Patnaik, A.K., and MacEwen, E.G. Canine hemangiosarcoma: retrospective analysis of 104 cases. *J Am Vet Med Assoc* 186:56-58, 1985.

Brunnert, S.R., Dee, L.A., Herron, A.J., et al. Gastric extramedullary plasmacytoma in a dog. *J Am Vet Med Assoc* 200:1501-1503, 1992.

Buerger, R.G. and Scott, D.W. Cutaneous mast cell neoplasia in cats: 14 cases (1975-1985). *J Am Vet Med Assoc* 190:1440-1443, 1987.

Calderwood Mays, M.B. and Bergeron, J.A. Cutaneous histiocytosis in dogs. *J Am Vet Med Assoc* 188:377-381, 1986.

Chastain, C.B., Turk, M.A.M., and O'Brien, D. Benign cutaneous mastocytomas in two litters of Siamese kittens. *J Am Vet Med Assoc* 193:959-960, 1988.

Clark, G.N., Berg, J., Engler, S.J., et al. Extramedullary plasmacytomas in dogs: results of surgical excision in 131 cases. *J Am Anim Hosp Assoc* 28:105-111, 1992.

Cotter, S.M. Oral pharyngeal neoplasms in the cat. *J Am Anim Hosp Assoc* 17: 917-920, 1981.

Coyne, M.J., Postorino Reeves, N.C., and Rosen, D.K. Estimated prevalence of infection-site sarcomas in cats during 1992. *J Am Vet Med Assoc* 210:249-251,1997.

Culbertson, M.R. Hemangiosarcoma of the canine skin and tongue. *Vet Pathol* 19:556-558,1982.

Davis, B.J., Page, R., Sannes, P.L., et al. Cutaneous mastocytosis in a dog. *Vet Pathol* 29:363-365, 1992.

Desnoyers, M. and St-Germain, L. What is your diagnosis? *Vet Clin Pathol* 23:89, 1994.

Doster, A.R., Tomlinson, M.J., Mahaffey, E.A., et al. Canine liposarcoma. *Vet Pathol* 23:84-87, 1986.

Esplin, D.G. and Carr, S.H. Cutaneous hemangiosarcoma in a cat. *Feline Practice* 16:38-40, 1986.

Frazier, K.S., Hines, M.E., Hurvitz, A.I., et al. Analysis of DNA aneuploidy and c-myc oncoprotein content of canine plasma cell tumors using flow cytometry. *Vet Pathol* 30:505-511, 1993.

Garma-Avina, J. Malignant fibrous histiocytoma of the giant cell type in a cat. *J Comp Pathol* 97:551-557, 1987.

Gibson, K.L., Blass, C.E., Simpson, M., et al. Malignant fibrous histiocytoma in a cat. *J Am Vet Med Assoc* 194:1443-1445, 1989.

Graham, J.C. and O'Keefe, D.A. Diagnosis and treatment of soft tissue sarcomas. *Compend Cont Ed Pract* 15:1627-1635, 1993.

Grindhem, C.B. and Riley, J. Myxosarcoma in a dog . *Vet Clin Pathol* 19:119-121,1990.

Hargis, A.M., Ihrke, P.J., Spangler, W.L., et al. A retrospective clinicopathologic study of 212 dogs with cutaneous hemangiomas and hemangiosarcomas. *Vet Pathol* 29:316-328, 1992.

Hause, W.R., Stevenson, S., Meuten, D.J., et al. Pseudohyperparathyroidism associated with adenocarcinomas of anal sac origin in four dogs. *J Am Anim Hosp Assoc* 17:373-379, 1981.

Hayden, D.W., Waters, D.J., Burke, B.A., et al. Disseminated malignant histiocytosis in a golden retriever: clinicopathologic, ultrastructural, and immunohistochemical findings. *Vet Pathol* 30:256-264, 1993.

Hendrick, M.J. and Brooks, J.J. Postvaccinal sarcomas in the cat: histology and immunohistochemistry. *Vet Pathol* 31:126-129, 1994.

Hendrick, M.J. and Goldschmidt, M.H. Do injection site reactions induce fibrosarcomas in cats? *J Am Vet Med Assoc* 199:968, 1991.

Kass, P.H., Barnes, W.G., Spangler, W.L., et al. Epidemiological evidence for a causal relation between vaccination and fibrosarcoma tumorigenesis in cats. *J Am Vet Med Assoc* 203: 396-405, 1993.

Kramek, B.A., Spackman, C.J., and Hayden, D.W. Infiltrative lipoma in three dogs. *J Am Vet Med Assoc* 186:81-82, 1985.

Lana, S.E., Ogilivie, G.K., Withrow, S.J., et al. Feline cutaneous squamous cell carcinoma of the nasal planum and the pinnae: 61 cases. *J Am Anim Hosp Assoc* 33:329-332,1997.

Legendre, A.M. and Krahwinkel, D.J. Feline ear tumors. *J Am Anim Hosp Assoc* 17:1035-1037, 1981.

Macy, D.W. Canine and feline mast cell tumours: biologic behaviour, diagnosis, and therapy. *Semin Vet Med Surg (Small Anim)* 1:72-83, 1986.

Madewell, B.R., Pool, R.R., Thelen, G.H., et al. Multiple subungual squamous cell carcinomas in five dogs. *J Am Vet Med Assoc* 180:731-734, 1982.

Marino, D.J., Matthiesen, D.T., Stefanacci , J.D., et al. Evaluation of dogs with digit masses: 117 cases (1981-1991). *J Am Vet Med Assoc* 207:726-728, 1995.

McChesney, A.E., Stephens, L.C., Lebel, J., et al. Infiltrative lipoma in dogs. *Vet Pathol* 17:316-322, 1980.

Messick, J.B. and Radin, M.J. Cytologic, histologic and ultra-structural characteristics of a canine myxoid liposarcoma. *Vet Pathol* 26:520-522, 1989.

Miller, M.A., Nelson, S.L., Turk, J.R., et al. Cutaneous neoplasia in 340 cats. *Vet Pathol* 28:389-395, 1991.

Miller, M.A., Ramos, J.A., and Kreeger, J.M. Cutaneous vascular neoplasia in 15 cats: clinical, morphologic, and immunohistochemical studies. *Vet Pathol* 29:329-336, 1992.

Moroff, S. *Case 17.* ASVCP Annual Case Review, ASVCP Annual Meeting, Phoenix, 1990.

Newlands, C., Vasconcelos, D., and Houston, D. *Case 17.* ASCVP Annual Slide Review, Annual Meeting, San Antonio, Texas, 1993.

O'Rourke, M. Multiple digital squamous-cell carcinomas in 2 dogs. *Mod Vet Pract* 66:644-645, 1985.

Oakes, M.G., Lewis, D.D., Hedlund, C.S., et al. Canine oral neoplasia. *Compend Cont Ed Pract* 15:15-31, 1993.

Pace, L.W., Kreeger, J.M., Miller, M.A., et al. Immunohistochemical staining of feline malignant fibrous histiocytomas. *Vet Pathol* 31:168-172, 1994.

Paradis, M., Scott, D.W., and Breton, L. Squamous cell carcinoma of the nail bed in three related giant schnauzers. *Vet Rec* 125:322-324, 1989.

Paterson, S., Boydell, P., and Pike, R. Systemic histiocytosis in the Bernese mountain dog *J Small Anim Pract* 36:233-236,1995.

Patnaik, A.K. and Mooney, S. Feline melanoma: a comparative study of ocular, oral and dermal neoplasms. *Vet Pathol* 25:105-112, 1988.

Peaston, A.E., Munn, R.J., and Madewell, B.R. Clinical vignette. *J Vet Intern Med* 7:101-103, 1993.

Pstotino, N.C., Berg, R.J., Powers, B.E., et al. Prognostic variable for canine hemangiopericytoma: 50 cases (1979-1984). *J Am Anim Hosp Assoc* 24:501-509, 1988.

Rakich, P.M., Latimer, K.S., Weiss, R., et al. Mucocutaneous plasmacytomas in dogs: 75 cases (1980-1987). *J Am Vet Med Assoc* 194:803-810, 1989.

Ramsey, I.K., McKay, J.S., Rudorf, I., et al. Malignant histiocytosis in three Bernese mountain dogs. *Vet Rec* 138:444-445,1996.

Richardson, R.C. Canine transmissible venereal tumor. *Compend Cont Ed Pract* 3:951-956, 1981.

Rogers, K.S. Diagnostic dilemma of extramedullary plasmacytomas. *Vet Cancer Soc Newsletter* 15:12-14, 1991.

Rosin, A., Moore, P., and Dublielzig, R. Malignant histiocytosis in Bernese mountain dogs *J Am Vet Med Assoc* 188:1041-1045,1986.

Ross, J.T., Scavelli, T.D., Matthiesen, D.T., et al. Adenocarcinoma of the apocrine glands of the anal sac in dogs: a review of 32 cases. *J Am Anim Hosp Assoc* 27:349-355, 1991.

Ruslander, D., Kaser-Hotz, B., and Sardias, J.C. Cutaneous squamous cell carcinoma in cats. *Compend Cont Ed Pract* 19:1119-1129, 1997.

Scavelli, T.D., Patnaik, A.K., Mehlhaff, C.J., et al. Hemangiosarcoma in the cat: a retrospective evaluation of 131 surgical cases. *J Am Vet Med Assoc* 187:817-819, 1985.

Schultze, A.E., Frank, L.A., and Hahn, K.A. Repeated physical and cytologic characterizations of subcutaneous postvaccinal reactions in cats. *Am J Vet Res* 58:719-724, 1997.

Scott, D.W. and Anderson, W.I. Canine sebaceous gland tumours: a retrospective analysis of 172 cases. *Canine Practice* 15:19-27, 1990.

Srebernik, N. and Appleby, E.C. Breed prevalence and sites of haemangioma and haemangiosarcoma in dogs. *Vet Rec* 129:408-409, 1991.

Strafuss, A.C., Cook, J.E., and Smith, J.E. Squamous cell carcinoma in dogs. *J Am Vet Med Assoc* 168:425-427, 1976.

Tanimoto, T., Shirota, K., Nakamura, Y., et al. Liposarcoma in an old cat. *Jpn J Vet Sci* 49:719-720, 1987.

Tyler, R.D., Cowell, R.L., and Meinkoth, J.H.. Cutaneous and subcutaneous lesions: masses, cysts, ulcers, and fistulous tracts. In *Diagnostic Cytology and Hematology of the Dog and Cat.* R.L. Cowell, R.D. Tyler, and J.H. Meinkoth (eds). Mosby, St Louis, 1999.

Vail, D.M., Withrow, S.J., Schwarz, P.D., et al. Perianal adenocarcinoma in the canine male: a retrospective study of 41 cases. *J Am Anim Hosp Assoc* 26:329-334, 1990.

vander Linde-Sipman, J.S., de Wit, M.M.L., van Garderen, E., et al. Cutaneous malignant melanomas in 57 cats: identification of (amelanotic) signet-ring and balloon cell types and verification of their origin by immunohistochemistry, electron microscopy and in situ hybridization. *Vet Pathol* 34:31-38, 1997.

Vos, J.H., van den Ingh, T.S.G.A.M., Ramaekers, F.C.S., et al. The expression of keratins, vimentin, neurofilament proteins, smooth muscle actin, neuron-specific enolase, and synaptophysin in tumours of the specific glands in the canine anal region. *Vet Pathol* 30: 352-361, 1993.

Walder, E.J. and Grosse, T.L. Neoplastic diseases of the skin. In *Veterinary Dermatopathology: A Macroscopic and Micoscopic Evaluation of Canine and Feline Skin Disease.* T.L. Gross, P.J. Ihrke, and E.J. Walder (eds). Mosby, St Louis, 1992.

Wilcock, B.P., Yager, J.A., and Zink, M.C. The morphology and behaviour of feline cutaneous mastocytomas. *Vet Pathol* 23:320-324, 1986.

Yager, J.A. and Wilcock, J.P. Tumours of the skin and associated tissues. In *Color Atlas and Text of Surgical Pathology of the Dog and Cat.* J.A. Yager and B.P. Wilcock (eds). St Louis, Mosby, 1994.

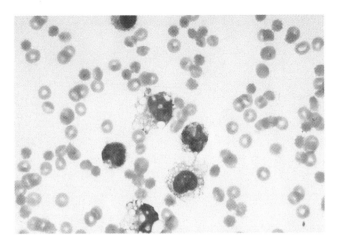

FIG. 4-1. Canine. Fine needle. Subcutaneous mass. Posttraumatic hematoma. Background of erythrocytes with mononuclear phagocytic cells showing various degrees of vacuolation and activation in response to recent hemorrhage. Erythrophagocytosis is expected at a later stage. (×250.)

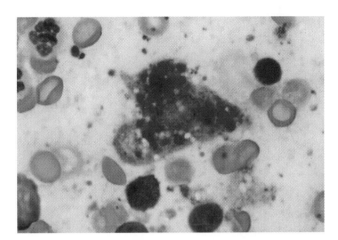

FIG. 4-2. Canine. Fine needle. Subcutaneous mass on trunk. Mononuclear inflammation. Mononuclear cells with intracytoplasmic vacuolation appear to be primarily monocyte/macrophages. Without further clinical information or stromal cells, including giant cells, cytological interpretation is limited to mixed inflammation. (×250.)

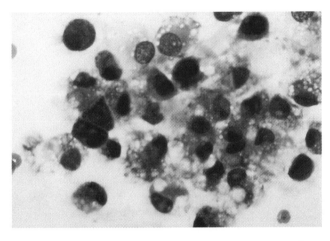

FIG. 4-3. Canine. Fine needle. Hematoma. Macrophages with intracytoplasmic hemoglobin breakdown products. Fresh red blood cells also present. (×500.)

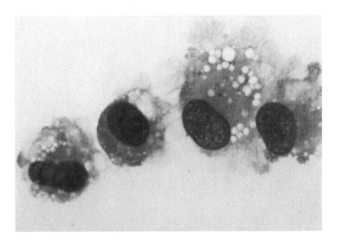

FIG. 4-4. Canine. Fine needle. Subcutaneous mass on trunk. Mononuclear inflammation. (Same case as Fig. 4-3.) Individual epithelioid macrophages or mononuclear phagocytic cells. (×500.)

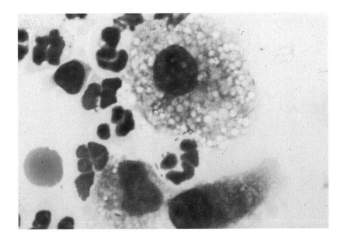

FIG. 4-5. Canine. Fine needle. Skin. Peripheral wall of abscess. The cells include poorly preserved neutrophils and macrophages with a few indistinct intracellular bacteria. The spindle-shaped cell suggests early fibroblast differentiation. (×400.)

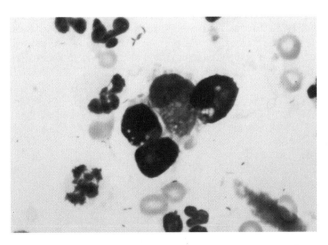

FIG. 4-6. Canine. Fine needle. Skin. Abscess. The mixed inflammatory cell population includes a macrophage, three plasma cells, and neutrophils, indicative of chronic inflammation. (×400.)

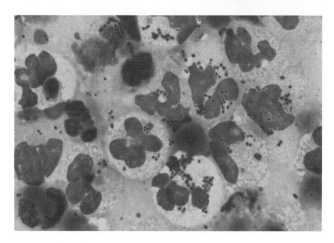

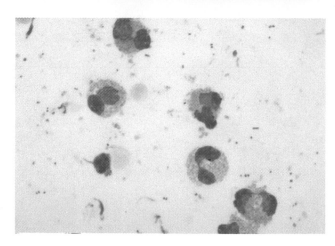

FIG. 4-7. Canine. Fine needle. Lumbar mass. Abscess. Dense background with numerous neutrophils undergoing chromatolysis. Intracellular and extracellular cocci are present. (×630.)

FIG. 4-8. Feline. Fine needle. Eosinophilic granuloma. Numerous lightly staining eosinophilic granules are visible in eosinophils and the extracellular space. (×400.)

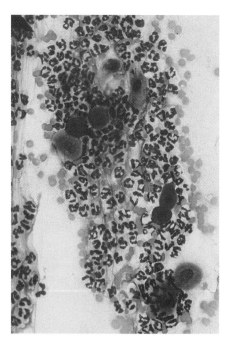

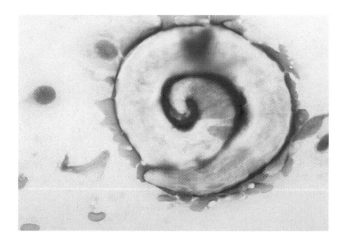

FIG. 4-9. Canine. Fine needle. Ear pustule. Pemphigus foliaceous. There are many well-preserved neutrophils without evidence of an etiological agent. The differentiating squamous epithelial cells are consistent with the acantholytic cells observed in autoimmune skin disorders. (×100.)

FIG. 4-10. Canine. Fine needle. Recurring mass on hind leg. Dracunculus larva. The coiled, light turquoise organism is typical for larva of *Dracunculus* spp. (×200.)

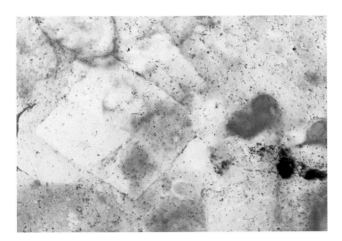

FIG. 4-11. Canine. Fine needle. Histological diagnosis: trichoepithelioma. Cytological diagnosis: epithelial inclusion cyst. Squamous epithelial debris, scattered melanin granules, and a few negative-staining cholesterol crystals are visible. Central versus peripheral origin of aspirate may result in marked differences in aspirate appearance and cellularity. (×200.)

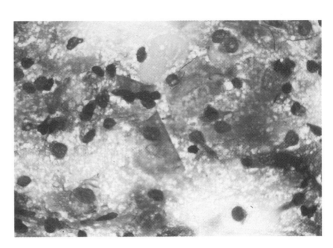

FIG. 4-12. Canine. Imprint. Epithelial inclusion cyst. Squamous epithelial cells and cellular debris without an inflammatory component are consistent with an inclusion cyst. (×100.)

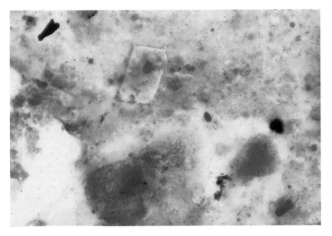

FIG. 4-13. Canine. Fine needle. Histological diagnosis: pilomatrixoma. Cytological diagnosis: epithelial inclusion cyst. Cholesterol crystals, a degenerating squamous epithelial cell, melanin granules, and amorphous cellular debris. (×250.)

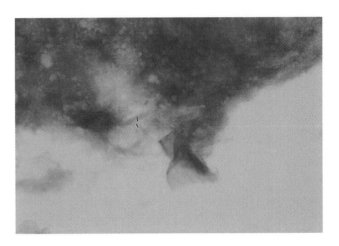

FIG. 4-14. Canine. Fine needle. Subcutaneous mass. Epithelial inclusion cyst. Background of blue amorphous material with a few superficial squamous epithelial cells. (×100.)

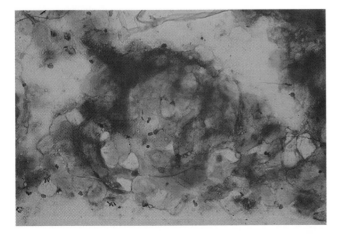

FIG. 4-15. Canine. Fine needle. Subcutaneous mass. Epithelial inclusion cyst. Background of blue amorphous material containing many intermediate to superficial squamous epithelial cells and a few erythrocytes. (×75.)

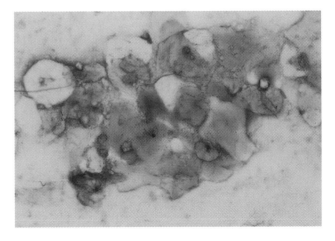

FIG. 4-16. Canine. Fine needle. Subcutaneous mass. Epithelial inclusion cyst. Squamous epithelial cells, with varying degrees of degeneration consistent with epithelial inclusion cyst. (×125.)

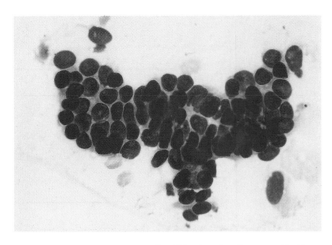

FIG. 4-17. Canine. Fine needle. Skin. Basal cell tumor. Uniform small, round cells with high N:C ratio and common adjoining cytoplasmic borders suggestive of epithelial cells. (×400.)

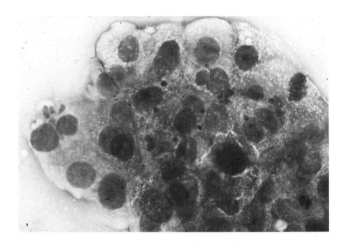

FIG. 4-18. Canine. Fine needle. Skin. Basal cell tumor. Ribbon of palisading cells characteristic of basal cell tumors. This palisading appearance is unusual in cytological preparations. (×250.)

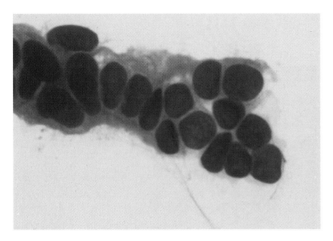

FIG. 4-19. Canine. Fine needle. Skin. Basal cell tumor. (Same case as Fig. 4-18.) Increased magnification of basilar epithelial cells. (×630.)

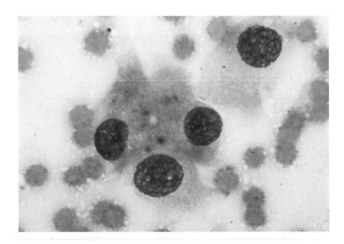

FIG 4-20. Canine. Fine needle. Dermal mass in a dog. Benign epithelial tumor with adnexal (sebaceous) differentiation. Cluster of cohesive epithelial cells with round to oval nuclei and light basophilic finely vacuolated cytoplasm. The cytological diagnosis is limited to basal cell tumor with sebaceous differentiation. Histopathological examination is required for identification. (×200.)

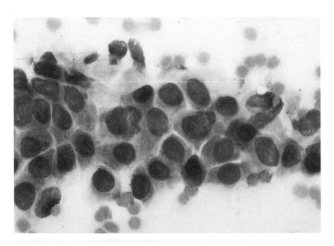

FIG 4-21. Canine. Fine needle. Skin mass. Histological diagnosis: focal epidermal hyperplasia. Cytological diagnosis: benign epithelial tumor of unknown origin. Cohesive sheet of uniform epithelial cells with round to oval nuclei and basophilic cytoplasm. (×250.)

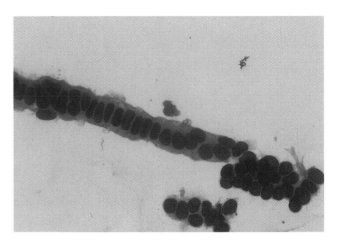

FIG. 4-22. Canine. Fine needle. Skin mass. Adenoma. (Same case as Fig. 4-21.) The blue-green intracytoplasmic pigment within the uniform benign-appearing cells suggests that the cells are melanophores, as frequently observed in aspirates from skin. (×400.)

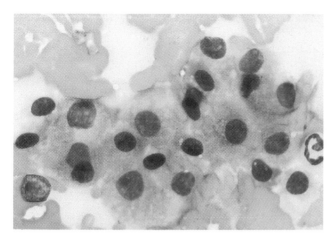

FIG. 4-23. Canine. Fine needle. Skin in perianal region. Perianal adenoma. The epithelial cells have abundant cytoplasm, low N:C ratio, a central nucleus, and indistinct small nucleoli. (×250.)

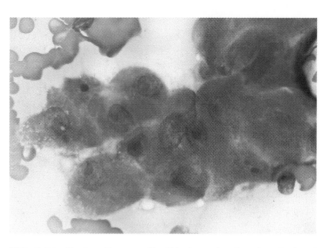

FIG. 4-24. Canine. Fine needle. Skin in perianal region. Perianal adenoma. Cohesive group of "hepatoid" epithelial cells with round to oval nuclei and distinct nucleoli. The cells have a low N:C ratio and a moderate amount of finely granular cytoplasm. (×250.)

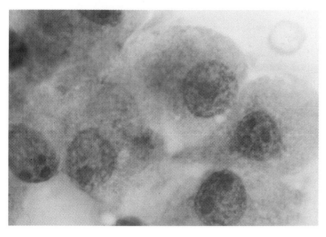

FIG. 4-25. Canine. Fine needle. Skin in perianal region. Perianal adenoma. Higher magnification of "hepatoid" epithelial cells illustrating round nuclei, several prominent nucleoli, and moderately dense light eosinophilic granular cytoplasm. (×400.)

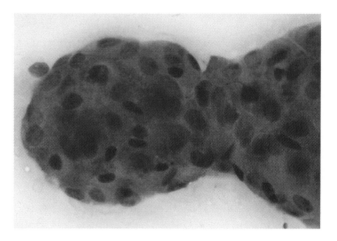

FIG. 4-26. Canine. Fine needle. Skin in perianal region. Perianal adenoma. Large polypoid arrangement of epithelial cells consisting primarily of larger "hepatoid" cells and a few basal (reserve) cells. The reserve cells are smaller and have small basophilic nuclei. (×250.)

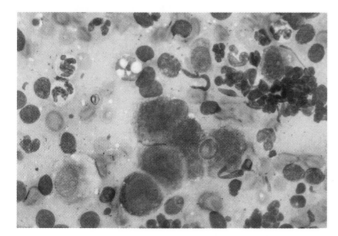

FIG. 4-27. Canine. Fine needle. Perianal gland carcinoma. Epithelial cells with a high N:C ratio and prominent nucleoli are surrounded by a mixed population of inflammatory cells. Differentiation of perianal carcinoma and adenoma may be difficult, either by cytological or histological examination. (×250.)

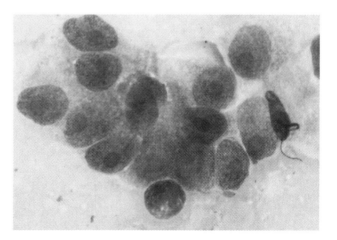

FIG. 4-28. Canine. Fine needle. Perianal gland carcinoma. The epithelial cells have a high N:C ratio with irregular prominent nucleoli. The "hepatoid" appearance is apparent. (×400.)

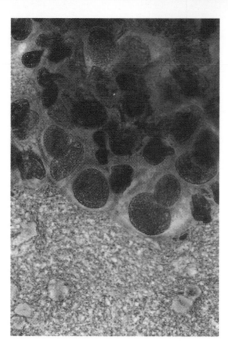

FIG. 4-29. Canine. Fine needle. Lateral thorax. Apocrine carcinoma. A cluster of epithelial cells with distinctive adjoining borders. Anisokaryosis is prominent. Nuclei are hyperchromatic and have a fine chromatin pattern and prominent variable-sized nucleoli supportive of malignant transformation. (×400.)

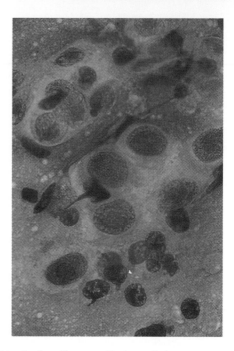

FIG. 4-30. Canine. Fine needle. Lateral thorax. Apocrine carcinoma. (Same case as Fig. 4-29.) Large, round cells with pale cytoplasm, dark anisokaryotic nuclei, and prominent nucleoli. Diffuse pink, finely granular background compatible with secretory product. (×400.)

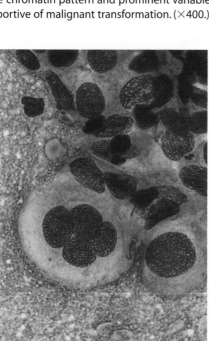

FIG. 4-31. Canine. Fine needle. Lateral thorax. Apocrine carcinoma. (Same case as Fig. 4-29.) Similar background and cells illustrating multinucleation and marked anisokaryosis. (×400.)

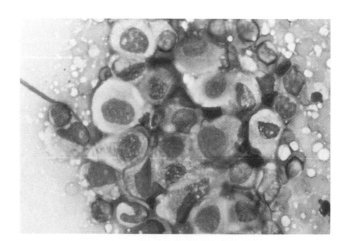

FIG. 4-32. Canine. Fine needle. Mandibular mass in a dog. Squamous cell carcinoma. Epithelial cells with moderate anisokaryosis, pale to lightly basophilic cytoplasm, and marked asynchrony of nuclear to cytoplasmic maturation. (×250.)

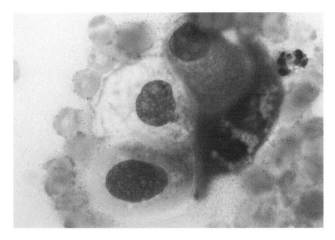

FIG. 4-33. Canine. Fine needle. Mandibular mass in a dog. Squamous cell carcinoma. (Same case as Fig. 4-32.) Three large squamous epithelial cells with asynchronous nuclear maturation and two smaller basophilic cells with distinctive perinuclear vacuolation typical for Wright's stained squamous epithelial cells. (×400.)

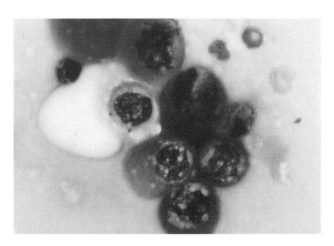

FIG. 4-34. Feline. Imprint. Nasal mass. Squamous cell carcinoma. Epithelial cells with moderate anisokaryosis, moderate to marked basophilic cytoplasm, and prominent perinuclear vacuolation. Note distinct adjoining cell borders at top of illustration. (×400.)

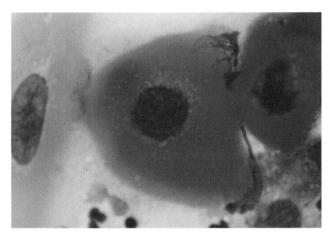

FIG. 4-35. Canine. Fine needle. Laryngeal mass. Squamous cell carcinoma. Cytoplasmic tinctorial properties and fine perinuclear cytoplasmic vacuolation characteristic of differentiating squamous epithelial cells. Although the N:C ratio appears low, it is high for keratinizing squamous epithelium. This nuclear cytoplasmic asynchrony is a feature of malignancy in squamous cell carcinomas. (×400.)

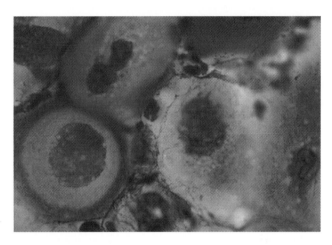

FIG. 4-36. Canine. Fine needle. Laryngeal mass. Squamous cell carcinoma. (Same case as Fig. 4-35.) Squamous epithelial cells with marked anisokaryosis, a high N:C ratio, and perinuclear cytoplasmic vacuolation. (×400.)

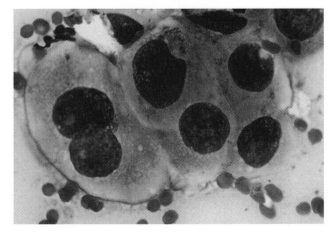

FIG. 4-37. Feline. Fine needle. Ear mass. Squamous cell carcinoma. Large squamous epithelial cells with limited cytoplasmic differentiation. Nucleoli are prominent. (×400.)

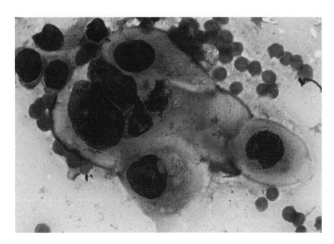

FIG. 4-38. Feline. Fine needle. Ear mass. Squamous differentiation. (Same case as Fig. 4-37.) Marked variation in nuclear size and shape. (×400.)

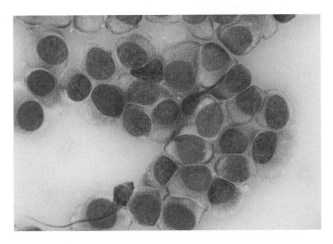

FIG. 4-39. Canine. Fine needle. Histiocytoma. Round cells with pale to basophilic cytoplasm, small nuclei with indistinct nucleoli, and chromatin pattern typical of histiocytoma. (×400.)

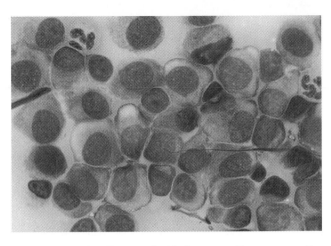

FIG. 4-40. Canine. Fine needle. Histiocytoma. (Same case as Fig. 4-39.) Round cells illustrating heterogeneity of cell morphology and anisokaryosis. There are a few lymphocytes, plasma cells, and neutrophils that are often indicators of tumor regression. (×400.)

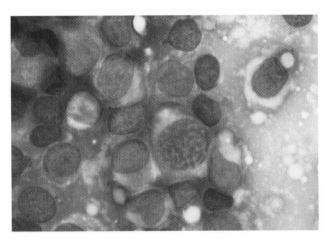

FIG. 4-41. Canine. Fine needle. Mass on neck. Histiocytoma. Typical pleomorphic round cells and lymphocytes. The prominent chromatin pattern in the large nucleus suggests mitotic activity. (×250.)

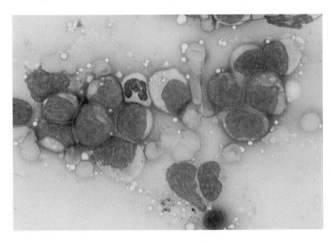

FIG. 4-42. Canine. Fine needle. Skin. Systemic histiocytosis. Note convoluted to round nuclei with moderate, pale cytoplasm but fewer small lymphocytes than reported for confirmed systemic histiocytosis. Diagnosis unconfirmed. History of recurring skin masses, oral lesions, and lymph node involvement over 18 months. Histological diagnoses included histiocytoma, atypical histiocytoma, possible reticulum cell sarcoma, and histiocytic lymphoma. (×250.)

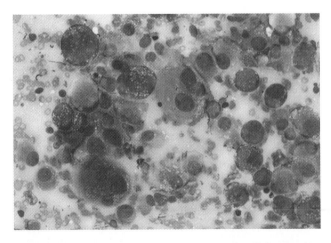

FIG 4-43. Canine. Fine needle. Lung. Rottweiler. Malignant histiocytosis. Large mononuclear cells, some multinucleated. Cytoplasm is basophilic with fine vacuolation. (×100.)

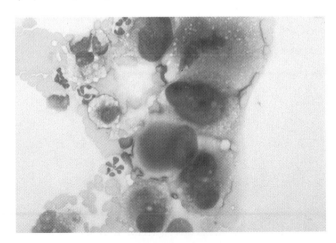

FIG. 4-44. Canine. Abdominal fluid. Mass on head with metastasis to liver and kidney. Malignant histiocytosis. Large mononuclear cells with marked anisokaryosis, binucleation, and a mitotic figure. Note size comparison with neutrophils and red blood cells. (×100.)

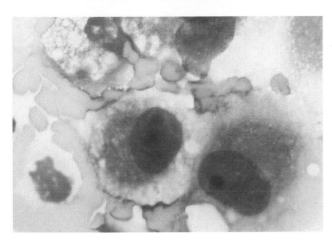

FIG. 4-45. Canine. Abdominal fluid. Malignant histiocytosis. (Same case as Fig. 4-44.) Large mononuclear cells with eccentrically located nuclei and prominent nucleoli. (×400.)

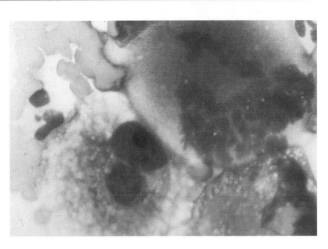

FIG. 4-46. Canine. Abdominal fluid. Malignant histiocytosis. (Same case as Fig. 4-44.) Large vacuolated mononuclear cells with aberrant mitotic figure. (×400.)

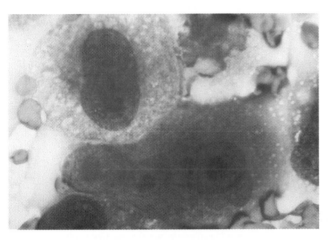

FIG. 4-47. Canine. Abdominal fluid. Malignant histiocytosis. (Same case as Fig. 4-44.) Large anaplastic mononuclear cells with large prominent nucleoli and multinucleation. (×400.)

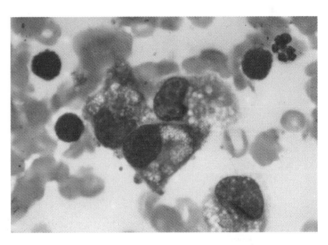

FIG. 4-48. Canine. Fine needle. Spleen. Malignant histiocytosis. Bernese mountain dog. Vacuolated histiocytic cells with occasional lymphocytes and a neutrophil. (×400.)

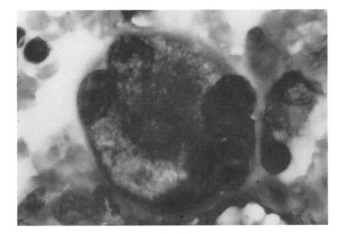

FIG. 4-49. Canine. Fine needle. Spleen. Malignant histiocytosis. A large, irregular, multinucleated cell and erythrocytophagy, as often observed in malignant histiocytosis. (×400.)

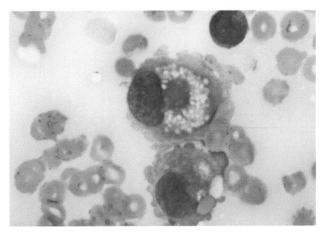

FIG. 4-50. Canine. Fine needle. Spleen. Malignant histiocytosis. Two large mononuclear cells with eccentrically located nuclei, vacuolated cytoplasm, and evidence of cytophagy and erythrocytophaagy. (×400.)

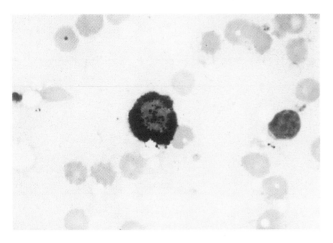

FIG. 4-51. Canine. Normal mast cell. Metachromatic granules often obscure nuclei. Mast cells may be present in most normal tissues. (×400.)

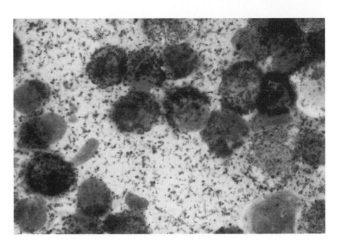

FIG. 4-52. Canine. Imprint. Skin mass. Mast cell tumor. Well-differentiated mast cells with intracytoplasmic and free metachromatic granules. Nuclear detail is obscured by granules. (×400.)

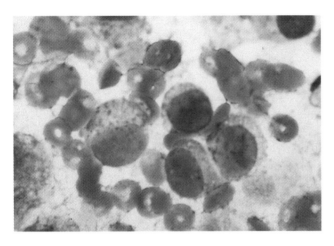

FIG. 4-53. Canine. Fine needle. Nasal mass. Mast cell tumor. The limited fine metachromatic granulation may indicate anaplasia or degranulation of the mast cells. There is greater nuclear detail visible. Anisokaryosis is mild. (×500.)

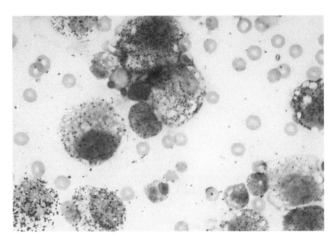

FIG. 4-54. Canine. Nasal wash. Nasal mass. Mast cell tumor. Mast cells with reduced amount of metachromatic granules and round to oval nuclei. Eosinophils are frequently associated with mast cell tumors. (×250.)

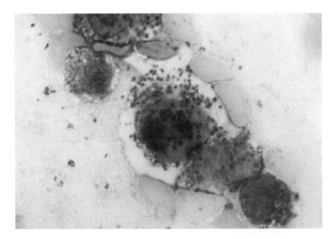

FIG. 4-55. Canine. Fine needle. Recurring skin mass. Mast cell tumor. Mast cells have decreased metachromatic granules and moderate to marked anisocytosis and anisokaryosis, suggesting anaplasia. The significance of these observations is uncertain because correlation between cytological grading and biological behavior is not yet confirmed. (×500.)

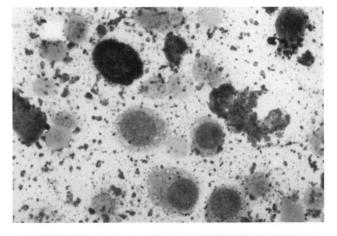

FIG. 4-56. Canine. Fine needle. Skin mass. Mast cell tumor. The round cells vary in the degree of metachromatic granulation, and there are numerous free granules in the background. (×400.)

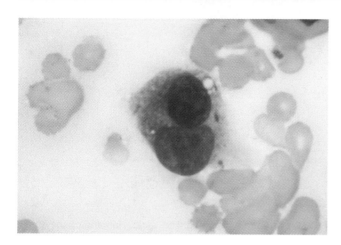

FIG. 4-57. Canine. Fine needle. Skin mass. Plasmacytoma. One large binuclear plasma cell. Binucleation is rare in benign plasma cell populations but is seen frequently in plasma cell tumors. (×400.)

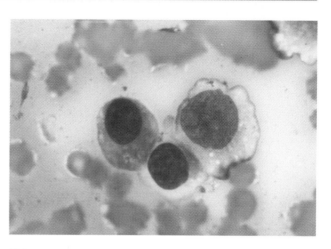

FIG. 4-58. Canine. Fine needle. Skin mass. Plasmacytoma. (Same case as Fig. 4-57.) Discrete round cells with eccentric round nuclei and light to moderate basophilic cytoplasm. (×500.)

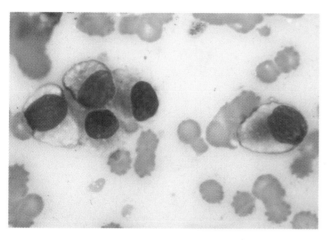

FIG. 4-59. Canine. Fine needle. Skin mass. Plasmacytoma. (Same case as Fig. 4-57.) A few round cells with eccentric nuclei and light basophilic cytoplasm. There is mild anisokaryosis. Differentiation from multiple myeloma depends on the site (skin), as well as the absence of bone lysis and/or gammopathy. (×400.)

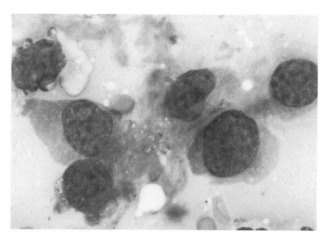

FIG. 4-60. Canine. Fine needle. Skin mass. Plasmacytoma. Several large plasmacytoid cells with moderate anisokaryosis, coarse chromatin, and prominent irregular nucleoli. This figure illustrates the variability possible within this tumor. (×500.)

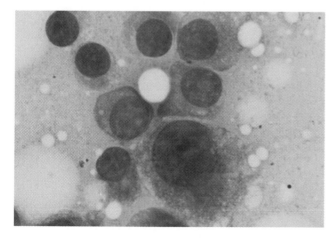

FIG. 4-61. Canine. Fine needle. Inguinal mass. Plasmacytoma. Anisokaryosis can be prominent within this tumor. (×630.)

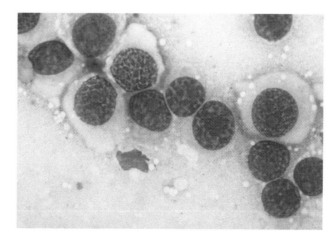

FIG. 4-62. Canine. Imprint. Preputial mass. Transmissible venereal tumor. Discrete cells with round nuclei; coarse chromatin; large, prominent, usually single nucleoli and a moderate amount of pale-staining cytoplasm. (×400.)

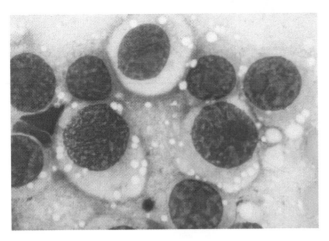

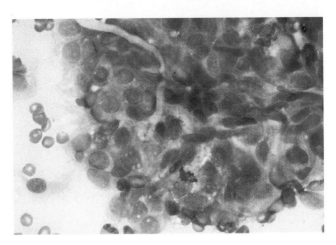

FIG. 4-63. Canine. Imprint. Preputial mass. Transmissible vene-real tumor. (Same case as Fig. 4-62.) Discrete cells with round nu-clei and a typical coarse chromatin pattern. A few small intracy-toplasmic vacuoles are observed within most cells. Mitotic figures, not present, are a common feature of this tumor. (×500.)

FIG. 4-64. Canine. Scraping. Leg mass. Hemangiopericytoma. Cluster of spindle-shaped cells with elongated nuclei and light basophilic cytoplasm. Fine-needle aspirates are often very cellu-lar and include many blood cells. (×200.)

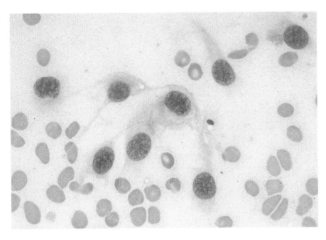

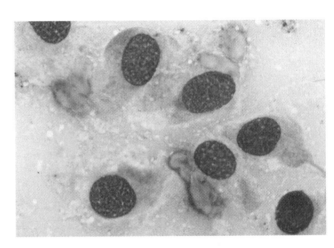

FIG. 4-65. Canine. Scraping. Leg mass. Hemangiopericytoma. Homogenous population of spindle-shaped cells with round to oval nuclei and light basophilic cytoplasm. (×250.)

FIG. 4-66. Canine. Fine needle. Left elbow mass. Hemangioperi-cytoma. Several uniform-appearing spindle-shaped cells inter-mixed with red blood cells. Nucleoli are small and indistinct. Fine-needle aspirates from hemangiopericytomas often have a higher cell yield than other stromal masses. (×400.)

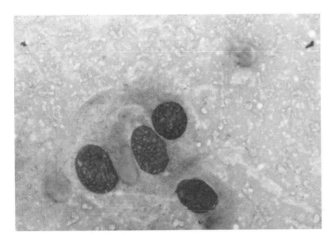

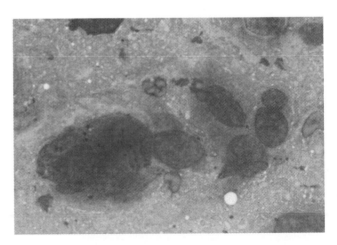

FIG. 4-67. Canine. Fine needle. Left elbow mass. Hemangioperi-cytoma. The swirling pattern observed in histological sections is suggested from the appearance of these cells. (×400.)

FIG. 4-68. Feline. Scraping. Distal hind limb mass. Malignant fi-brous histiocytoma. Spindle-shaped cells and a multinucleated cell are present. The pink background suggests matrix produc-tion. (×400.) (Courtesy Jeff McCartney, 1993.)

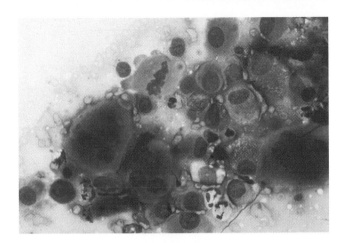

FIG. 4-69. Feline. Scraping. Distal hind limb mass. Malignant fibrous histiocytoma. Histological diagnosis: malignant fibrous histiocytoma. Cytological diagnosis: malignant mesenchymal neoplasm with multinucleated giant cells. (Same case as Fig. 4-68.) Large multinucleated cells are surrounded by mononuclear cells. These large giant cells resemble osteoclasts. (×100.)

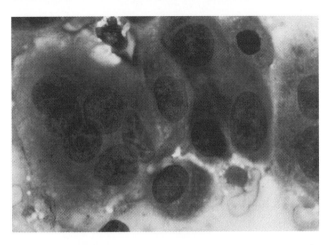

FIG. 4-70. Feline. Scraping. Distal hind limb mass. Malignant fibrous histiocytoma. (Same case as Fig. 4-68.) Large multinucleated cell contains fine to coarse red cytoplasmic granulation. (×400.)

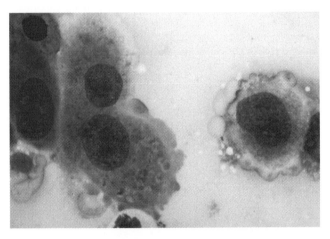

FIG. 4-71. Feline. Scraping. Distal hind limb mass. Malignant fibrous histiocytoma. (Same case as Fig. 4-68.) Histiocytic-like cells with prominent red cytoplasmic granular material, likely extracellular matrix precursor. (×400.)

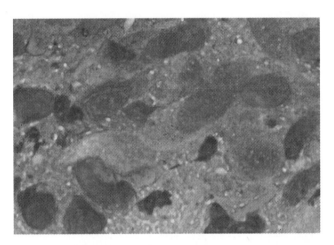

FIG. 4-72. Feline. Scraping. Distal hind limb mass. Malignant fibrous histiocytoma. (Same case as Fig. 4-68.) The cells have a distinct stromal appearance with a prominent extracellular pink matrix. Pleomorphism is common in this tumor. (×400.)

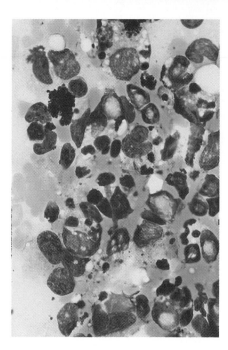

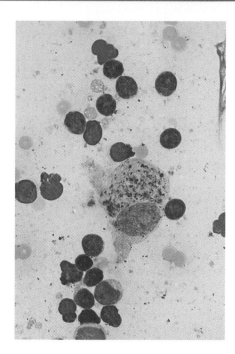

FIG. 4-73. Canine. Fine needle. Subcutaneous mass near scapula. Vaccine reaction. Mixed mononuclear cell population. Free and phagocytized bright red granular material, likely residual product from vaccine. (×400.)

FIG. 4-74. Canine. Fine needle. Subcutaneous mass. Vaccine reaction. (Same case as Fig. 4-73.) Nucleated cells are predominantly lymphocytes. The large central macrophage contains finely dispersed granular material presumably of similar vaccine origin. (×400.)

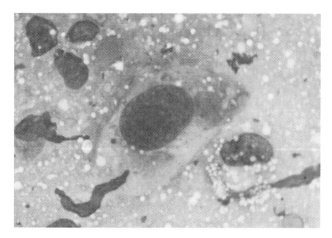

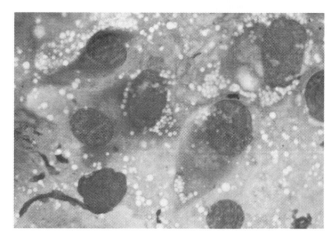

FIG. 4-75. Feline. Fine needle. Mass in axilla. Fibrosarcoma. Large spindle-shaped cell with oval nucleus and prominent nucleolus. Intracytoplasmic pink granules may represent matrix secretory product. Free nuclei and cellular debris are also observed. (×400.)

FIG. 4-76. Feline. Fine needle. Mass in axilla. Fibrosarcoma. (Same case as Fig. 4-75.) Spindle-shaped cells with oval-shaped nuclei, marked anisokaryosis, blue-gray cytoplasm and intracytoplasmic vacuoles. Nucleoli are multiple and irregular. (×400.)

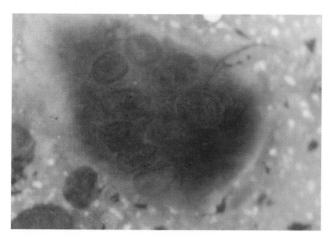

FIG. 4-77. Feline. Fine needle. Mass in axilla. Fibrosarcoma. (Same case as Fig. 4-75.) Multinucleated cell with prominent nucleoli. Multinucleated giant cells can be observed in any stromal mass. (×400.)

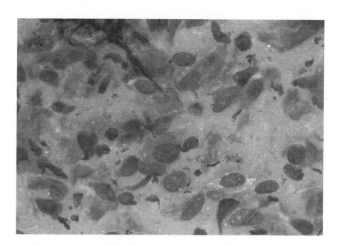

FIG. 4-78. Canine. Fine needle. Lymph node. Fibrosarcoma. Pleomorphic stromal cells embedded in light pink extracellular matrix. Higher cellularity is expected in the less-differentiated stromal cell populations. (×250.)

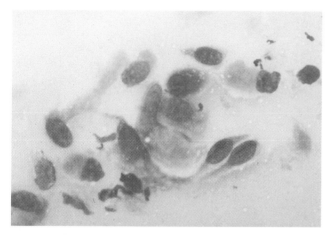

FIG. 4-79. Canine. Fine needle. Lymph node. Fibrosarcoma. (Same case as Fig. 4-78.) Spindle-shaped cells with oval nuclei and moderate anisokaryosis. Observing these moderately differentiated spindle cells within the lymph node, without other evidence for stromal reaction or inflammation, indicates metastatic origin. (×250.)

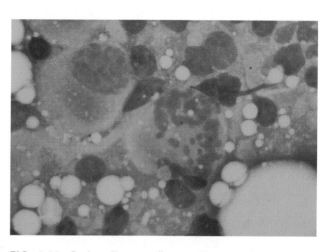

FIG. 4-80. Canine. Fine needle. Lymph node. Fibrosarcoma. (Same case as Fig. 4-78.) Large stromal cells in a lymph node. Note mitosis. (×400.)

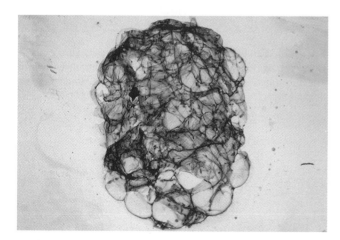

FIG. 4-81. Canine. Fine needle. Skin mass. Lipoma. Large cluster of adipocytes. Accidental aspiration of normal fatty tissue must be considered when adipocytes are aspirated. (×100.)

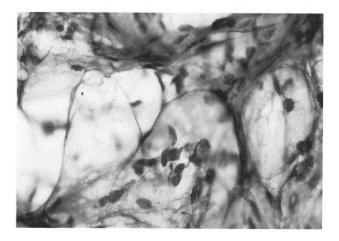

FIG. 4-82. Canine. Fine needle. Subcutaneous neck mass. Lipoma. A cluster of adipocytes with peripheralized small round to oval nuclei and abundant nonstaining cytoplasm outlined by a thin cell membrane. (×100.)

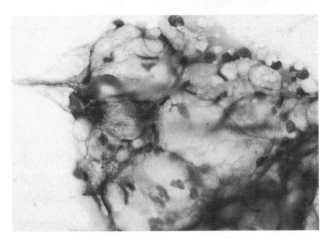

FIG. 4-83. Canine. Fine needle. Subcutaneous neck mass. Lipoma. A cluster of adipocytes. Aspirates of fatty tissue are clear and do not dry easily. Cells may not adhere to the slide during the staining procedure. As a result this degree of cellularity is not always obtained. (×100.)

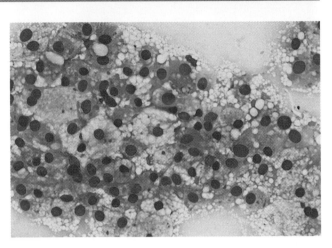

FIG. 4-84. Canine. Fine needle. Axillary mass. Liposarcoma. Many well-preserved cells of similar origin. The abundant cytoplasm varies from amorphous dense basophilic to highly vacuolated. There is marked variation in nuclear size and density. (×100.)

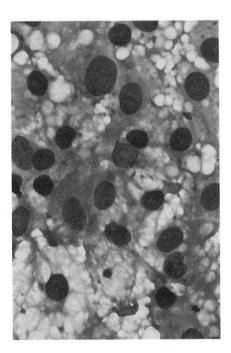

FIG. 4-85. Canine. Fine needle. Axillary mass. Liposarcoma. (Same case as Fig. 4-84.) The degree of anisokaryosis and hyperchromasia supports the interpretation of malignant transformation of lipocytes. (×400.)

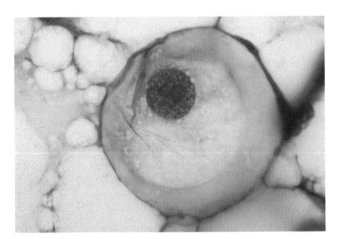

FIG. 4-86. Canine. Fine needle. Mediastinal mass. Liposarcoma. One large adipocyte with a high N:C ratio for a mature lipocyte. The nucleolus is prominent. This cell illustrates the importance of evaluating N:C ratio relative to the tumor type. (×500.)

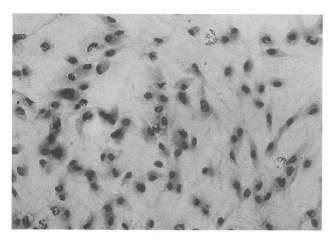

FIG. 4-87. Canine. Fine needle. Shoulder mass. Myxosarcoma. Moderate number of spindle-shaped cells with a background of light pink amorphous material. The eosinophilic background is suggestive of mucin. (×100.)

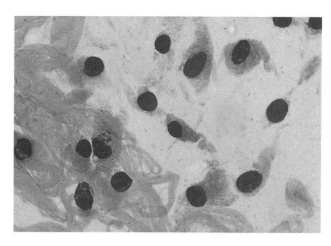

FIG. 4-88. Canine. Fine needle. Shoulder mass. Myxosarcoma. (Same case as Fig. 4-87.) Spindle cell population with minimal criteria of malignancy. (×400.)

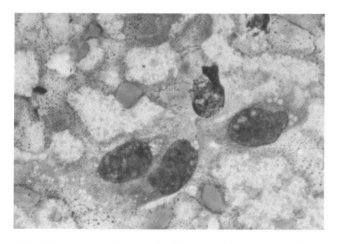

FIG. 4-89. Canine. Fine needle. Skin mass. Myxosarcoma. Three large stromal cells with several large indistinct nucleoli. Pink mucin in background. (×400.)

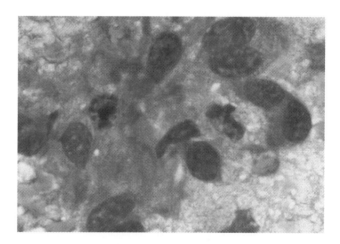

FIG. 4-90. Canine. Fine needle. Skin mass. Myxosarcoma. (Same case as Fig. 4-89.) Spindle-shaped cells with hyperchromatic nuclei, prominent nucleoli, marked anisokaryosis, and dense pink extracellular matrix. (×400.)

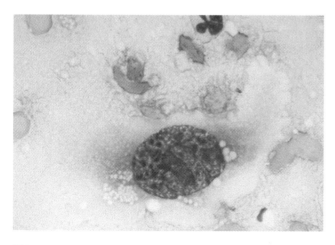

FIG. 4-91. Canine. Fine needle. Skin mass. Myxosarcoma. (Same case as Fig. 4-89.) One stromal cell with a large nucleus and bipolar cytoplasm with indistinct cytoplasmic borders. Although this cell was from a myxosarcoma, such a cell could be found in many malignant stromal tumors. Without further evidence for differentiation, such as matrix production, cytological diagnosis is often limited to "malignant tumor of soft tissue." (×400.)

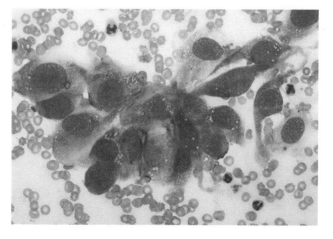

FIG. 4-92. Canine. Fine needle. Axillary mass. Hemangiosarcoma. Irregular cluster of hyperchromatic, very large, oval to spindle cells with round to oval nuclei and multiple nucleoli. Highly cellular aspirates from stromal masses may be an indicator of anaplasia. (×100.)

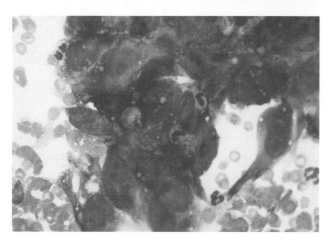

FIG. 4-93. Canine. Fine needle. Skin masses. Hemangiosarcoma. (Same case as Fig. 4-92.) Large, irregular cluster of spindle cells. N:C ratio is high and cytoplasmic basophilia is prominent, as is anisokaryosis. (×200.)

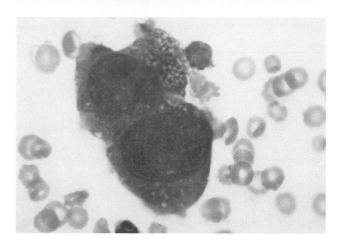

FIG. 4-94. Canine. Fine needle. Skin masses. Hemangiosarcoma. (Same case as Fig. 4-92.) Two large, bizarre stromal cells with high N:C ratio illustrate the extremes in morphology often observed with hemangiosarcoma. (×400.)

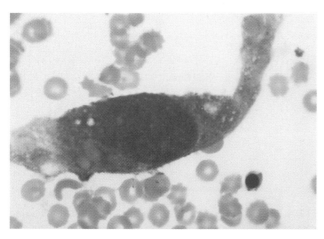

FIG. 4-95. Canine. Fine needle. Skin masses. Hemangiosarcoma. (Same case as Fig. 4-92.) Large, spindle-shaped cell with oval nucleus and marked cytoplasmic basophilia. Erythrocytophagy is a feature of hemangiosarcoma cells. Because of the vascularity, nucleated cell harvest may be poor. (×400.)

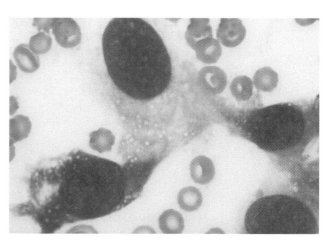

FIG. 4-96. Canine. Fine needle. Axillary mass. Hemangiosarcoma. Poorly differentiated stromal cells with marked anisokaryosis. (×200.)

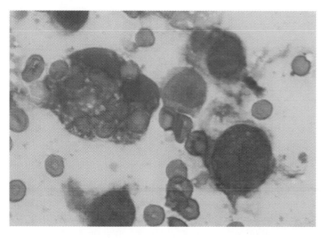

FIG. 4-97. Feline. Fine needle. Skin mass. Hemangiosarcoma. Anaplastic stromal cells, one with fresh erythrocytophagy. (×400.)

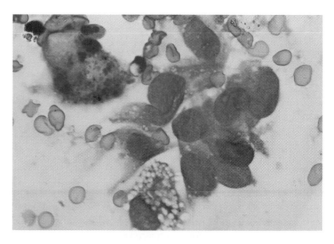

FIG. 4-98. Feline. Fine needle. Skin mass. Hemangiosarcoma. (Same case as Fig. 4-97.) Cluster of anaplastic stromal cells, one with intracytoplasmic hemosiderin. (×400.)

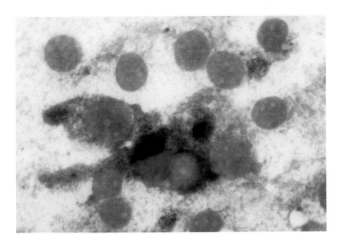

FIG. 4-99. Canine. Fine needle. Oral mass. Melanoma. A cluster of cells with abundant intracytoplasmic and extracellular brown-black melanin granules, round nuclei, and indistinct multiple nucleoli. (×400.)

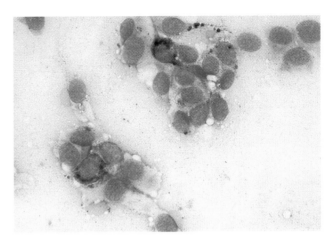

FIG. 4-100. Canine. Fine needle. Skin mass. Melanoma. Polygonal to spindle-shaped cells with round to oval nuclei. Intracytoplasmic melanin granules are indistinct to prominent. (×200.)

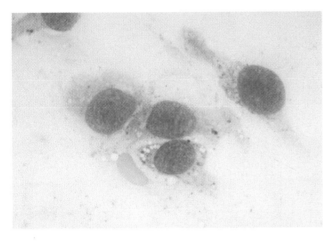

FIG. 4-101. Canine. Fine needle. Skin mass. Melanoma. (Same case as Fig. 4-100.) Spindle-shaped cells with moderate anisokaryosis. Fine to coarse intracytoplasmic brown granules (melanin pigment) are visible. (×400.)

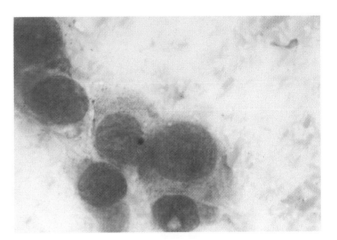

FIG. 4-102. Canine. Fine needle. Skin mass. Melanoma. (Same case as Fig. 4-100.) Round cells with moderate anisokaryosis. These cells have a blue-gray "dusty" appearing cytoplasmic granulation often seen in melanomas. Frequently, when melanin granules are not prominent, this indistinct cytoplasmic granulation is the primary indicator of cell type and thus tumor identification. A single large granule consistent with melanin is present. (×500.)

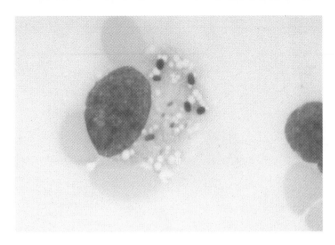

FIG. 4-103. Canine. Fine needle. Gingiva. Melanoma. A single polygonal-shaped cell with an eccentrically located nucleus and several granules consistent with melanin. (×630.)

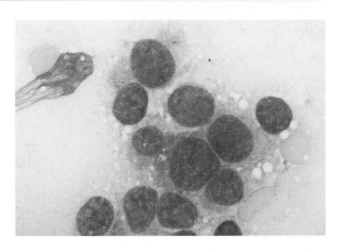

FIG. 4-104. Canine. Impression. Toe. Melanoma. Cluster of cohesive cells with marked anisokaryosis and prominent nucleoli. The cytoplasmic borders are poorly defined. Cells may vary in morphology from mesenchymal to epithelial in appearance within different areas of a melanosarcoma. (×400.)

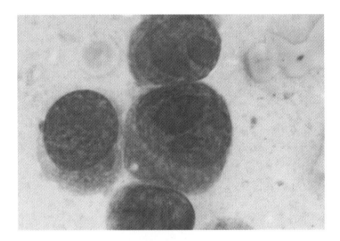

FIG. 4-105. Canine. Fine needle. Skin mass. Melanoma. Round to oval single cells with high N:C ratio and large, prominent, variable-sized nucleoli. Although melanin granules are not visible, the blue-gray cytoplasm and the indistinct granulation are strongly supportive of melanosarcoma differentiation. (×630.)

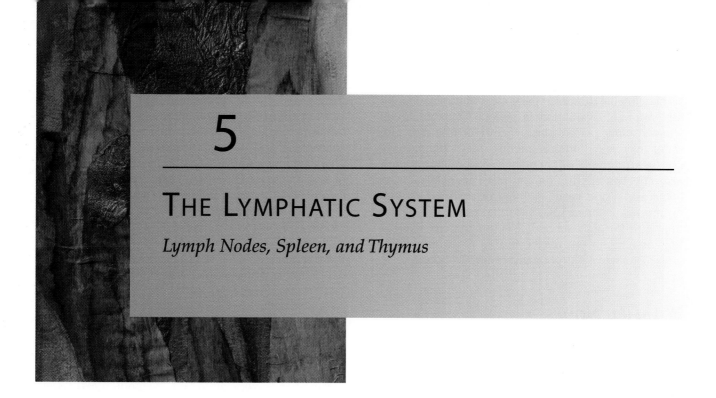

5

THE LYMPHATIC SYSTEM

Lymph Nodes, Spleen, and Thymus

Lymph node enlargement is a frequently encountered problem in veterinary patients. Lymphadenopathy may be localized or generalized, depending on the underlying cause. FNA is particularly useful in the diagnosis of lymphoid disorders. Enlarged peripheral lymph nodes are readily palpable and immobilized for optimal specimen collection. Aspiration biopsy produces rapid and reliable diagnostical information with excellent cytological detail. In many cases it is the preferred method for assessing lymphocyte morphology and identification and classification of the cell types. It is a relatively simple and inexpensive way of differentiating benign and malignant lymphoid disease and should be performed routinely in any patient presenting with one or more enlarged lymph nodes. If the diagnosis cannot be confirmed on the cytological sample, lymph node biopsies or node excisions should be submitted for histopathological evaluation.

TECHNIQUES

Insufficient sampling or inadequate quality of lymph node smears may result in an equivocal cytological diagnosis. Lymph node aspirates should be taken before therapeutic intervention. The lympholytic effect of chemotherapeutics results in intranodal cell necrosis, which reduces the diagnostical value of the biopsy. For best cytological detail, thin smears must be made. If air-dried smears are too thick, inadequate Romanowsky's staining will make cytological evaluation difficult to impossible. The aspirated material must be dispensed onto and spread over the slides very gently because lymphoid cells are very fragile. Smears should be prepared using the spreader technique rather than using a

crush method to preserve cell integrity. Disruption of cells results in bare nuclei or isolated strands of deoxyribonucleic acid (DNA) and precludes cell identification. Multiple lymph nodes should be biopsied in cases of generalized lymphadenopathy. If a single node is enlarged, care must be taken to obtain representative samples. Gentle redirection of the needle will assist sampling of various areas of the affected node while minimizing hemorrhage and tissue.

Excess fluid or tissue obtained from a diseased node may be flushed into transport media for cytocentrifugation or flow cytometry. This will facilitate further processing, such as immunocytochemistry or cytochemical staining, which has been reported useful in distinguishing between B cells and T cells, and in the detection of different cell types of canine lymphomas (Caniatti, 1996; Raskin, 1992). In cases of suspected septic lymphadenitis, aspirated material may be placed directly onto blood agar plates or into enrichment broth for microbial isolation (Mills, 1989). Aspirated material may be fixed with 3% glutaraldehyde and processed for ultrastructural evaluation, or in the case of clotted aspirates, fixation in 10% formalin will facilitate histological processing and H&E staining (Akhtar, 1980). Impression smears may be made from excisional biopsies to confirm benign or malignant lymphoid disease and as an adjunct to lymph node histopathology.

Romanowsky's stains are preferred for air-dried lymphoid smears. Diff-Quick stains provide less adequate staining of nuclear and cytoplasmic details. Staining techniques should be modified in the case of thick smears to ensure adequate cell staining. This may require prolonged or repeated stages in the staining procedure. Papanicolaou's stain, requiring wet fixation, may be preferred in cases of suspected metastasis of epithelial tumors to the node, but it is inadequate for lymphoid evaluation in general (Magnol, 1994). Gram's stains, periodic acid–Schiff, or toluidine blue stains may be required to identify intranodal bacteria, mycoses, or poorly differentiated mast cell infiltration, respectively. Rehydration and fast Papanicolaou's, or hematoxylin and eosin, staining of air-dried aspirate or impression smears has potential value, in conjunction with Wright's-stained cells, for the characterization of lymphocyte nuclei and to assist correlation with histological morphological classifications.

■ LYMPH NODES

NORMAL LYMPH NODE (Figs. 5-1 to 5-9 and Boxes 5-1 and 5-2)

Normal lymph nodes characteristically have a heterogeneous population of lymphoid and nonlymphoid cells within a clear background. The lymphoid cells are predominantly small, well-differentiated lymphocytes with nuclear diameters equivalent to one red

blood cell. The nuclear chromatin is condensed, deeply basophilic with prominent aggregation of DNA or chromocenters, and scant, pale, basophilic cytoplasm. These cells are generally referred to as *small lymphocytes* and may be of either T- or B-cell origin. There are low numbers of medium-sized lymphocytes, or *centrocytes*, and rarer immature cells, or *centroblasts*. Centrocytes are small or large and have cleaved nuclei, dense chromatin, and indistinct nucleoli. Small cleaved cells are one to two red cells in diameter. The centroblasts are larger cells (nuclear diameters average three red blood cells), with pale, finely stippled chromatin and multiple small nucleoli that are peripheralized in the nucleus (Magnol, 1994). The largest of the lymphoid cells, the *B-immunoblasts*, have nuclear diameters of four or more red blood cells with abundant, sometimes vacuolated basophilic cytoplasm and pale, stippled chromatin, with single to multiple prominent nucleoli. *T-immunoblasts* are far fewer, with paler cytoplasm that is very abundant (Magnol, 1994). Small noncleaved lymphocytes have a nuclear diameter equivalent to one to two red cells, a complete rim of visible cytoplasm, and coarsely clumped or aggregated chromatin. Lymphoblasts have a nuclear diameter equivalent to one to two red cells and fine to amorphous chromatin with occasional nucleoli. Together, the lymphoid cells represent 95% to 98% of the nodal

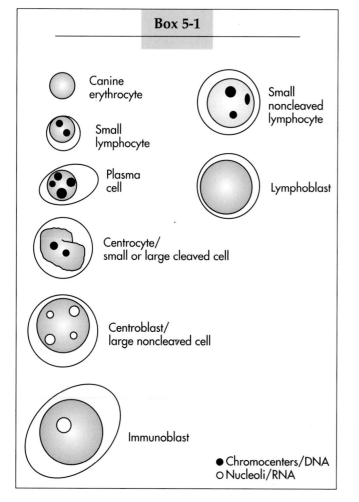

Box 5-1

Canine erythrocyte

Small lymphocyte

Plasma cell

Centrocyte/ small or large cleaved cell

Centroblast/ large noncleaved cell

Immunoblast

Small noncleaved lymphocyte

Lymphoblast

● Chromocenters/DNA
○ Nucleoli/RNA

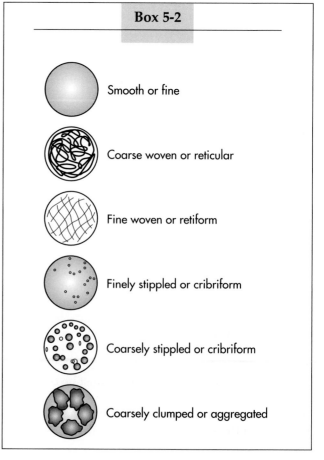

Box 5-2

Smooth or fine

Coarse woven or reticular

Fine woven or retiform

Finely stippled or cribriform

Coarsely stippled or cribriform

Coarsely clumped or aggregated

population. Plasma cells are present in very low numbers (0% to 4.7%) (Lucas, 1955). They feature small, condensed, eccentric nuclei with aggregated chromatin, moderate N:C ratios, and a pale perinuclear area compatible with the Golgi apparatus.

The nonlymphoid component consists of neutrophils, eosinophils, mast cells, and macrophages and supportive cells, such as interdigitating cells and follicular dendritic cells. There are few inflammatory cells in a normal, or nonstimulated, node. In a study of normal canine lymph nodes, the following were reported (mean + SD): 0.1 + 0.1% neutrophils, 0.3 + 0.7% eosinophils, 0.04 + 0.04% macrophages, and 0.02 + 0.03% mast cells (Gosset, 1987). Feline lymph nodes have a higher proportion of mast cells, even in the absence of eosinophils.

NONNEOPLASTIC DISEASE (Figs. 5-10 to 5-16)

CLINICAL DIAGNOSIS

Benign lymph node hyperplasia is a frequent clinical finding in the dog and to a lesser extent in the cat. It may occur in a single node or as generalized lymphadenopathy. Causes are variable but range from isolated disease within the region drained by the lymph node to severe systemic infections. The node is classified as benign reactive or hyperplastic when there is clinical evidence of lymph node enlargement with little, if any, modification in the cytological appearance. Submandibular and mesenteric lymph nodes frequently are reactive, presumably because of chronic antigenic exposure from the mouth and intestine, respectively. For this reason, aspiration of these nodes should be less of a priority because hyperplasia may confound the cytological diagnosis. Lymph nodes that are hyperplastic are often nonpainful; those with lymphadenitis are often painful on palpation.

CYTOLOGICAL DIAGNOSIS

The cytological appearance of lymphoid hyperplasia may be indistinguishable from a normal node. There is a heterogeneous appearance to the node, which may be accompanied by an increase in plasma cells, centroblasts, or immunoblasts. Plasmacytic hyperplasia is associated with chronic antigenic stimulation; hypergammaglobulinemia; and some cases of focal infiltrative disease, such as metastatic carcinomas or sarcomas. A few plasma cells may contain intracytoplasmic, pale to lightly basophilic vacuoles, or *Russell bodies.* They represent accumulations of immunoglobulins (Ig) within vesicles derived from rough endoplasmic reticulum, although some studies have raised questions as to their true nature (Hsu, 1982; Matthews, 1983). Plasma cells containing Russell bodies are known as *Mott cells.* A partial or complete block of Ig secretion is the proposed underlying defect responsible for the formation of Mott cells (Alanen, 1985). In cats, infections by retroviruses, such as feline immun-

odeficiency virus (FIV) and feline leukemia virus (FeLV), may incite follicular hyperplasia, characterized by an abundant, heterogeneous population of predominantly centroblasts, some immunoblasts, centrocytes, plasma cells, and macrophages (Magnol, 1994).

Follicular hyperplasia may be difficult to distinguish cytologically from a well-differentiated B-cell lymphoma because both are characterized by a monotonous population of small cells with condensed nuclei and scant peripheral cytoplasm in the absence of obvious plasma cells or other nonlymphoid components. Immunophenotyping may help distinguish between benign T-cell hyperplasia and B-cell lymphoma (Magnol, 1994).

Lymphadenitis is routinely encountered in the dog and cat. It may be localized to one node or may involve multiple nodes, depending on the underlying cause. It is usually characterized by the predominant inflammatory cell type or types observed on cytology. Lymph nodes affected by suppurative lymphadenitis have a heterogeneous population of lymphoid cells with a predominance of small, well-differentiated lymphocytes. There are increased neutrophils and a mild increase in lymphoblasts, plasma cells, and immunoblasts. Macrophages may also be increased, and there may be evidence of cell necrosis. Suppurative lymphadenitis may be a secondary response to fungal infections; rapidly expanding metastatic or lymphoid tumors; infarction; immune vasculitis; and other infections, such as salmonellosis and toxoplasmosis (Mills, 1989). Intracellular or extracellular organisms should be identified when possible.

Lymphadenitis with a more prominent macrophage or monocyte component and increased neutrophils and plasma cells (granulomatous or pyogranulomatous lymphadenitis) may be seen with disorders such as leishmaniasis, mycobacteriosis (Fournel, 1994), fungal infections, *Neorickettsia helminthoeca* (i.e., salmon poisoning), chronic immune diseases (e.g., systemic lupus erythematosus), vasculitis, and chronic nonsuppurative infections (Mills, 1989). Dermatopathic lymphadenopathy results from chronic skin disease or cutaneous hypersensitivity and features a heterogeneous inflammatory component, usually with increased eosinophils and mast cells. Melanin-containing macrophages (melanophages) are frequently observed with dermatopathic lymphadenopathy. Eosinophilic lymphadenitis may also be observed as part of the feline eosinophilic granuloma complex (Magnol, 1994), with eosinophilic myositis (Valli, 1993), and microfilaremic heartworm infections (Gossett, 1987).

Myeloid metaplasia may be observed in lymph nodes in association with chronic bone marrow insufficiency. Cytologically, the node features a range of hematopoietic progenitors and their progressive stages of synchronous maturation. There may be an associated plasmacytic and centroblastic hyperplasia (Magnol, 1994)

NEOPLASTIC DISEASE

METASTATIC LYMPH NODE NEOPLASIA (Figs. 5-17 to 5-26)

Clinical Diagnosis

Malignant tumors frequently spread via the hematogenous or lymphatic route to local draining lymph nodes. A variety of tumors have this potential, but those most often diagnosed include carcinomas, mast cell tumors, and malignant melanomas. Sarcomas, such as hemangiosarcomas, will occasionally spread via the lymphatic route (Magnol, 1994). The clinical findings at the time of presentation will vary depending on the biological behavior and site of the primary mass, duration of disease, and the presence or absence of paraneoplastic syndromes. If regional lymphadenopathy is detected in the cancer patient, cytological specimens should be collected. If metastatic involvement cannot be confirmed by cytology, histopathology is recommended because early or focal infiltration may reduce the sensitivity of cytological examination.

Cytological Diagnosis

Cytological examination of lymph nodes with metastatic disease may reveal a heterogeneous background of lymphocytes that resemble those in a normal node. There may be variable plasmacytic hyperplasia. In instances in which the metastatic tumor is rapidly expanding, resulting in loss of normal architecture and disruption of the normal vascular supply, there may be significant lymphadenitis (neutrophilic or granulomatous) with abundant cell necrosis and amorphous globular debris. There may be a diluted edematous background. Obliteration of normal node elements with complete replacement by neoplastic cells can be seen with metastatic mast cell tumors or melanomas.

Identification of cells that are foreign to the nonaffected nodal population is supportive of infiltrative disease. Carcinomas may be identified by the observation of cohesive nests, sheets, or acini of cells with malignant criteria. With anaplastic tumors, single cells may be dispersed focally throughout the node, making the cytological diagnosis more difficult. These cells may be difficult to distinguish from the indigenous dendritic cells or epithelioid macrophages. A review of the cytological features of the primary mass may assist in definitive identification of metastatic cells within the node.

Hematopoietic nonlymphoid tumors may infiltrate lymph nodes. Acute myelogenous leukemia (AML) and malignant histiocytosis (MH) may be identified on cytological examination of affected nodes. In all cases a current hemogram and bone marrow evaluation are essential to confirm the diagnosis (Magnol, 1994). Cytological findings of poorly differentiated blast cells within a heterogeneous background of lymphocytes is supportive of infiltration with AML. Cytochemical stains may be helpful but are dependent on the differentiation of the neoplastic cell line. A population of poorly differentiated, large, round cells with variable N:C ratios and frequent multinucleation is a characteristic finding in nodes with malignant histiocytosis. The histiocytic cells have very irregularly shaped and convoluted nuclei with reticular, pale-staining chromatin and abundant, pale to intensely basophilic, finely vacuolated cytoplasm. Erythrocytophagy is a characteristic of malignant histiocytosis. Examination of bone marrow, various soft tissues (e.g., lung, kidneys, liver), and other lymphoid organs (e.g., spleen) may be needed to establish the diagnosis (Brown, 1994).

LYMPHOMA (Figs. 5-27 to 5-41)

Clinical Diagnosis

Hematopoietic and lymphoid tumors are among the most commonly diagnosed neoplasms in veterinary medicine. Canine lymphosarcoma is detected in 0.36% of all dogs presented for veterinary care, accounting for 83% of all canine hematological tumors (Couto, 1985). This is twice the incidence in humans and approximately two-thirds the incidence in cats (MacEwen, 1992). An underlying etiology for canine lymphoma has not been established. Increased levels of reverse transcriptase in some lymphoma cell lines has implicated a role for a retrovirus (Armstrong, 1981). Genetic predisposition, immunological dysfunction, and exposure to environmental toxins are considered potential alternative causes. The average age at diagnosis is 6 to 7 years (range 6 months to 15 years or older). A relationship between lymphoma type (morphological or phenotypical) and age or breed of dogs has yet to be established (Teske, 1994).

In dogs, lymphomas are classified according to the anatomical location of the tumor. The most common is the multicentric form. Some 80% of dogs with lymphoma present with painless, peripheral lymphadenopathy but may be otherwise asymptomatic. Approximately 40% of dogs with multicentric lymphoma present with weight loss, lethargy, anorexia, and pyrexia (MacEwen, 1992). Concurrent hepatosplenomegaly, bone marrow infiltration, or extranodal involvement may be detected. The thymic, or mediastinal, form involves the cranial mediastinal lymph nodes and is often associated with hypercalcemia, polyuria, and polydipsia. The alimentary form has focal or diffuse gastrointestinal involvement, with or without hepatosplenomegaly or mesenteric node involvement. Extranodal forms include sites such as the eye, kidney, CNS, heart, and skin.

Domestic cats have the highest incidence of lymphoma. Hematopoietic tumors represent one third of feline neoplasms, with lymphoma identified in 90% of these cases (Dorn, 1968). Most cats with lymphoma (70%) are infected with FeLV (Moore, 1995; Moulton, 1990). FIV may have an indirect role in lymphomagenesis because of the potential for malignant transformation during polyclonal B-cell activation (Callanan, 1996). In contrast to dogs, peripheral lymphadenopathy occurs less frequently in cats with lymphoproliferative disease. Thymic, cranial mediastinal lymph node, intestinal, or renal involvement is more common. In a study of 103 cases of feline lymphoma, only 9% of cats presented with peripheral lymphadenopathy (Mooney, 1989).

Classification of Lymphoma

Nuclear diameter, N:C ratio, and nuclear details, including chromatin pattern, visibility of nucleoli, and nuclear cleavage, can be markedly influenced by the methods used for cell fixation and staining. Comparisons between cytological, air-dried or alcohol-fixed specimens and histological classification schemes usually do not address these effects, thus contributing to apparent contradictions and confusion, especially when using diameter of nuclei relative to red cells or visibility of nuclear cleavage for classifying lymphocytes.

Current attempts to correlate the morphological, immunological, and genetic categorizations of human non-Hodgkin's lymphoma (NHL) with disease outcome are well ahead of veterinary medicine (Harris,

1994). There are well-established correlations between tumor cell types and clinical behavior in human NHL (National Cancer Institute, 1982; Tindle, 1984).

Numerous classification schemes have been applied to lymphoid tumors in dogs (Table 5-1). Categorizations based on histology (Carter, 1986; Carter, 1988; Gray, 1984; Greenlee, 1990; Parodi, 1988; Weller, 1980), cytology (Fournel-Fleury, 1997; Magnol, 1994), ultrastructural features (Madewell, 1990), cytochemistry (Carter, 1986; Raskin, 1992), immunophenotype (Appelbaum, 1984; Caniatti, 1996; Carter, 1986; Ferrer, 1993; Fournel-Fleury, 1997; Greenlee, 1990; Ruslander, 1997; Teske, 1994), and proliferative rate (Fournel-Fleury, 1997) have been reported. Unfortunately, the terminology used in the classification schemes is often confusing and dependent on the inherent morphological basis of the scheme (histology versus cytology). There are inconsistencies of classification that are dependent on differences such as fixation and staining techniques, the specificity of immunologic markers, and differences based on individual pathologists' interpretation. Classification systems are continually being revised as newer genetic and immunological techniques are applied. Some categories of lymphoma are easily recognized, such as lymphoblastic and immunoblastic cell types, whereas others remain indefinite because of tumor variability.

The two major histomorphological classifications of canine lymphoma include the Working formulation and Kiel's classification (Carter, 1986; Greenlee, 1990;

Table 5-1

Classification of Canine Lymphoma

International Formulation (Working Formulation)*	Kiel Formulation (After Lennert)*	Cytological Classification (Magnol, 1994)†
Low Grade	**Low Grade**	**Low Grade**
Diffuse small lymphocytic	Lymphocytic	Lymphocytic
Follicular, predominantly small cleaved cells	Lymphoplasmacytic/ Lymphoplasmacytoid	Lymphoplasmacytic
Follicular, mixed (small cleaved + large cells)	Centrocytic, follicular	Centrocytic
	Centroblastic/centrocytic, follicular, small cells	Small-cell variants
		Mycosis fungoides
Intermediate Grade	**Intermediate Grade**	**Intermediate or High Grade**
Follicular, predominantly large	Centroblastic/centrocytic, follicular, large cells	Centroblastic/centrocytic
Diffuse, small cleaved	Centrocytic, diffuse	Medium-sized, irregular, multinucleolated cells
Diffuse, mixed (small cleaved + large cells)	Centroblastic/centrocytic, diffuse, small cells	Homogeneous, medium-sized, macronucleolated cells
Diffuse, large cleaved	Centrocytic, diffuse, large cells	Heterogeneous, with a centroblastic component
Diffuse, large, noncleaved	Centroblastic monomorphous	Homogeneous, centroblastic
High Grade	**High Grade**	**High Grade**
Immunoblastic	Immunoblastic	Immunoblastic
Lymphoblastic (convoluted or round nuclei)	Lymphoblastic	Lymphoblastic
Small noncleaved (Burkitt or non-Burkitt)	Lymphoblastic	Blastic, small cells

From Fournel-Fleury, C., Magnol, J.P., and Guelfi, J.F. The lymph node. In *Colour Atlas of Cancer Cytology of the Dog and Cat.* Conference Nationale des Veterinaries Specialises en Petits Animaux, 1994.
*Alcohol fixation, histologic specimens.
†Air-dried fixation, cytologic specimens.

Magnol, 1994). A recent cytomorphological classification has been proposed (Magnol, 1994). Demonstration of a correlation between any one classification scheme and disease remission and survival times remains elusive in the veterinary literature. The predictive value of the classification of lymphoma based on cell type is not well established with respect to canine lymphoproliferative disease (Carter, 1986; Teske, 1996; Weller, 1980).

Canine lymphomas differ from human NHL when lymph node architecture and mitotic index are considered. In dogs, the predominant feature of lymphomas is a diffuse pattern of infiltration (Carter, 1986; Fournel-Fleury, 1997; Teske, 1984; Teske, 1994). The diffuse or focal nodal architecture cannot be confirmed based on cytological examination alone. Most canine lymphomas have a high grade of malignancy. In a study of 285 cases of lymphoma, high-grade tumors accounted for 66.3% of surveyed cases with high-grade malignancy defined as 6 or more mitoses per 400× field on histological specimens (Carter, 1986). Identification of mitoses on cytological specimens is much less reliable as a result of the variability in the specimens. However, for cytological biopsies, mitoses are quantitated by the average number of mitotic figures observed per field, with the suggestion that 2 to 3 mitoses per 400× field is indicative of a high-grade tumor (Carter, 1986). Another cytological study reported the mitotic index as the average number of mitoses found in 5 fields observed at 50× magnification. Mitotic indexes were reported as low (0-1), medium (2-4), and high (>5 mitoses/50×) (Fournel-Fleury, 1997).

Canine lymphomas are predominantly B-cell tumors. Carter (1986) reported in a study of 285 dogs with lymphoma that 70% of the tumors were of B-cell origin, 25% were of T-cell origin, and 5% expressed no distinct immunophenotype. This is remarkably consistent with other studies (Ferrer, 1993; Fournel-Fleury, 1997; Ruslander, 1997). Teske (1994) reported a higher percentage of T-cell tumors (37.9%) in a series of 95 immunophenotyped canine lymphomas. Higher rates of relapse and shorter survival times are consistently associated with T-cell phenotype, whereas B-cell lymphomas are a large and heterogeneous group both clinically and morphologically.

Feline lymphomas have been less intensively studied with respect to cell classification, perhaps because of the rarity of peripheral lymph node involvement in this species. Immunophenotypical, cytochemical, and histological studies have been conducted on limited numbers of feline cases (Callanan, 1996; Rojko, 1989). Given its frequent association with lymphoproliferative disease, it may be that FeLV status is a more significant determinant of survival than cell type (Mooney, 1989).

CYTOLOGICAL DIAGNOSIS

Lymphomas are characterized by the maturational arrest of a malignant clone of lymphoid cells. With progression of the disease, the normal node architecture is completely replaced by tumor cells. This is characterized by a monotypical, homogenous, or heterogenous population of lymphocytes, depending on the cell type, and usually devoid of the few inflammatory cells found in a normal node. Macrophages with densely staining remnants of DNA (tingible body macrophages) may be prominent because of increased cytorrhexis. There may be numerous rounded-up and variably sized fragments of cytoplasm evident in the background (lymphoglandular bodies); these are not pathognomonic for lymphoma and may be seen with benign hyperplasia or lymphadenitis. They have been reported in higher frequency with B-cell and high-grade tumors than in T-cell tumors (Teske, 1994). With focal node involvement, or in early tumor infiltration, the residual heterogeneous population of lymphocytes may make the cytological diagnosis of lymphoma difficult to impossible.

Cytological evaluation, based on air-dried fixation, includes assessment of the following (see Boxes 5-1 and 5-2):

1. *Cell size* is estimated by comparing an average lymphocyte nuclear diameter to the size of a nondistorted red cell. Lymphocytes with nuclear diameters averaging 1 to 2 erythrocytes are labeled small lymphocytes, whereas cells with nuclear diameters of 3 or more erythrocytes are labeled large lymphocytes.
2. *Nuclear shape* is determined to be cleaved or noncleaved, round or convoluted.
3. *Nuclear chromatin* is described as fine, pinpoint, stippled or cribriform, aggregated or clumped, woven or reticular. The absence or presence of chromocenters is noted.
4. *Nucleolar features* such as size, number, and location within the nucleus.
5. *Cytoplasmic features* including volume, basophilic intensity, positioning around the nucleus, vacuolation, and presence of granules.
6. *Mitotic index* usually subjectively estimated based on the average number observed per 400× or oil field.

Large Granular Lymphoma (Fig. 5-42)

CLINICAL AND CYTOLOGICAL DIAGNOSES

A rare subtype of lymphoma known as large granular lymphoma (LGL) characterized by large cells with prominent azurophilic cytoplasmic granules has been identified in both dogs and cats (Helfand, 1995; Kariya, 1997). The cells have been classified phenotypically as cytotoxic T cells or natural killer (NK) cells and have perforin-like immunoreactivity. Clinically, these cells have been identified in the gastrointestinal tract and associated lymph nodes; in the peripheral blood; and in various other sites, such as the skin, spleen, heart, and CNS (Darbes, 1998; Wellman, 1992). In cats, proviral genome of FeLV has been identified in a cell line derived from a cat with alimentary LGL (Goitsuka, 1993). In another study, 9 of 11 cats with LGL were seronegative when tested for FeLV (Wellman, 1992).

Thymic Lymphoma

CLINICAL DIAGNOSIS

In a recent study of thymic pathology, thymic lymphoma was the most commonly documented disorder in 19 of 30 cats (63%) and 12 of 36 dogs (33%) (Day, 1997). The mean age of affected cats and dogs was 4.07 and 5.79 years, respectively. FeLV was associated in 4 of 8 cats tested. Clinically, dyspnea, regurgitation, or both were recognized in both cats and dogs, whereas lethargy, anorexia, weight loss, polydipsia, vomiting, and diarrhea were also occasionally reported in the latter species. Involvement with other intrathoracic or extrathoracic nodes, liver, kidney, spleen, lung, bone marrow, and intercostal muscles were reported concurrently.

CYTOLOGICAL DIAGNOSIS

In both species, there was some variability to the cytological evaluation of the neoplastic lymphocytes, which ranged from well-differentiated small lymphocytes to lymphoblastic and histiocytic types (Day, 1997). Most cases had the lymphoblastic form with round to oval pale nuclei, often with a single central nucleolus. The mitotic index in both species was high.

Gastrointestinal Lymphoma (Fig. 5-43)

CLINICAL DIAGNOSIS

Primary gastrointestinal lymphoma is less common than the multicentric forms and represents less than 10% of canine lymphoproliferative disease (MacEwen, 1989). Alimentary lymphoma is the third most common form of feline lymphoproliferative disease following thymic and multicentric extranodal forms. FeLV serology is usually negative in these patients. Weight loss, vomiting, diarrhea, and signs of malabsorption are common in both species.

CYTOLOGICAL DIAGNOSIS

Intestinal lymphoma may be difficult to distinguish from lymphocytic gastroenteritis as a result of the small sample size and the uniformity of the lymphocytes in both specimens. There is a monotypic population of small cells with coarsely condensed nuclear chromatin and scant cytoplasm. Histopathology may be more helpful in unraveling the underlying architecture of the intestinal lymphoid infiltrate. In some cases, alimentary lymphoma may resemble plasma cell tumors (MacEwen, 1992).

Cutaneous Lymphoma (Fig. 5-45)

CLINICAL DIAGNOSIS

Cutaneous lymphoma is uncommon in dogs and cats. Lymphoid tumors of the skin may be of primary cutaneous origin or a component of multicentric lymphoma (Day, 1995). The disease is slowly progressive and occurs in aged animals, usually over 10 years of age. The mean ages of dogs with epitheliotropic and nonepitheliotropic lymphoma were 10.6 ± 2.6 years and 8.0 ± 2.9 years, respectively. Cats with cutaneous lymphoma had a mean age of 11.5 ± 2.9 years (Day, 1995). The presenting signs are quite variable, ranging from single to multiple discrete nodular eruptions, erosive mucocutaneous or footpad lesions, to generalized exfoliative dermatitis with pruritus, erythema, and alopecia. It may closely mimic such skin disorders as solitary tumors or granulomas and immune-based (such as systemic or discoid lupus) or hypersensitivity diseases (e.g., drug eruption). Lymph node involvement may be detected at the time of initial diagnosis, or lymphadenopathy may develop during the course of the disease. Cutaneous lymphoma is ultimately fatal, although a rare patient has survived with a single skin lesion that had been surgically excised. As with other types of lymphoma, a relationship between clinical behavior of cutaneous lymphoma, immunohistopathology, and mitotic rate has not been established. In cats, circulating FeLV antigen has not been identified in association with cutaneous lymphoid tumors (Caciolo, 1984). However, polymerase chain reaction has demonstrated integrated FeLV provirus in some tumor DNA (Tobey, 1994).

CYTOLOGICAL DIAGNOSIS

The hallmark finding of cutaneous lymphoma is a monotypic population of lymphocytes that have abundant, pale-staining cytoplasm and nuclei that show cytological atypia ranging from deep clefting to multilobulation or bizarre convolutions, sometimes described as "cerebriform." Nests, or clusters, of these cells form the so-called Pautrier's microabscesses, which are recognizable in histological sections. In other cases the cytological appearance of the lymphocytes may vary from small, well-differentiated cells to plasmacytoid or even lymphoblastic. The mitotic rate is variable. Cutaneous lymphoma has been classified as epitheliotropic (or epidermotropic), nonepitheliotropic (or nonepidermotropic), or of plasma cell origin. Epitheliotropic is more common in canine primary cutaneous lymphoma (Day, 1995; Teske, 1994). Day (1995) reported nonepitheliotropic lymphoma to be predominantly of T-cell origin (8 of 10 canine cases, 5 of 6 feline cases). The distinction between epitheliotropic and nonepitheliotropic is made on the basis of immunocytochemistry and histopathology. Diffuse dermal and subcutaneous lymphoid infiltration characterizes the nonepitheliotropic form.

MULTIPLE MYELOMA (Figs. 5-46 to 5-49)

CLINICAL DIAGNOSIS

Multiple myeloma is an uncommon malignancy of plasma cells reported in dogs and cats (Sheafor, 1996; Villiers, 1998; Weber, 1998). It accounts for less than 1% of all canine malignancies, 3.6% of all bone tumors, and approximately 8% of hematopoietic tumors. In dogs, clinical signs associated with plasma cell tumors include anorexia, vomiting, polyuria or polydipsia, neuromuscular weakness, ataxia, blindness, and coagulopathies. The clinical signs in cats are vague and include anorexia, lethargy, vomiting, splenomegaly, and polydipsia.

Bone marrow infiltration is variable. Malignant plasma cells may occupy 5% to 90% of the total nucleated cell mass (Magnol, 1994). Infiltration of other hemolymphatic tissues (spleen, liver, lymph nodes) may be present. Other criteria, such as monoclonal or biclonal gammopathy, light-chain proteinuria, and osteolytic lesions, are helpful in establishing the diagnosis (Peterson, 1997; Sheafor, 1996). Gammopathies may be absent in the rare nonsecretory form of myeloma (Marks, 1995).

CYTOLOGICAL DIAGNOSIS

An increased number of plasma cells may be identified on aspiration of bone marrow or other soft tissues. In bone marrow aspirates especially, this may be difficult to confirm because of the discrete focal nature of the tumor. The cytomorphology of the cells may be normal, or the plasma cells may have more atypical features. Ovoid, eccentric, hyperchromatic nuclei with multiple nucleoli and abundant amphophilic ("flame cells") to deeply basophilic cytoplasm may be punctuated by prominent perinuclear Golgi zones. Increased N:C ratios with reticular nuclear chromatin may be seen in immature plasma cells. Mott cells distended with Russell bodies may be increased in number. Multinucleation, binucleation, and increased mitotic activity are frequent findings. Prominent anisokaryosis or anisocytosis and erythrophagocytosis has been noted (Magnol, 1994; Marks, 1995).

■ *THYMUS*

Diseases of the thymus are uncommon in the dog and rare in the cat. Recognition of thymic tissue and neoplastic conditions of the thymus are important in the differential diagnosis of lesions in the neck and thoracic region.

TECHNIQUE

Purposeful aspiration of the thymus is never done clinically. However, thymic masses may be aspirated when investigating lesions in the thoracic cavity. Aspiration of thoracic masses follow the same procedures as previously outlined. Handling of any tissues with suspect lymphatic origin must be done with extreme care because of the naturally fragile nature of the cells.

NORMAL THYMUS (Figs. 5-50 to 5-54)

Two distinct cell populations are visible in imprints of normal thymic tissue. The first is a population of benign small and large lymphocytes with small lymphocytes predominating. Mitosis is common. The second population consists of large epithelioid cells with pale, lightly basophilic, abundant cytoplasm. Nuclei are approximately two red blood cells in diameter with coarse cribriform chromatin and small, indistinct nucleoli.

NONNEOPLASTIC DISEASE

CYTOLOGICAL DIAGNOSIS

In dogs and cats, inflammatory diseases involving the thymus are not well characterized. If suspect, imaging techniques should be used to direct aspiration of representative cells.

NEOPLASTIC DISEASE

Thymoma (Figs. 5-55 to 5-57)

CLINICAL DIAGNOSIS

In humans, thymomas are associated with myasthenia gravis, polymyositis, myocarditis, and dermatitis. Dogs and cats with thymomas frequently present with coughing, dyspnea, pleural effusion, and generalized malaise (Bellah, 1983; Carpenter, 1982). Myasthenia gravis was reported in seven dogs with thymoma (Aronsohn, 1984). Dyspnea, pleural effusion, polymyositis, myocarditis, and dermatitis were reported in cats with thymoma (Carpenter, 1982).

In dogs and cats, thymomas are rare and usually benign (Bellah, 1983; Carpenter, 1982; Hauser, 1984; Middleton, 1985). Thymomas are tumors derived from thymic epithelial components. Thymomas are usually heavily encapsulated (Valli, 1993) and appear in the cranial portion of the mediastinum (Carpenter, 1982). Thymomas are classified as lymphoid, epithelial, or mixed, based on the predominant cell type. Because of the poor correlation between clinical behavior and histological or cytological appearance, *noninvasive* and *invasive* are suggested alternative terms for benign and malignant thymoma, respectively (Bellah, 1983; Carpenter, 1982). Malignancy is confirmed with observation of malignant cells in pleural effusions, infiltrative patterns, pleural implants, and distant metastasis.

Thymomas must be differentiated from mediastinal lymphoma, thymic lymphoma, and benign lymphoid proliferation. Because of the great differences in prognosis, it is especially important to differentiate benign thymoma from malignant mediastinal lymphoma (Carpenter, 1982; Simpson, 1992).

Based on a limited number of cases, well-encapsulated thymomas that are easily resectable have a good prognosis (Bellah, 1983).

CYTOLOGICAL DIAGNOSIS

Aspirate smears from thymomas characteristically contain epithelial cells and lymphocytes. The epithelial cells are considered to be malignant and typically polygonal but may be round, oval, or spindle-shaped. Small, benign lymphocytes often exceed the epithelial cells in aspirate smears.

Cytological features from nine dogs and four cats with histologically confirmed thymoma indicate the good potential for identification of canine and feline thymomas using aspiration biopsies (Rae, 1989). Cytological features were not separated for dogs and cats. Seven of nine FNA smears contained both lymphocytes and epithelial-like cells, whereas in two cases there was only evidence for hemorrhage and/or necrosis, although impression smears and histological sections contained both lymphocytes and epithelial cells (Rae, 1989). The epithelial-like cells predominated in four tumors, whereas the lymphocyte was the predominant cell in nine tumors (Rae, 1989). In one thymoma, large sheets of epithelial cells were prominent (Rae, 1989). The epithelial cells were three to five red blood cells in diameter and were present in sheets or small clumps (Rae, 1989). In 10 tumors the epithelial cells were polygonal, and in three tumors they included both spindle and polygonal cells (Rae, 1989). The epithelial nuclei were eccentric and round to oval. The cytoplasm was pale, abundant, and gray-blue with occasional vacuoles (Rae, 1989). Nucleoli were small and insignificant. Small lymphocytes predominated in seven tumors, but in three tumors there were more large than small lymphocytes (Rae, 1989). No cytological preparation contained structures suggestive of Hassall's corpuscles. Mast cells were present in five cases (Rae, 1989). Most tumors contained less than 10% foamy macrophages, which frequently exhibited cytophagy and contained hemosiderin or melanin pigment (Rae, 1989). Aspiration smears of a lytic lesion in the scapula of a dog with metastatic thymoma contained large polygonal epithelial cells with irregular large nuclei and coarse nuclear chromatin (Bellah, 1983).

Histological but not cytological features were reported for 11 cats with thymoma (Carpenter, 1982). One was malignant. Lymphocytes and distribution of epithelial cells varied between tumors. In six cases, tumors contained cysts that varied in number and size. Necrosis was observed in eight tumors (Carpenter, 1982). Of six cats with dyspnea, five had pale yellow to milky pleural effusions (Carpenter, 1982). The lymphocytes were mature and not suggestive of lymphoma (Carpenter, 1982). In one cytology report of canine thymoma the epithelial cells had round to oval nuclei and indistinct nucleoli (Andreason, 1991) The N:C ratio was low to moderate. Epithelial cells were oval to polyhedral and were often found in thick clusters. Lymphocytes were interspersed throughout the slide, as were cells resembling mast cells. Homogeneous eosinophilic extracellular material was present in the background (Andreason, 1991).

Thymic Lymphoma

Thymic lymphoma is described earlier in this chapter.

■ SPLEEN

The spleen is a hemolymphatic organ that is affected by many hematological and systemic inflammatory disorders. Extramedullary hematopoiesis; lymphosarcoma; some leukemias and anemias; mast cell tumors; and systemic inflammatory conditions, such as histoplasmosis and cytauxzoonosis, can induce splenomegaly. Fine-needle splenic biopsy is considered if the cause is not discernible from blood or bone marrow examination. Unless a diffuse lesion is expected, ultrasound-directed aspirations have a greater probability for success. Coagulation parameters should be confirmed if suspect before aspiration.

TECHNIQUE

Fine-needle aspirates of the spleen are performed with the animal in right lateral or dorsal recumbency (O'Keefe, 1987). The spleen is localized with one hand while FNAs are made as previously described. Cell concentration is often diluted as a result of organ vascularity. For the same reason, when making impression smears of a freshly cut surface of the spleen, the surface must be repeatedly blotted with absorbent material to remove blood and plasma; otherwise, significant cells will not be transferred to the glass slide. FNA or scrapings should be considered for surgically removed organs.

NORMAL SPLEEN (Figs. 5-58 to 5-62)

A heavy background of red blood cells is expected on all aspirates and impression smears of the spleen. Small lymphocytes predominate in cytology preparations (Swischer, 1955), with low numbers of nucleated erythrocytes and occasional megakaryocytes. Macrophages, sometimes laden with hemosiderin, and plasma cells may be observed. There may be occasional interspersed endothelial-lined capillaries and stromal types of endothelial cells.

NONNEOPLASTIC AND NEOPLASTIC DISEASE

Splenomegaly

CLINICAL AND CYTOLOGICAL DIAGNOSES

Most abnormalities associated with splenomegaly can potentially be diagnosed with aspiration biopsy, although many authors suggest that aspiration biopsy of splenic masses should be made with caution (Johnson, 1989; O'Keefe, 1987; Osborne, 1974). The primary concern arises from the danger of tumor seeding along the needle tract. However, because the median survival time for dogs with splenic hemangiosarcoma after splenectomy is only 13 weeks (Johnson, 1989), the absolute risk is minimal. Tumor seeding for any needle biopsy has been a subject of discussion. There is some confusion in the literature resulting from the fact that an 18-gauge needle is a "fine needle" in comparison with the larger-core biopsy needle used for histopathology biopsies. We recommend 22-gauge needles, which are unlikely to cause seeding, although there is some risk for induction of splenic rupture. Hematomas and hemangiosarcomas may contain large cavities filled with blood, hemorrhage, or necrotic tissue. These cavities are subject to rupture at the time of biopsy (Osborne, 1974). Nonneoplastic lesions were identified as the cause for localized splenomegaly in 51% of dogs that underwent splenectomy for suspect neoplastic disease (Neer, 1996). A total of 497 cases were considered (Neer, 1996). In the cat, 37% of localized splenic diseases were neoplastic in origin (Spangler, 1992).

Hemangiosarcoma is the most common primary splenic neoplasm, accounting for 51 of 123 surgical splenic submissions (Spangler, 1994) and responsible for 50% of the splenectomies done in dogs (Johnson, 1989). In 100 dogs with splenomegaly, determined on surgical biopsy or at necropsy, 66 had splenic neoplasia and 44 of these had hemangiosarcoma (Johnson, 1989). In 28 dogs with diffuse splenomegaly examined by FNA biopsy, 24% had extramedullary hematopoiesis and 24% had hematopoietic neoplasms (O'Keefe, 1987). Dogs with localized splenic masses were excluded from the study (O'Keefe, 1987). All cytological diagnosis correlated well with the histological diagnosis, and no complications from the cytological procedure were observed (O'Keefe, 1987).

In five cats with splenomegaly investigated using splenic aspiration, one biopsy was suggestive of carcinoma, one indicated feline eosinophilic syndrome, one was due to erythremic myelosis, and two were normal (O'Keefe, 1987). It was concluded that FNA biopsy of the spleen was useful in the differentiation of causes of splenomegaly (O'Keefe, 1987).

FNA biopsies are useful in confirming neoplasia but cannot be used to rule out neoplasia because of the sampling error that may occur; that is, an erroneous diagnosis of hematoma is possible when the true lesion is hemangiosarcoma. Generalized disease is more likely to be diagnosed than localized disease when using FNA biopsy (Neer, 1996). Even when using histopathology, multiple sections are frequently required for confirmation or differentiation of hematoma (Osborne, 1974). A cytological investigation for suspect hemangiosarcoma can be very cost-beneficial, especially when surgical biopsy cannot be done because of cost or risk to the patient. The cytological appearance of hemangiosarcoma is described in Chapter 4.

References

Akhtar, M., Ali, M.A., Owen, E., et al. A simple method for processing fine-needle aspiration biopsy specimens for electron microscopy. *J Clin Pathol* 33:1214, 1980.

Alanen, A., Pira, U., Lassila, O., et al. Mott cells are plasma cells defective in immunoglobulin secretion. *Eur J Immunol* 15:235-242, 1985.

Andreasen, C.B., Mahaffey, E.A., and Latimer, K.S. What is your diagnosis? *Vet Clin Pathol* 20:15-16, 1991.

Applebaum, F.R., Sale, G.E., Storb, R., et al. Phenotyping of canine lymphoma with monoclonal antibodies directed at cell surface antigens: classification, morphology, clinical presentation and response to chemotherapy. *Haematol Oncol* 2:151-168, 1984.

Armstrong, S.J., Thomley, F.M., Nunes deSouza, P.A., et al. Reverse transcriptase activity associated with canine leukemia and lymphosarcoma. In *Advances in Comparative Leukemia Research*. D.S. Yohn, J.R. Blakeslee (eds). pp 411-414, 1981.

Aronsohn, G.G., Schunk, K.L., Carpenter, J.L., et al. Clinical and pathologic features of thymoma in 15 dogs. *J Am Vet Med Assoc* 184:1355-1362, 1984.

Bellah, J.R., Stiff, M.E., and Russell, R.G. Thymoma in the dog: two case reports and review of 20 additional cases. *J Am Vet Med Assoc* 183:306-311, 1983.

Brown, D.E., Thrall, M.A., Getzy, D.M., et al. Cytology of canine malignant histiocytosis. *Vet Clin Pathol* 23:118-122, 1994.

Caciolo, P.L., Nesbitt, G.H., Patnaik, A.K., et al. Cutaneous lymphosarcoma in the cat: a report of nine cases. *J Am Anim Hosp Assoc* 20:491-496, 1984.

Callanan, J.J., Jones, B.A., Irvine, J., et al. Histologic classification and immunophenotype of lymphosarcomas in cats with naturally and experimentally acquired feline immunodeficiency virus infections. *Vet Pathol* 33:264-272, 1996.

Caniatti, M., Roccabianca, P., Scanziani, E., et al. Canine lymphoma: immunocytochemical analysis of fine-needle aspiration biopsy. *Vet Pathol* 33:204-212, 1996.

Carpenter, J.L. and Holzworth, J. Thymoma in 11 cats. *J Am Vet Med Assoc* 181:248-251, 1982.

Carter, R.F. and Valli, V.E.O. Advances in the cytologic diagnosis of canine lymphoma. *Semin Vet Med Surg (Small Anim)* 3:167-175, 1988.

Carter, R.F., Valli, V.E.O., and Lumsden, J.H. The cytology, histology and prevalence of cell types in canine lymphoma classified according to the National Cancer Institute working formulation. *Can J Vet Res* 50:154-164, 1986.

Couto, C.G. Canine lymphomas: something old, something new. *Compend Cont Ed Pract* 7:291-302, 1985.

Darbes, J., Majzou, M., Breuer, W., et al. Large granular lymphocyte leukemia/lymphoma in six cats. *Vet Pathol* 35:370-379, 1998.

Day, M.J. Immunophenotypic characterization of cutaneous lymphoid neoplasia in the dog and cat. *Can J Comp Pathol* 112:79-96, 1995.

Day, M.J. Review of thymic pathology in 30 cats and 36 dogs. *J Small Anim Pract* 38:393-403, 1997.

Dorn, C.R., Talor, D.O.N., Schneider, R., et al. Survey of animal neoplasms in Alameda and Contra Costa Counties, California II. Cancer morbidity in dogs and cats from Alameda County. *J Natl Cancr Inst* 40:307-318, 1968.

Ferrer, L., Fondeuila, D., Rabanal, R., et al. Immunohistochemical detection of CD3 antigen (pan-T marker) in canine lymphomas. *J Vet Diagn Invest* 5:616-620, 1993.

Fournel, C. *Lymph node cytology in veterinary dermatopathology.* 11th Annual Congress of the ESVD, Bordeaux, France, 1994.

Fournel-Fleury, C., Magnol, J.P., Bricaire, P., et al. Cytohistological and immunological classification of canine malignant lymphomas: comparison with human non-Hodgkin's lymphomas. *J Comp Pathol* 117:35-59, 1997.

Fournel-Fleury, C., Magnol, J.P., Chabanne, L., et al. Growth fractions in canine non-Hodgkin's lymphomas as determined *in situ* by the expression of the Ki-67 antigen. *J Comp Pathol* 117:61-72, 1997.

Goitsuka, R., Ohno, K., Matsumoto, Y., et al. Establishment and characterization of a feline large granular lymphoma cell line expressing interleukin 2 receptor alpha-chain. *J Vet Med Sci* 55: 863-865, 1993.

Gosset, K.A., Root, C.R., and Cleghorn, B. Effects of heartworm and intestinal parasitic infections on hematology and peripheral lymph node cytology in Louisiana dogs. *Vet Clin Pathol* 16:97-101, 1987.

Gray, K.N., Raulston, G.L., Geiser, C.A., et al. Histologic classification as an indication of therapeutic response in malignant lymphoma of dogs. *J Am Vet Med Assoc* 184:814-817, 1984.

Greenlee, P.G., Filippa, D.A., Quimby, F.W., et al. Lymphomas in dogs: a morphologic, immunologic, and clinical study. *Cancer* 66:480-490, 1990.

Harris, N.L., Jaffe, E.S., Stein, H., et al. A revised European-American classification of lymphoid neoplasms: a proposal from the International Lymphoma Study Group. *Blood* 84:1361-1392, 1994.

Hauser, B. and Mettler, F. Malignant thymoma in a cat. *J Comp Pathol* 94:311-313, 1984.

Helfand, S.C., Modiano, J.F., Moore, P.F., et al. Functional interleukin-2 receptors are expressed on natural killer-like leukemic cells from a dog with cutaneous lymphoma. *Blood* 8:636-645, 1995.

Hsu, S.M., Hsu, P.L., McMillan, P.N., et al. Russell bodies: a light and electron microscopic immunoperoxidase study. *Am J Clin Pathol* 77:26-31, 1982.

Johnson, K.A., Powers, B.E., Wothgrow, S.J., et al. Splenomegaly in dogs. *J Vet Med* 3:160-166, 1989.

Kariya, K., Konno, A., and Ishida, T. Perforin-like immunoreactivity in four cases of lymphoma of large granular lymphocytes in the cat. *Vet Pathol* 34:156-159, 1997.

Lennert, K. *Histopathology of Non-Hodgkin's Lymphomas (Based on the Kiel Classification).* Springer, Berlin, 1981.

Lucas, P.F. Lymph node smears in the diagnosis of lymphadenopathy: a review. *Blood* 10:1030, 1955.

MacEwen, E.G. and Young, K.M. Canine lymphoma and lymphoid leukemias. In *Clinical Veterinary Oncology.* S.J. Withrow (ed). WB Saunders, Philadelphia, 1992.

Madewell, B.R. and Munn, R.J. Canine lymphoproliferative disorders: an ultrastructural study of 18 cases. *J Vet Intern Med* 4:63-70, 1990.

Magnol, J.P., Fournel-Fleury, C., and Guelfi, J.F. The lymph node. In *Colour Atlas of Cancer Cytology of the Dog and Cat.* Conference Nationale des Veterinaires Specialises en Petits Animaux, 1994.

Marks, S.L., Moore, P.F., Taylor, D.W., et al. Nonsecretory multiple myeloma in a dog: immunohistologic and ultrastructural observations. *J Vet Intern Med* 9:50-54, 1995.

Matthews, J.B. The immunoglobulin nature of Russell bodies. *Br J Pathol* 64:331-335, 1983.

Middleton, D.J., Ratcliffe, R.C., and Xu, F.N. Thymoma with distant metastases in a cat. *Vet Pathol* 22:512-514, 1985.

Mills, J.N. Lymph node cytology. *Vet Clin North Am* 4: 696-717, 1989.

Mooney, S.C., Audrey, A.H., MacEwen, G., et al. Treatment and prognostic factors in lymphoma in cats: 103 cases (1977-1981). *J Am Vet Med Assoc* 194:696-699, 1989.

Moore, A.S. and Mahony, O.M. Treatment of feline malignant lymphoma. In *Current Veterinary Therapy XII, Small Animal Practice.* R.W. Kirk (ed). WB Saunders, Philadelphia, 1995.

Moore, P.F. Utilization of cytoplasmic lysozyme immunoreactivity as a histiocytic marker in canine histiocytic disorders. *Vet Pathol* 23:757-762, 1986.

Moulton, J.E. and Harvey, J.W. Tumors of the lymphoid and hematopoietic tissues. In *Tumors in Domestic Animals.* ed 3. J.E. Moulton (ed). University of California Press, Berkeley, Calif, 1990.

National Cancer Institute sponsored study of classification of Non Hodgkin's Lymphomas: summary and description of a working formulation for clinical usage. *Cancer* 49: 2112-2135, 1982.

Neer, T.M. Clinical approach to splenomegaly in dogs and cats. *Compend Cont Ed Prac* 18:35-46,1996.

O'Keefe, D.A. and Guillermo Couto, C. Fine-needle aspiration of the spleen as an aid in the diagnosis of splenomegaly. *J Vet Intern Med* 1:102-109, 1987.

Osborne, C.A., Perman, V., and Stevens, J.B. Needle biopsy of the dog. *Vet Clin North Am (Small Anim)* 4:311-316, 1974.

Parodi, A.L., Dargen, F., and Crespeau, F. Histological classification of canine malignant lymphomas. *J Am Vet Med Assoc* 35:178-182, 1988

Peterson, E.N. and Meininger, A.C. Immunoglobulin A and immunoglobulin G biclonal gammopathy in a dog with multiple myeloma. *J Am Anim Hosp Assoc* 33:45-47, 1997.

Rae, C.R., Jacobs, R.M., and Couto, C. A comparison between the cytological and histological characteristics in thirteen canine and feline thymomas. *Can Vet J* 30:497-500, 1989.

Raskin, R.E. and Nipper, M.N. Cytochemical staining characteristics of lymph nodes from normal and lymphoma-affected dogs. *Vet Clin Path* 21:62-67, 1992.

Rojko, J.L., Kociba, G.J., Abkowitz, J.L., et al. Feline lymphomas: immunological and cytochemical characterization. *Cancer Res* 49:345-351, 1989.

Ruslander, D.A., Gebhard, D.H., Tompkins, M.B., et al. Immunophenotypic characterization of canine lymphoproliferative disorders. *In Vivo* 11:169-172, 1997.

Sheafor, S.E., Gamblin, R.M., and Couto, C.G. Hypercalcemia in two cats with multiple myeloma. *J Am Anim Hosp Assoc* 32:503-508, 1996.

Simpson, R.M., Waters, D.J., Gebhard, D.H., et al. Case report: massive thymoma and medullary differentiation in a dog. *Vet Pathol* 29:416-419, 1992.

Spangler, W.L. and Culbertson, M.R. Prevalence and type of splenic diseases in cats: 455 cases (1985-1991). *J Am Vet Med Assoc* 201:773-776, 1992.

Spangler, W.L., Culbertson, M.R., and Kass, P.H. Primary mesenchymal (nonangiomatous/nonlymphomatous) neoplasms occurring in the canine spleen: anatomic classification, immunohistochemistry, and mitotic activity correlated with patient survival. *Vet Pathol* 31:37-47, 1994.

Swischer, S.N. and Dale, D.A. Splenic aspiration biopsy in the dog. *Blood* 10:812-819, 1955.

Teske, E. Canine malignant lymphoma: a review and comparison with human non-Hodgkin's lymphoma. *Vet Quarterly* 16:209-219, 1994.

Teske, E. and Van Heerde, P. Diagnostic value and reproducibility of fine-needle aspiration cytology in canine malignant lymphoma. *Vet Quarterly* 18:112-115, 1996.

Teske, E., Wisman, P., Moore, P.F., et al. Histologic classification and immunophenotyping of canine non-Hodgkin's lymphomas: unexpected high frequency of T cell lymphomas with B cell morphology. *Exp Hematol* 22:1179-1187, 1984.

Tindle, B.H. Teaching monograph: malignant lymphomas. *Am J Pathol* 116:115-174, 1984.

Tobey, J.C., Houston, D.M., Breur, G.J., et al. Cutaneous T-cell lymphoma in a cat. *J Am Vet Med Assoc* 204:606-609, 1994.

Valli, V.E.O. and Parry, B.W. The hematopoietic system. In *Pathology of Domestic Animals, vol 3.* ed 4. K.V.F. Jubb, P.C. Kennedy, and N. Palmer (eds). Academic Press, San Diego, 1993.

Villiers, E. and Dobson, J. Multiple myeloma with associated polyneuropathy in a German shepherd dog. *J Small Anim Pract* 39:249-251, 1998.

Weber, N.A. and Tebeau, C.S. An unusual presentation of multiple myeloma in two cats. *J Am Anim Hosp Assoc* 34:477-483, 1998.

Weller, R.E., Holmberg, A.C., Theilen, G.H., et al: Histologic classification as a prognostic criterion for canine lymphosarcoma. *Am J Vet Res* 41:1310-1314, 1980.

Wellman, M.L., Hammer, A.S., DiBartola, S.P., et al. Lymphoma involving large granular lymphocytes in cats: 11 cases (1982-1991). *J Am Vet Med Assoc* 201:1265-1269, 1992.

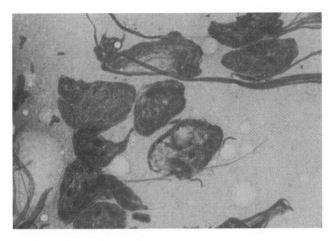

FIG. 5-1. Canine. Fine needle. Lymph node. There is poor cell integrity, many bare nuclei, strands of DNA, and too few intact lymphocytes for satisfactory interpretation. (×500.)

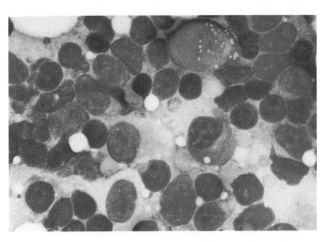

FIG. 5-2. Canine. Fine needle. Normal lymph node. There is a predominance of small lymphocytes, one plasma cell, and a large lymphocyte. The larger lymphocyte, which may represent a T cell immunoblast, has pale abundant cytoplasm and a nuclear diameter of 4 or more red cells. (×312.)

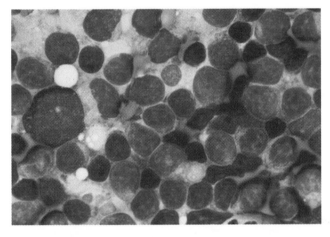

FIG. 5-3. Canine. Fine needle. Normal lymph node. There is a heterogeneous population of lymphocytes with a single large centroblast showing fine chromatin, multiple small nucleoli, and a scant rim of intensely basophilic cytoplasm. (×400.)

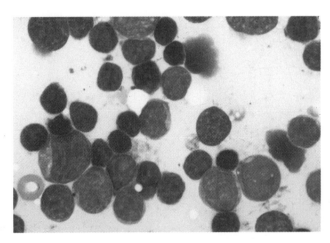

FIG. 5-4. Canine. Imprint. Normal peripheral lymph node. Small, medium, and large lymphocytes illustrating the degree of pleomorphism expected within normal node of a young dog. Some large lymphocytes with prominent nucleoli are acceptable within a normal-sized node. (×400.)

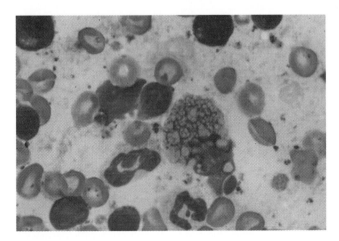

FIG. 5-5. Canine. Fine needle. Benign lymph node. Round cell containing many pale basophilic, variably sized vacuoles, or Russell bodies, sometimes called a Mott cell. The vacuoles may represent intracytoplasmic accumulations of immunoglobulins. (×312.)

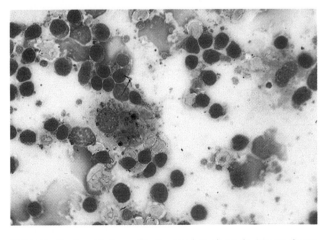

FIG 5-6. Canine. Fine needle. Benign lymph node. Macrophage containing melanin pigment (melanophage). These are observed in darkly pigmented animals or in dermatopathic lymphadenopathy and may be difficult to distinguish from hemosiderin-laden macrophages. (×100.)

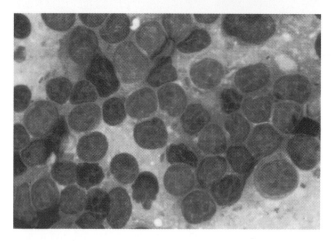

FIG. 5-7. Canine. Imprint. Normal mesenteric lymph node. Lymphocytes illustrate high N:C ratio with indistinct coarse chromatin and small nucleoli. (×400.)

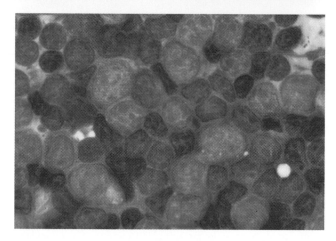

FIG. 5-8. Canine. Imprint. Normal mesenteric lymph node. Pleomorphic population of lymphocytes. (×400.)

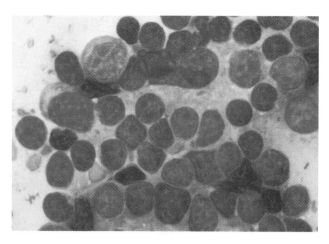

FIG. 5-9. Canine. Imprint. Normal mesenteric lymph node. Pleomorphic population of lymphocytes. The diameter of most nuclei is greater than 2 erythrocytes, there is an indistinct chromatin pattern, and nucleoli are visible. (×400.)

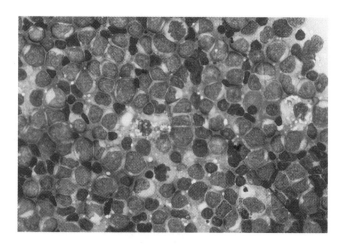

FIG. 5-10. Canine. Fine needle. Hyperplastic lymph node. The node is palpably enlarged, but the cytological presentation is consistent with a normal node. (×200.)

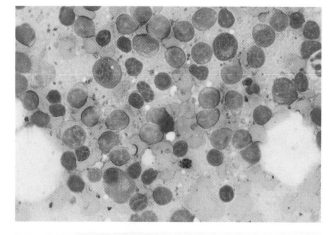

FIG. 5-11. Canine. Fine needle. Lymph node with plasmacytic hyperplasia. Plasma cells constitute less than 5% of the nucleated cells within a normal node. They may be increased with metastatic disease, local lymphadenopathy, or any chronic antigenic stimulus. (×200.)

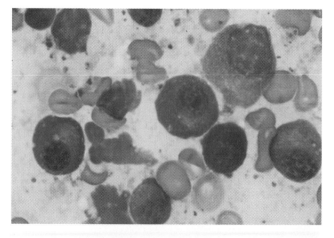

FIG. 5-12. Canine. Fine needle. Lymph node with plasmacytic hyperplasia. (Same case as Fig. 5-11.) There are multiple plasma cells with mild to moderate anisocytosis and anisokaryosis. (×500.)

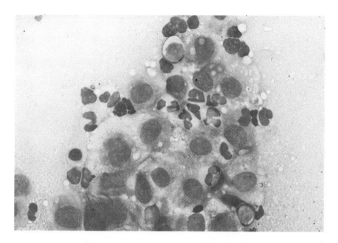

FIG. 5-13. Canine. Fine needle. Lymph node. Granulomatous lymphadenitis. There are numerous histiomonocytic cells and increased numbers of neutrophils showing moderate karyolysis. These cells are displacing the normal lymphoid population. (×200.)

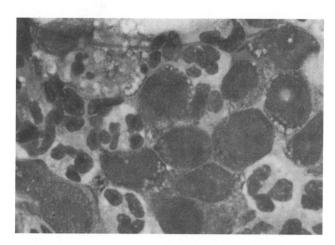

FIG. 5-14. Canine. Fine needle. Lymph node. Suppurative lymphadenitis. Large lymphocytes with fine to aggregated chromatin, indistinct nucleoli, and basophilic cytoplasm. There are increased neutrophils with varying degrees of karyolysis and one phagocytized by a macrophage. (×500.)

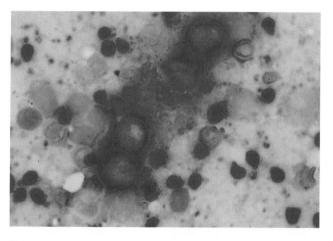

FIG. 5-15. Canine. Fine needle. Lymph node. Blastomycosis. There are numerous refractile, thick-walled, basophilic budding organisms. Frequently there is an accompanying suppurative or mixed lymphadenitis with this fungal infection. (×312.)

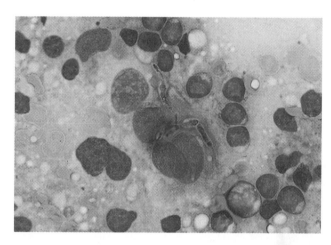

FIG. 5-16. Canine. Fine needle. Lymph node. Fungal lymphadenitis. Lymphocytes and septate branching hyphae of *Aspergillus* spp. The typical mixed inflammatory reaction is not evident in this slide. (×500.)

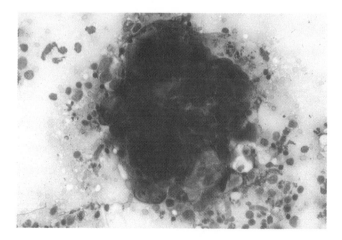

FIG. 5-17. Feline. Fine needle. Lymph node. Metastatic squamous cell carcinoma. A large cluster of malignant epithelial cells with high N:C ratio, hyperchromasia, and irregular nucleoli. Their presence in the lymph node confirms malignancy. (×100.)

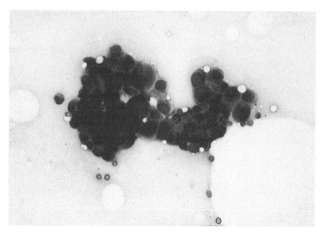

FIG. 5-18. Canine. Fine needle. Popliteal lymph node. Metastatic carcinoma. The sheet of cells with distinct intercellular borders readily identifies these cells as foreign to the site and of epithelial origin. (×62.5.)

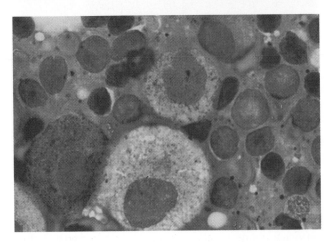

FIG. 5-19. Feline. Fine needle. Lymph node. Metastatic mast cell tumor. Mast cells surrounded by lymphocytes. The mast cells have variable degrees of cytoplasmic granulation and convoluted to cleft nuclear outlines. There is mild anisocytosis and anisokaryosis. (×500.)

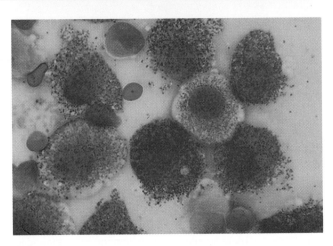

FIG. 5-20. Canine. Fine needle. Lymph node. Metastatic mast cell tumor. Numerous mast cells are showing a higher degree of cytoplasmic granulation than in Fig. 5-19. Small lymphocytes and a plasma cell are present in the background. (×500.)

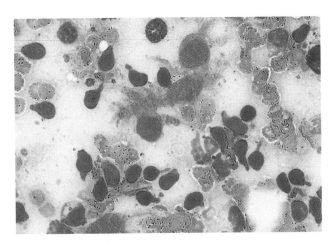

FIG. 5-21. Canine. Fine needle. Lymph node. Metastatic fibrosarcoma. There are several large anaplastic spindle cells with finely stippled chromatin and pale-staining gray cytoplasm. These may be difficult to differentiate from follicular dendritic cells that are normally found in low numbers in benign nodes. Review of the cytology from the primary tumor may assist identification of intranodal metastatic tumor cells. (×312.)

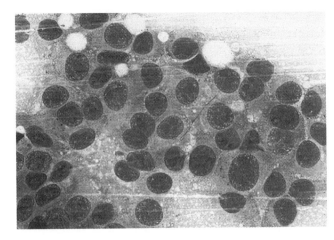

FIG. 5-22. Canine. Fine needle. Submandibular lymph node. Metastatic amelanotic melanoma. The tumor cells are showing prominent anisocytosis and anisokaryosis. Fine green-black intracytoplasmic pigment is visible in a few cells. Diff-Quick. (×312.)

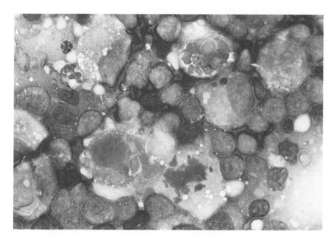

FIG. 5-23. Canine. Fine needle. Lymph node. Malignant histiocytosis. There are many large histiocytic cells with abundant pale-staining gray cytoplasm, fine nuclear chromatin, nuclear pleomorphism, and a high mitotic rate. Erythrocytophagy is prominent. (×312.)

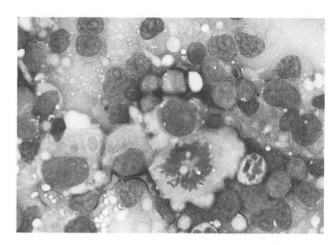

FIG. 5-24. Canine. Fine needle. Lymph node. Malignant histiocytosis. There is prominent anisocytosis and anisokaryosis of the malignant cells. Multiple nodes were involved, and cystic splenic masses were noted on ultrasound. (×312.)

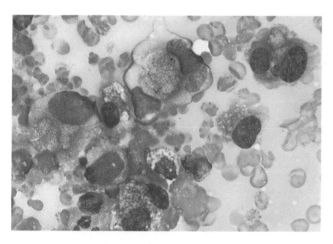

FIG. 5-25. Canine. Fine needle. Spleen. Malignant histiocytosis. There is marked atypia and pleomorphism among the neoplastic cells. (×312.)

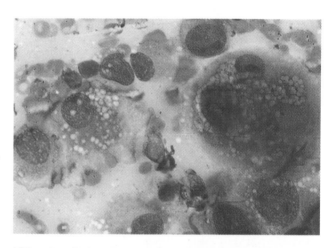

FIG. 5-26. Canine. Fine needle. Lung. Malignant histiocytosis. Anisocytosis and anisokaryosis are prominent. This marked variation, in conjunction with multinucleation, is associated with malignant histiocytosis. (×312.)

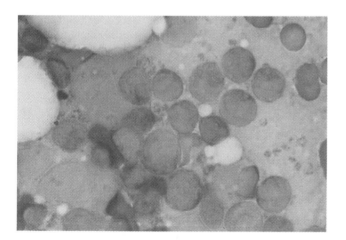

FIG. 5-27. Canine. Fine needle. Lymph node. Lymphoma. Cell staining and detail are inadequate because of excessive thickness of smear. (×500.)

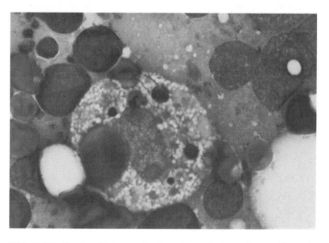

FIG. 5-28. Canine. Fine needle. Lymph node. Lymphoma. There is one macrophage filled with pyknotic cell debris, indicating cytophagy. These are known as *tingible body macrophages* and frequently give a "starry sky" appearance to the aspirate when present in high numbers. (×500.)

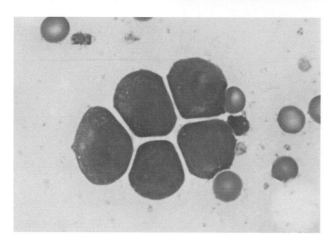

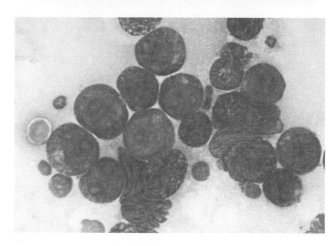

FIG. 5-29. Canine. Fine needle. Lymph node. Lymphoma. The lymphocytes are large cells based on the nuclear diameters averaging 2 to 3 red cells. The nuclei have a fine chromatin pattern, one or two nucleoli, and intensely basophilic cytoplasm. These lymphocytes are consistent with *centroblastic* type (Magnol, 1994) or *immunoblastic* type (Carter, 1986). Some cells have a perinuclear clearing indicating Golgi apparatus. (×312.)

FIG. 5-30. Canine. Fine needle. Lymph node. Lymphoma. Lymphocyte nuclear diameter averages 1 to 2 red cells. The nuclei are eccentric and contain single macronucleoli. There is granular basophilic cytoplasm. Most of these are B-cell tumors. Occasional Golgi zones are noted. C*entroblastic* or *immunoblastic lymphoma*. (×312.)

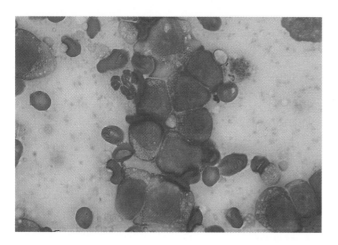

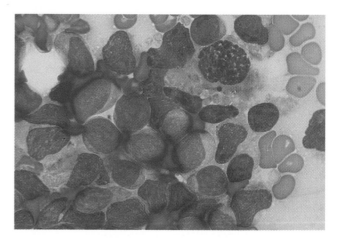

FIG. 5-31. Canine. Fine needle. Lymph node. Lymphoma. Large cells with prominent anisocytosis, abundant pale cytoplasm, and fine nuclear chromatin with indistinct nucleoli in most cells. Mitotic index was moderate to high. *Heterogeneous with a centroblastic component* (Magnol, 1994) or *large noncleaved cell lymphoma* (Carter, 1986). (×312.)

FIG. 5-32. Canine. Fine needle. Lymph node. Lymphoma. Primarily noncleaved small nuclei, 1 to 1.5 red blood cells in diameter, with fine to reticular chromatin, indistinct nucleoli, and unipolar, lightly basophilic cytoplasm. These are mostly high-grade T-cell tumors and are frequently associated with hypercalcemia, mediastinal masses, and a poor prognosis. There is good agreement between the cytological and histological classification for this tumor type. *Lymphoblastic lymphoma.* (×312.)

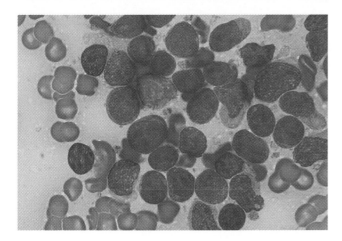

FIG. 5-33. Canine. Fine needle. Lymph node. Lymphoma. (Same case as Fig. 5-32.) Small cells with thin rim of more basophilic cytoplasm than in previous figure. There is greater clumping of chromatin and prominent chromocenters. This morphology is more consistent with *small noncleaved* or *blastic small cell lymphoma* but illustrates the apparent variation in phenotypic expression, effects of fixation and staining, or the difficulty encountered in the differentiation of cell types within the same tumor. (×312.)

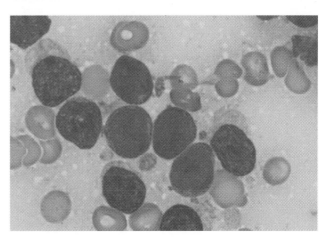

FIG. 5-34. Canine. Fine needle. Lymph node. Lymphoma. These are small cells and have more basophilic cytoplasm than noted in the previous figure. There are abundant lymphoglandular bodies in the background. *Lymphoblastic lymphoma.* (×500.)

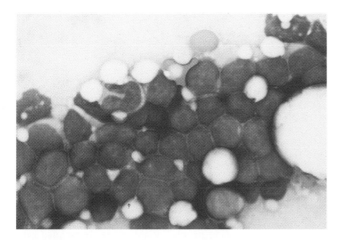

FIG. 5-35. Canine. Fine needle. Lymph node. Lymphoma. Small cells with fine nuclear chromatin and one to several small nucleoli. *Lymphoblastic lymphoma.* (×500.)

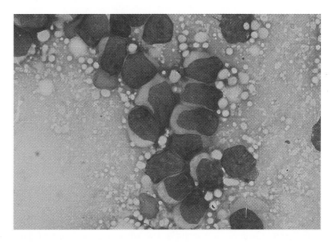

FIG. 5-36. Canine. Fine needle. Lymph node. Lymphoma. Small cells, nuclear diameters averaging 1 to 1.5 red blood cells, stippled to irregularly condensed chromatin, multiple nucleoli, and variable amounts of lightly basophilic cytoplasm. *Blastic small cell lymphoma* (Magnol, 1994) or *small noncleaved lymphoma* (Carter, 1986). (×312.)

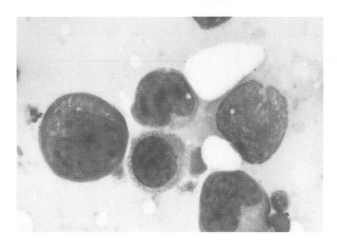

FIG. 5-37. Canine. Fine needle. Lymph node. *Convoluted lymphoma.* Note the variability within cells, large cells with multiple nucleoli, fine chromatin, and distinct nuclear indentations. Abundant cytoplasm is moderate to very basophilic. (×312.)

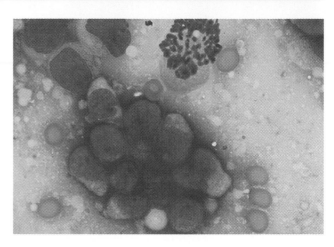

FIG. 5-38. Canine. Fine needle. Lymph node. *Convoluted lymphoma.* On a cytological basis this may also be classified as *heterogeneous lymphoma with a centroblastic component.* There are many small and medium lymphocytes intermixed with larger cells, prominent nuclear indentations, multiple nucleoli, and fine stippled to irregularly condensed chromatin. The mitotic figure indicates the moderate to high mitotic index usually observed. (×312.)

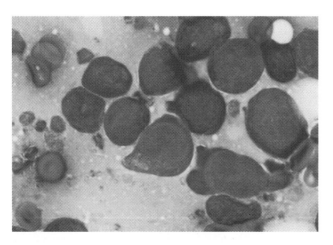

FIG. 5-39. Canine. Fine needle. Lymph node. *Convoluted lymphoma (heterogeneous lymphoma with a centroblastic component).* Note the variability in cell size. (×500.)

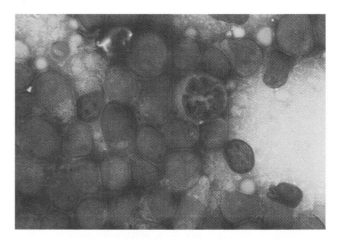

FIG. 5-40. Canine. Fine needle. Lymph node. *Convoluted lymphoma (heterogeneous lymphoma with a centroblastic component).* Distinct nuclear clefts and mitotic figures. (×312.)

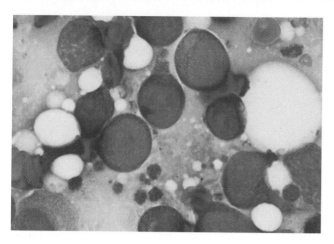

FIG. 5-41. Canine. Fine needle. Lymph node. *Convoluted lymphoma (heterogeneous lymphoma with a centroblastic component).* The irregular nuclear periphery may be evident by single to multiple deep clefts or indentations in the nuclear outline. Rare cells have distinct Golgi zones within the highly basophilic cytoplasm. (×500.)

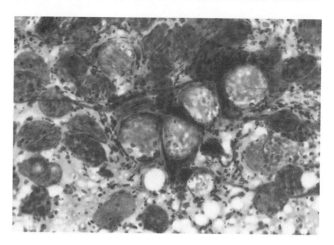

FIG. 5-42. Feline. Scraping. Anterior mediastinal mass. Large granular lymphoma. Discrete round mononuclear cells with eccentric oval to indented nuclei; uniform granular chromatin; and faintly basophilic cytoplasm containing round azurophilic 1-μ granules. (×400.) (Courtesy D.J. Honour, 1985.)

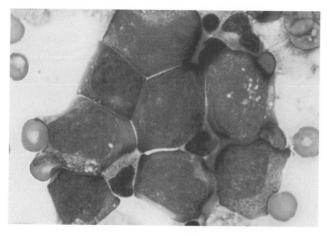

FIG. 5-43. Canine. Fine needle. Abdominal fluid. Gastrointestinal lymphoma. Large cells with moderately basophilic cytoplasm, coarsely woven to clumped chromatin, and single to multiple nucleoli. Some cells have nuclear indentations. (×500.)

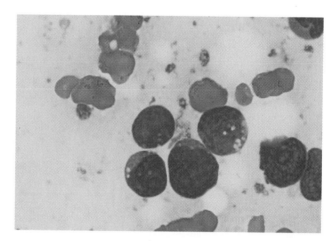

FIG. 5-44. Feline. Fine needle. Kidney. Lymphoma. Four intact large lymphocytes, one distinctly cleaved. FNA of the feline kidney is possible because of its accessibility. (×500.)

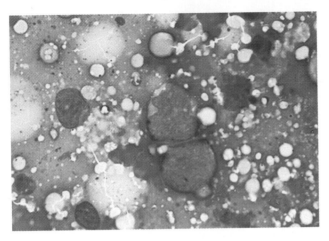

FIG. 5-45. Canine. Fine needle. Skin. Cutaneous lymphoma. These lymphocytes are variably sized with finely woven or reti-form chromatin and indistinct nucleoli. The nuclear outline is ir-regular in some cells with multiple indentations to prominent and often bizarre convolutions. Nuclear convolutions suggest T-cell origin. (×312.)

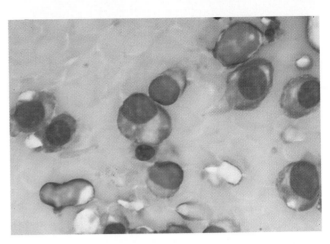

FIG. 5-46. Canine. Imprint. Spleen. Multiple myeloma. Plasma cells with mild anisokaryosis and anisocytosis. Cytological atypia may be minimal, as seen here. (×312.)

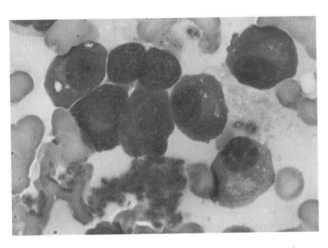

FIG. 5-47. Canine. Imprint. Spleen. Multiple myeloma. A cluster of plasma cells with minimal cytological atypia. Clinical history and the presence of gammopathy are essential when determin-ing the significance of increased plasma cells. (×500.)

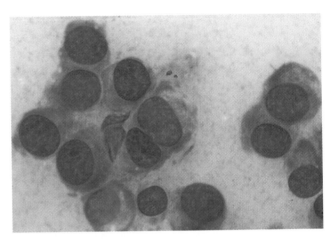

FIG. 5-48. Canine. Fine needle. Skin mass. Myeloma with bone and skin lesions and gammopathy. Round cells with round to oval eccentrically located nuclei and very basophilic cytoplasm with some suggestion of perinuclear clearing indicative of a Golgi region. There is moderate anisokaryosis. (×400.)

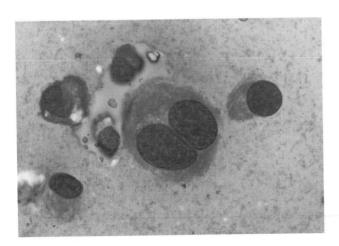

FIG. 5-49. Canine. Fine needle. Skin mass. Myeloma. (Same case as Fig. 5-48.) Small, well-differentiated cells surround a large bin-ucleated plasma cell. Binucleation, rare within benign plasma cells, supports malignancy. (×400.)

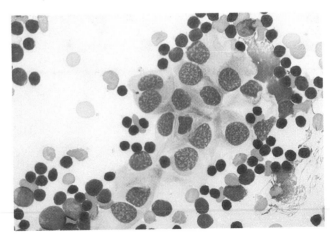

FIG. 5-50. Canine. Imprint. Normal thymus of a 4-month-old puppy. Two distinct cell populations including small lympho-cytes and larger epithelial cells. (×200.)

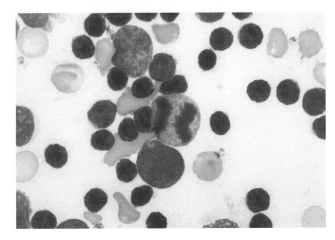

FIG. 5-51. Canine. Imprint. Normal thymus. Background of small lymphocytes and three large mononuclear cells consistent with lymphocytes, including one in mitosis. (×400.)

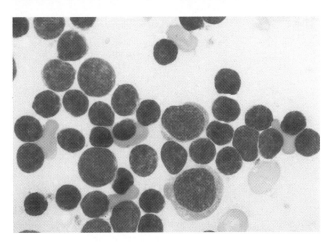

FIG. 5-52. Canine. Imprint. Normal thymus. Heterogeneous population of lymphocytes. (×400.)

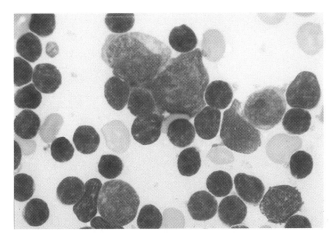

FIG. 5-53. Canine. Imprint. Normal thymus. Further illustration of the heterogeneous lymphoid cells, possibly related to young age of animal. (×400.)

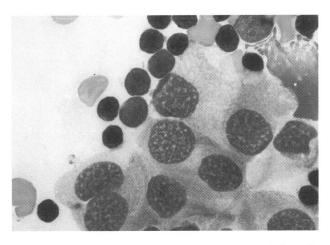

FIG. 5-54. Canine. Imprint. Normal thymus. Large epithelial cells with abundant pale, lightly basophilic cytoplasm and nuclei greater than 2 erythrocytes in diameter. The nuclei have coarse cribriform chromatin and small indistinct nucleoli. (×400.)

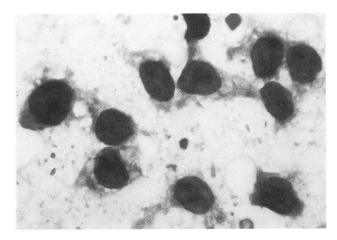

FIG. 5-55. Canine. Fine needle. Chest mass. Thymoma. The cells aspirated from a confirmed thymoma vary in shape, have limited basophilic cytoplasm, a high N:C ratio, and are consistent with neoplasia. Diff-Quick stain. (×400.)

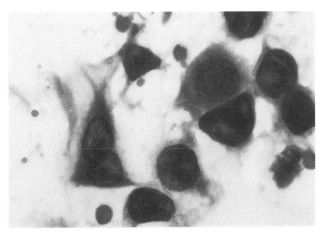

FIG. 5-56. Canine. Fine needle. Chest mass. Thymoma. (Same case as Fig. 5-55.) Polygonal, slightly cohesive epithelial cells with large nuclei, high N:C ratio, moderate anisokaryosis, and some binucleation. Diff-Quick stain. (×500.)

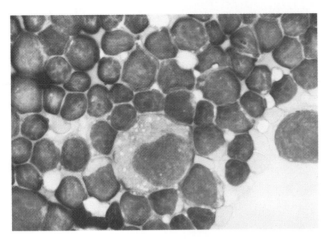

FIG. 5-57. Feline. Imprint. Mediastinal mass. Thymoma. Variably sized lymphoid cells with a single large epithelial cell. The presence of variably sized lymphoid cells is useful when differentiating thymoma from mediastinal lymphoma. (×400.) (Courtesy S.M. Shelly, 1986.)

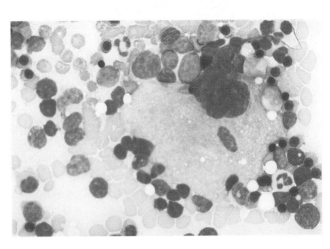

FIG. 5-58. Canine. Imprint. Normal spleen of a 4-month-old puppy. There are many bare nuclei and a heterogeneous population of cells, including rubricytes, at various stages of differentiation. The rubricytes and the megakaryocyte are consistent with extramedullary hematopoiesis. (×200.)

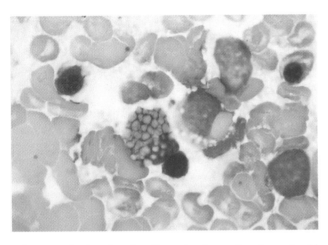

FIG. 5-59. Canine. Imprint. Normal spleen of a 4-month-old puppy. Central cell contains large blue-green spherules, often called Russell bodies, as observed in "pregnant" plasma cells. (×250.)

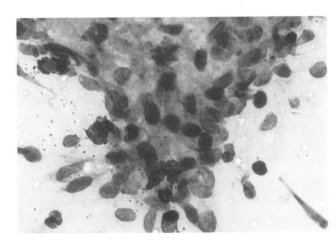

FIG. 5-60. Canine. Imprint. Normal spleen of a 4-month-old puppy. Cluster of cells with indistinct cytoplasmic and nuclear details from the stromal or dendritic components. Mast cells are visible. (×250.)

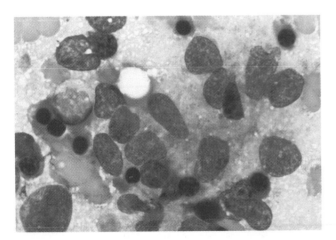

FIG. 5-61. Canine. Imprint. Normal spleen of a 4-month-old puppy. Background cells include erythrocytes and rubricytes. Cluster of cells with indistinct cytoplasmic borders and large irregular round to oval nuclei with small nucleoli illustrating dendritic origin. (×400.)

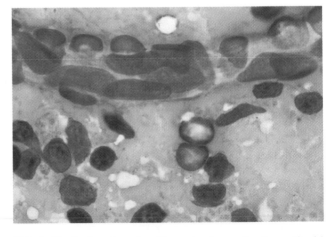

FIG. 5-62. Canine. Scraping. Normal spleen of a 4-month-old puppy. Background of erythrocytes and lymphocytes. A small blood vessel lined by endothelial cells is present. (×400.)

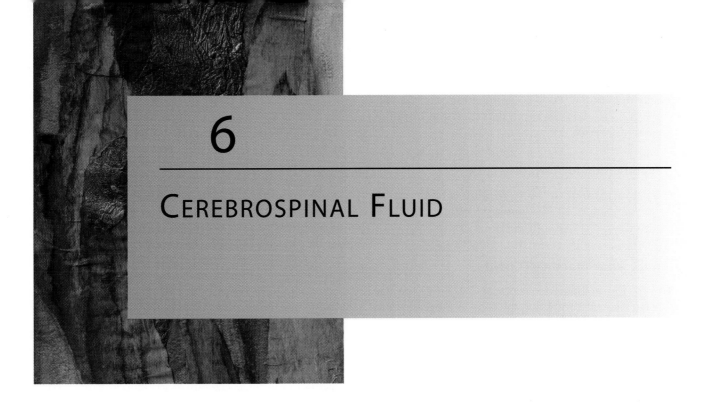

6

CEREBROSPINAL FLUID

Cerebrospinal fluid is routinely examined in dogs and cats with neurological abnormalities. Collection and processing procedures are critical to obtaining adequate representative cells for cytological examination. For many CNS disorders the clinician relies on an increase or change in total protein and changes in cell concentration or type for collation with history and clinical examination in order to make reliable diagnoses. A normal cerebrospinal fluid (CSF) can rule out many disease processes.

TECHNIQUE

Cisternal Tap

General anesthesia is required for obtaining CSF. The skin is prepared aseptically from the occipital protuberance to the axis. The patient is placed on the right side and the head is flexed at a 90-degree angle to the spine. A 20- to 22-gauge spinal needle is inserted in the dorsal midline depression at the intersection of lines drawn down the midline and perpendicular to the cranial wings of the atlas (Allen, 1991; Bailey, 1997). The needle is advanced slowly, stopping to check occasionally for fluid production. A decrease in resistance may be felt as the subarachnoid space is entered. Fluid is collected by gravity into vials containing EDTA. EDTA enhances cellular preservation and prevents clotting if fibrinogen accumulation caused by inflammation is present.

Lumbosacral Tap

Lumbar punctures are technically more difficult because the spinal cord is usually penetrated when fluid is collected from the subarachnoid space. The needle causes a small area of myelomalacia, which is not usually associated with detectable neurological dysfunction (Allen, 1991). The animal is placed in lateral recumbency with the thoracolumbar spine parallel to the table. The fore and hind limbs are brought together, slightly flexing the caudal spine. A needle is inserted between lumbar vertebrae 5 and 6 at the cranial border of the dorsal spinal process. The needle is advanced perpendicular to the spine and into the subarachnoid space. If no fluid is obtained, the needle is inserted through to the ventral spinal floor and then retracted into the ventral subarachnoid space. If CSF is not obtained, the needle is redirected and the procedure is repeated (Allen, 1991).

SAMPLE PROCESSING

CSF should be processed within 30 minutes of collection because of the fragility of cells in CSF and the rapid deterioration in cellular morphology. The fragility is partly related to the low normal CSF protein and lipid concentrations that in other fluids contribute to stabilization of cell membranes. Because of the fragility, cells in CSF must be concentrated onto glass slides at the site of collection unless there is immediate access to alternative laboratory facilities. Laboratory examination of CSF includes the following procedures:

1. Examination for Xanthochromia

When xanthochromia is present as a result of subarachnoid hemorrhage, the CSF is pink to orange tinged. The color peaks at 24 hours and disappears by

4 to 8 days (Jamison, 1988). The supernatant is clear after centrifugation if blood contamination is iatrogenic. However, fresh red cells begin to lyse within 1 hour of collection (Jamison, 1988).

2. Examination for Turbidity

A visual increase in turbidity requires a minimum of 200 leukocytes $\times$ 10^6/L (Jamison, 1988) or 700 red blood cells $\times$ 10^6/L (Rand, 1995).

3. Total White Blood Cell Count

The very low cellularity of normal CSF limits the use of electronic cell counters, which have a background count of up to 500 cells $\times$ 10^6/L. A hemocytometer must be used. Both chambers of a Neubauer hemocytometer are charged with well-mixed CSF. The chamber is placed in a humidified environment (e.g., under a Petri dish with damp tissue) for up to 15 minutes to allow cells to settle to the surface of the glass. Total cells in the nine large squares on each side of the chamber are counted. The calculations are performed using the average of the two sets of nine squares.

$$\text{Number of cells} \times 10 \div 9 = \text{cells/}\mu\text{l } or \text{ cells/mm}^3 \text{ } or$$
$$\text{cells} \times 10^6\text{/L}$$

Reported normal values for canine cisternal and lumbar taps are 1.5 $\times$ 10^6/L and 0.5 $\times$ 10^6/L, respectively (Bailey, 1985). The upper reference limit for canine CSF cisternal taps obtained from 40 clinically and histologically normal healthy dogs was 1 $\times$ 10^6/L (Jamison, 1992). The mean WBC count in feline cisternal fluid was 0.1 $\times$ 10^6/L (Rand, 1990a). Of 33 normal cats, none had a count that exceeded 2.0 $\times$ 10^6/L (Rand, 1990a).

4. Total Red Blood Cells

In properly collected CSF from healthy dogs and cats, erythrocytes should not exceed 30 $\times$ 10^6/L (Jamison, 1992; Rand, 1990a). The human literature reports that nucleated cell and protein concentrations may be increased by iatrogenic blood contamination if the CSF erythrocyte count exceeds 30 $\times$ 10^6/L (Sornas, 1972). However, no effect was seen on white blood cell numbers in CSF from six cats having up to 500 $\times$ 10^6 red blood cells/L. (Rand 1990a). It is reported that in both clinically normal dogs and dogs with neurological diseases, iatrogenic blood contamination contributing up to 13,200 $\times$ 10^6 /L erythrocytes did not significantly alter CSF nucleated cell and protein concentrations (Hurtt, 1997). Frequent attempts have been made to correlate red blood cell contamination with corrections for white blood cell counts (Rand, 1995; Wilson, 1977). Correction for blood contamination is considered to be unreliable according to most studies.

5. Preparation of Slides

Because of the low cellularity and the fragility of CSF cells, a standard centrifuge is not used to concentrate cells. Where a cytocentrifuge is not available, such as in a clinical setting, a sedimentation chamber can be fabricated for concentrating cells. The chamber is made by cutting off 2 cm from the end of a 15-mm diameter centrifuge tube (Jamison, 1988). The smooth end of the cylinder is dipped in heated Vaseline and set on a clean glass slide, thus sealing it to the slide as the Vaseline cools. These chambers can be prepared and stored in a clean, dry environment until required. Approximately 0.5 ml of CSF is pipetted into the chamber. After 30 minutes the supernatant is gently removed with a Pasteur pipette. The supernatant can be used for protein analysis. The cylinder is removed, the slide is tilted slightly, excess fluid is absorbed using filter paper, and the slide is waved rapidly to enhance drying of the cells. The air-drying step is critical to ensure good cellular preservation and must be completed quickly. The slide is stained using a standard Romanowsky's stain or sent unstained to a diagnostic laboratory for evaluation.

Most diagnostic laboratories use a cytocentrifuge to concentrate cells from CSF and other body fluids. Excellent cellular morphology is obtained, although there is increased vacuolation of cells and alterations in morphology, particularly of macrophages. Cells are concentrated from 200 μl of CSF in many laboratories. Because of limitations of cell fragility and access to a cytocentrifuge, this procedure is usually restricted to referral clinics or teaching institutions.

6. Differential Cell Counts (Figs. 6-1 to 6-4)

In dogs and cats, mononuclear cells predominate in CSF from healthy animals. The exact identification can be difficult, resulting in considerable variation in criteria and thus classification schemes used for nucleated CSF cells. At the Ontario Veterinary College, mononuclear cells are assigned to one of four categories. Lymphocytes are small, round cells with scant cytoplasm and dark, clumped nuclear chromatin. At the other extreme in size are the large, foamy mononuclear cells, or macrophages, with a round to oval nucleus and abundant foamy cytoplasm. The mononuclear cells not included in these readily identified end groups can be subdivided into small and large monocytoid cells. Small monocytoid cells have a nuclear diameter less than two erythrocytes, and large monocytoid cells have a nuclear diameter greater than two erythrocytes (Jamison, 1988; Rand, 1990a). Although many of these monocytoid cells appear to be lymphoid or monocytoid in origin, many cannot be reliably differentiated. This results in significant variation when 100 or even 200 nucleated cells are classified by the same cytopathologist or by different cytopathologists. The above classification scheme allows for greater reproducibility, although there is loss of detail, which can be compensated for within the written report.

Results of cisternal taps from 40 clinically healthy dogs are described (Jamison, 1992). Large mononuclear cells and small mononuclear cells accounted for 53% and 37%, respectively, of the total nucleated cells (Jamison, 1992). Small lymphocytes accounted for 4% of the total and large foamy mononuclears 6% (Jamison, 1992).

In healthy cats, when using this classification scheme, monocytoid cells accounted for 69% to 100% of the normal cell population (Rand, 1995; Rand, 1989). The majority of these monocytoid cells were large monocytoid as previously defined (Rand, 1990a). Neutrophils were absent or rare and when present often correlated closely with red blood cell contamination (Rand, 1990a). The occasional neutrophil observed was often degenerate with nuclear aging changes of hyperchromasia and hypersegmentation (Rand, 1990a). Eosinophils were rarely present and usually correlated with the degree of red blood cell contamination (Rand, 1990a). Lymphocytes contributed 0% to 27% of the total white blood cells. Most of these were lymphocytes with prominent pale-staining cytoplasm (Rand, 1995). Distribution of cell types in the dog and cat are presented in Table 6-1.

Occasionally, large clumps of cells originating from the choroid plexus are seen. These cells have a low N:C ratio with abundant foamy cytoplasm. Bone marrow cells have also been identified in cytocentrifuge preparations from lumbar punctures (Christopher, 1992) and must be considered as a potential interference when interpreting CSF cytology. Rarely, normal neurons and myelin may be seen in CSF samples (Fallin, 1996; Mesher, 1996). The myelin was associated with acute myelomalacia in a dog (Mesher, 1996).

7. CSF Total Protein

Because of the low protein concentration in normal CSF, special methods for determination are required. Many diagnostic laboratories use sensitive dye binding assays. A minimum of 50 μl may be requested. The CSF sample can be submitted fresh, frozen, or refrigerated, but protocol should be prearranged with the laboratory.

In the dog, normal CSF protein is reported as 0.12 to 0.16 g/L in cisternal taps (Bailey, 1985) and 0.27 to 0.31 g/L in lumbar taps (Bailey, 1985). Protein concentration was not significantly altered in 74 samples containing up to 13,230 cells $\times$ 10^6/L red blood cells from iatrogenic contamination (Hurtt, 1997). In the cat, lumbar tap protein concentration averaged 0.41 to 0.47 g/L (Hochwald, 1967). In contrast, in 33 clinically healthy cats, cisternal tap mean protein concentration was 0.18 g/L with an upper limit of 0.36 g/L (Rand, 1995).

Semiquantitative tests, such as the Pandy test or Nonne-Apelt test, estimate globulin concentrations. The sensitivity of these tests is approximately 0.50 g/L. Some experience is recommended for setting up and interpreting the results. Urine dipstick methods have been compared with sensitive dye-binding methods as a screening test for CSF protein in clinical cases (Jacobs, 1990). Protein concentration greater than 1 g/L is easily detected. However, protein concentrations between 0.3 and 1.0 g/L can be missed when using the dipstick method (Jacobs, 1990). Although most healthy dogs have a negative or trace CSF dipstick protein reading (Jacobs, 1990), in one study, 28% of normal dogs had a dipstick reading of +1 (Jacobs, 1990). Most normal cats test negative or trace for CSF protein when screened using urine dipsticks (Rand, 1995). Provided the limitations of urinary dipsticks are understood, they can be used as an ancillary aid in a practice setting.

Table 6-1

Reference Values for WBC in CSF—Total Cell Count and Differential

Species	Total WBC	Sample size	Small lymphocytes %	Small mononuclear	Large mononuclear	Large foamy macrophages	Neutrophils %	Degenerate (other) %
Canine*	0-2 $\times$ 10^6/L	n = 50 (cytocentrifuge sample)	4 (0-61)	36.7 (0-73)	53 (18-89)	6.0 (0-46)	—	—
Feline†	0-1 $\times$ 10^6/L	n = 20 (sedimented sample)	9 (0-27)	84‡ (74-100)	6 (0-13)	0 (0-3)	1 (0-9)	0 (0-5)
Feline†	0-2 $\times$ 10^6/L	n = 22 (cytocentrifuge)	14 (0-25)	54‡ (0-100)	27 (0-100)	3 (0-33)	2 (0-25)	1 (0-11)

*Jamison, E.M. *A study of cerebrospinal fluid in dogs with central nervous system disease.* Thesis. University of Guelph, 1992.

†Rand, J.S., Parent, J., Jacobs, R., et al. Reference intervals for feline cerebrospinal fluid: cell counts and cytologic features. *Am J Vet Res* 51:1044-1048, 1990.

‡The cells classified as lymphomono are included in small mononuclear for the purposes of this table.

In-depth analysis of CSF protein using electrophoresis and various protein ratios has been reviewed extensively elsewhere (Bichsel, 1984; Chrisman, 1992; Jamison, 1992; Sorjonen, 1987; Sorjonen, 1989).

CYTOLOGICAL INTERPRETATION OF CSF
(Figs. 6-15 to 6-31)

Variation in cellular response is characteristic of most CNS diseases. The cytological changes observed with common canine and feline CNS disorders are described.

NONNEOPLASTIC DISEASE

Bacterial Meningoencephalitis

CLINICAL AND CYTOLOGICAL DIAGNOSES
Bacterial meningoencephalitis is uncommon in the dog and cat. Clinical signs often reflect a widespread inflammatory reaction. The cellular response is predominantly neutrophilic; however, bacteria are rarely observed in concentrated CSF preparations, and they are often difficult to culture. With treatment the cellular response can become mononuclear and can be difficult to differentiate from other inflammatory or neoplastic disorders of the CNS (Chrisman, 1992).

Documented cases of bacterial meningoencephalitis in the dog and cat are uncommon. In 10 dogs, total leukocyte counts varied from 13 to 465 cells $\times$ 10^6/L and the percentage of neutrophils varied from 60% to 95% (Sarfaty, 1986). In one of the dogs, 86% of nucleated cells were lymphocytes (Sarfaty, 1986). In two dogs with *Staphylococcus aureus* meningitis, nucleated cell counts were approximately 2550 $\times$ 10^6/L with 80% to 90% neutrophils and protein concentrations of approximately 1.75 g/L (Kornegay, 1978; Kornegay, 1981a). In two dogs with confirmed bacterial meningoencephalitis, CSF nucleated counts were 335 and 74 cells $\times$ 10^6/L with protein concentrations of 1.06 and 2.48 g/L, respectively (Bullmore, 1978). In one cat with *Bacterioides* infection involving the CSF, the nucleated cell count was 107 $\times$ 10^6/L with 85% neutrophils, 15% mononuclear cells, and a protein concentration of 4.3 g/L (Dow, 1988). In one cat with bacterial emboli caused by *Pseudomonas* sp., the CSF nucleated cell count was 900 $\times10^6$/L with 55% neutrophils, 15% lymphocytes, and 30% mononuclear cells. Protein concentration was 0.94 g/L (Rand, 1994a).

Canine Distemper Virus

CLINICAL DIAGNOSIS
Canine distemper, a *Morbillivirus* infection, presents with many clinical and histopathological manifestations. Severity of the disease is more pronounced in young dogs. Mortality frequently depends on the IgG antibody response (Johnson, 1987). Clinical signs vary depending on the immune response and age at time of infection. Symptoms relative to the nervous, gastrointestinal, or respiratory system may predominate. Analysis of CSF may be of some assistance in ruling out other multisystemic diseases.

CYTOLOGICAL DIAGNOSIS
In 13 dogs with acute demyelinating distemper, nucleated cell counts ranged from normal to 27 $\times$ 10^6/L with a predominantly mononuclear cellular response (Bichsel, 1984). In another 25 dogs, nucleated cell counts were less than 25 $\times$ 10^6/L in all but two dogs (Vandevelde, 1977). These two dogs had massive encephalomalacia and CSF counts of 501 and 288 $\times$ 10^6/L (Vandevelde, 1977). Lymphocytes accounted for 61% of the cells, with mononuclear cells at 33% and neutrophils at 4% (Vandevelde, 1977). CSF protein varied from normal to a maximum of 1.36 g/L with a mean of 0.37 g/L. In two dogs, cell counts were 29 and 56 $\times$ 10^6/L with 80% lymphocytes (Sarfaty, 1986). Five other dogs had CSF cellularity ranging from 1 to 31 cells $\times$ 10^6/L and 60% to 90% lymphocytes (Sorjonen, 1989b). Intranuclear inclusions were reported in the CSF mononuclear cells in one dog with peracute distemper (Alleman, 1992). The CSF nucleated cell count in this dog was normal, and cells were 63% monocytic and 36% lymphocytic (Alleman, 1992). In 15 of 32 dogs with noninflammatory distemper, CSF was normal (Tipold, 1995). In one study, decreased lymphocytes and elevated CSF albumin concentration correlated with a poor prognosis early in the disease, whereas later in the disease course or during recovery lymphocytic pleocytosis correlated with an improved prognosis (Johnson, 1987).

Rabies

CLINICAL AND CYTOLOGICAL DIAGNOSES
Rabies is associated with a typical viral CSF response, although published reports of CSF analysis in dogs clinically affected with rabies are rare (Chrisman, 1992). A mild increase in CSF nucleated cells with a lymphocyte predominance is classical for viral infection (Chrisman, 1992). In two cats with vaccine-induced rabies the CSF protein concentration was 0.55 and 0.80 g/L and nucleated cell counts were 5 $\times$ 10^6/L and 17 $\times$ 10^6/L with predominantly lymphocytes (Esh, 1982). Nucleated cell counts of 5 and 17 $\times$ 10^6/L were seen in two other cats with vaccine-induced rabies (Kornegay, 1981b). CSF protein concentration in these cats was 0.55 and 0.80 g/L, respectively (Kornegay, 1981b).

Feline Infectious Peritonitis

CLINICAL AND CYTOLOGICAL DIAGNOSES
Feline infectious peritonitis (FIP), caused by coronavirus infection, is a multisystemic fatal disease in cats. Neurological involvement is seen in up to 30% of

affected cats (Kornegay, 1981b). CSF from one affected cat revealed a CSF nucleated cell count of 2000 cells $\times$ 10^6/L with 80% to 90% neutrophils (Shepherd, 1980). Four cats with FIP had CSF nucleated cell counts ranging from 37 to 1160 $\times$ 10^6/L and protein concentrations of 1.05 to 4.15 g/L (Kornegay, 1981b). Neutrophils were 39% to 76% of the total cellularity (Kornegay, 1981b). In 11 cats with FIP, all had increased CSF protein and in 10 of 11 cats the protein exceeded 2.8 g/L. Nucleated cells ranged from 1 to 2500 $\times$ 10^6/L with a mean of 510, of which 85% were neutrophils (Rand, 1994b). Ten cats with suspect viral disease other than FIP had mean nucleated cell counts of 5 cells $\times$ 10^6/L and a mean total protein of 0.28 g/L (Rand, 1994b).

Rocky Mountain Spotted Fever

CLINICAL AND CYTOLOGICAL DIAGNOSES

Rickettsia rickettsii, an obligate intracellular parasite, is the tickborne causative agent of Rocky Mountain spotted fever (RMSF) in dogs (Greene, 1986). Young dogs are more commonly affected. Clinical signs are multisystemic, including fever, depression, anorexia, diarrhea, vomiting, hemorrhage, and neurological signs (Green, 1986; Sellon, 1995). Reports of CSF examination in infected dogs are rare. In one infected dog a pleocytosis of 82% neutrophils and 18% mononuclear was reported (Green, 1985). This predominance of neutrophils appears to differentiate RMSF from ehrlichiosis, in which lymphocytes predominate (Greene, 1986). CSF cellularity and protein concentration in infected dogs has also been reported to be normal (Greene, 1985).

Toxoplasmosis

CLINICAL AND CYTOLOGICAL DIAGNOSES

Toxoplasma gondii is a protozoan infection that can affect dogs of any age or breed, but the clinically severe forms are more common in young or immunosuppressed animals (Meric, 1988). The disease usually has an acute progressive course, with either respiratory and gastrointestinal signs or neuromuscular disease (Meric, 1988). In 100 cats with histologically confirmed toxoplasmosis, only seven had neurological signs (Dubey, 1996). Reports of examination of CSF in dogs and cats with toxoplasmosis are rare. Mixed cell pleocytosis is reported, but lymphocytes can predominate and eosinophils have been reported (Dubey, 1990). In one dog the CSF nucleated cell count was 26 $\times$ 10^6/L (Vandevelde, 1977). Nucleated cells were 14% neutrophils, 26% lymphocytes, and 58% mononuclear cells (Vandevelde, 1977). In a 4-month-old puppy the CSF nucleated cell count was 38 $\times$ 10^6/L with 100% mononuclear cells. Protein was increased to 0.82 g/L (Kornegay, 1981a). Rarely are toxoplasmosis organisms found in cells of the CSF.

Neosporosis

CLINICAL AND CYTOLOGICAL DIAGNOSES

Neospora caninum is a recently described protozoan that has probably been previously confused with toxoplasmosis (Dubey, 1990). Clinically, signs are similar to toxoplasmosis with neurological deficits and muscular abnormalities (Dubey, 1990). Both old and young dogs are susceptible, with the most severe lesions seen in young puppies (Dubey, 1990). A progressive ascending paralysis of young dogs is typical (Dubey, 1990; Greig, 1995). One dog presented with overwhelming respiratory infection, and organisms were detected on bronchial lavage (Greig, 1995). Reported CSF abnormalities include a mild increase in protein (0.20-0.50 g/L) with total nucleated cells of 10 to 50 cells $\times$ 10^6/L that are primarily mononuclear (Dubey, 1990). *N. caninum* organisms found within the cytoplasm of affected cells are not separated by a parasitophorous vacuole as seen in toxoplasmosis (Dubey, 1990). *Neospora* and *Toxoplasma* cannot be differentiated with light microscopy alone (Greig, 1995).

Ehrlichiosis

CLINICAL AND CYTOLOGICAL DIAGNOSES

In one puppy with neurological dysfunction and ehrlichiosis the CSF had 83 $\times$ 10^6/L nucleated cells with 87 % lymphocytes and 13% neutrophils (Greene, 1985).

Prototheca

CLINICAL AND CYTOLOGICAL DIAGNOSES

Although colitis and ophthalmological abnormalities are the most common presentations of prototheciasis in the dog, CNS involvement occurs in about 40% of the cases (Tyler, 1990). Clinical signs in the dog include depression, ataxia, and paresis (Tyler, 1990). One dog with disseminated prototheciasis had a normal CSF (Rakich, 1984). In one dog, CSF nucleated cell concentration was 6182 $\times$ 10^6/L with 85% eosinophils, 5% neutrophils, and 10% mononuclear cells (Tyler, 1980). In the cat, only cutaneous involvement has been reported (Dillberger, 1988).

Hepatozoon canis

CLINICAL AND CYTOLOGICAL DIAGNOSES

Hepatozoon canis–infected dogs in the United States typically present with gait abnormalities, decreasing body condition, and generalized pain (Vincent-Johnson, 1997). Elevated body temperature and extremely high peripheral white blood cell counts (20,000-80,000 $\times$ 10^6/L) are common (Vincent-Johnson, 1997). CSF changes were reported for an infected 10-month-old puppy. There was a CSF pleocytosis of 320 cells $\times$ 10^6/L with 56% neutrophils, 32% lymphocytes, and 12% plasma cells. The protein concentration was

1.14 g/L (Baker, 1988). CSF analysis was performed on five affected dogs from the Georgia/Alabama area (Macintire, 1997). One of five affected dogs had a lymphocytic pleocytosis, and the other four had no significant abnormalities (Macintire, 1997).

Cuterebra

CLINICAL AND CYTOLOGICAL DIAGNOSES

Aberrant parasite migration is occasionally documented. In one young dog, migration of a *Cuterebra* larva resulted in a progressive localized inflammatory lesion in the brain (Macdonald, 1976). The CSF nucleated cell count was $280 \times 10^6/L$ with 84% neutrophils and 16% mononuclear cells. Total protein was reported at 0.98 g/L (Macdonald, 1976). Feline ischemic encephalopathy has been linked to aberrant migration of *Cuterebra* larva (Williams, 1998).

Blastomycosis

CLINICAL AND CYTOLOGICAL DIAGNOSES

In the dog, the lung, skin, and lymph node are the most frequent sites of blastomycosis infection (Nafe, 1983). Hematogenous spread after pulmonary involvement or acute systemic fulminating disease may infrequently result in CNS involvement with generalized neurological symptoms reported (Nafe, 1983). In two cases reported in dogs, CSF nucleated cell counts were 6 and $283 \times 10^6/L$ with 50% and 24% neutrophils, respectively, without visible organisms (Nafe, 1983). Another affected dog had a CSF nucleated cell count of $235 \times 10^6/L$ with 61% neutrophils and identified blastomycosis organisms (Vandevelde, 1977). Two cases are reported in cats in which the nucleated cell counts were 11 and $39 \times 10^6/L$ with 95% mononuclear cells, and in each case the protein concentration was greater than 1.0 g/L (Kornegay, 1981a).

Cryptococcosis

CLINICAL AND CYTOLOGICAL DIAGNOSES

Cryptococcosis occurs in both the dog and cat, but it is the most common systemic mycosis in the cat, with CNS involvement reported occasionally (Medleau, 1989). Upper respiratory, skin, and lymph node infections are most common (Medleau, 1989). CNS involvement presents with variable neurological signs (Medleau, 1989). CSF cell counts are often high with neutrophils usually predominating (Cook, 1991). One dog with cryptococcal organisms within the CSF had a very high estimated nucleated cell count (not counted) with many neutrophils (Cook, 1991). One affected dog had a CSF nucleated cell count of $433 \times 10^6/L$ with 80% eosinophils (Vandevelde, 1977). In two cases involving cats the nucleated cell count was normal to slightly increased and protein concentrations were 0.38 and 0.66 g/L (Kornegay, 1981b).

Pug and Maltese Encephalitis

CLINICAL AND CYTOLOGICAL DIAGNOSES

A syndrome of extensive nonsuppurative cerebral cortical necrosis has been documented in pug dogs (Bailey, 1997; Cordy, 1989). The disease affects adolescent and mature dogs and can follow an acute or chronic clinical course (Cordy, 1989). Signs are referable to the cerebrum and meninges, with seizures, ataxia, and depression. Analysis of CSF from 12 affected pugs revealed a mean increase in nucleated cells to $374 \times 10^6/L$ (SD = 178) with 71% to 98% small lymphocytes and a mean protein concentration of 1.22 g/L (Cordy, 1989).

A similar syndrome is reported in Maltese dogs (Stalis, 1995). A history of seizures is a consistent clinical sign (Stalis, 1995). CSF abnormalities in three affected dogs included pleocytosis (cell counts ranged from 50 to $247 \times 10^6/L$) and increased total protein (0.33-1.26 g/L). The differential cell count varied from primarily lymphocytic to primarily neutrophilic (Stalis, 1995).

Necrotizing Encephalitis in Yorkshire Terriers

CLINICAL AND CYTOLOGICAL DIAGNOSES

Several reports of necrotizing encephalitis in Yorkshire terriers exist (Jull, 1997; Tipold, 1993). Affected dogs present with gait abnormalities and seizures (Tipold, 1993). The disease is chronic and progressive (Tipold, 1993). CSF from five affected dogs revealed a pleocytosis of lymphocytes and monocytes in four of the dogs. The cell count ranged from 12 to $76 \times 10^6/L$ (Tipold, 1993). Protein was increased in four of five dogs based on the Pandy reaction (Tipold, 1993).

White-Shaker Dog Syndrome (Fig. 6-32)

CLINICAL AND CYTOLOGICAL DIAGNOSES

A syndrome of generalized tremors in white hair coat dogs is described (Bagley, 1993) with Maltese most commonly affected (Bagley, 1993). Treatment with prednisolone is reported to cause remission of clinical signs (Bagley, 1993). In seven dogs, CSF abnormalities varied between dogs. Total cellularity was increased in six of nine CSF samples and cell counts ranged from 1 to $282 \times 10^6/L$. In eight of nine samples, lymphocytes predominated. In one sample, neutrophils accounted for 50% of the total cell population (Bagley, 1993). Total protein ranged from 0.21 to 0.66 g/L.

Beagles and Bernese Mountain Dogs with Necrotizing Vasculitis

CLINICAL AND CYTOLOGICAL DIAGNOSES

A syndrome of necrotizing vasculitis of the spinal pachyleptomeningeal arteries in Bernese mountain dog littermates has been reported. Affected dogs were less than 1 year of age, and most presented with fever and cervical pain (Meric, 1985). CSF examination revealed a nucleated cell count of 3240 to 12600 $\times$ 10^6/L, of which 70% to 95% were neutrophils (Meric, 1986). Protein concentrations were 1.14 to 2.74 g/L (Meric, 1986). A similar syndrome with polyarteritis was reported in eight beagles in which there was a mean CSF nucleated cell count of 2868 $\times$ 10^6/L consisting primarily of neutrophils (Harcourt, 1978). Necrotizing vasculitis has also been reported in German short-haired pointers (Meric, 1988).

Granulomatous Meningoencephalitis (Figs. 6-33 to 6-45)

CLINICAL AND CYTOLOGICAL DIAGNOSES
Granulomatous meningoencephalitis (GME) is an acute, progressive, idiopathic CNS disease that affects adult dogs (Bailey, 1986). Histological lesions are predominantly in the white matter of the brain and spinal cord (Kipar, 1998). Clinical signs depend on the area affected, which can vary greatly from dog to dog (Bailey, 1986). There is considerable variation in CSF cellularity. In 10 affected dogs, cisternal CSF nucleated cell counts ranged from normal to 260 $\times$ 10^6/L. Cells varied from predominantly neutrophils to predominantly mononuclear cells (Sorjonen, 1990). In the CSF of three dogs, no lymphocytes were seen (Sorjonen, 1990). CSF protein was increased in all dogs with a mean of 1.54 g/L (Sorjonen, 1989a; Sorjonen, 1990). Five affected dogs had a mean CSF protein of 2.50 g/L, but nucleated cell counts were not reported (Sorjonen, 1987). In CSF from 18 of 22 dogs with GME, the nucleated cell count was 800.8 $\times$ 10^6/L (SD = 300) in the cisternal tap (n = 18 dogs) and 533 $\times$ 10^6/L (SD = 256) in the lumbar fluid (n = 4 dogs) (Bailey, 1986a). Cells were predominantly lymphocytic, but the mean neutrophil percentage was 18.6 $\pm$ 5.3%. Lymphocytes accounted for 62% of the nucleated cells in the cisternal taps and 80% in the lumbar taps (Bailey, 1986a). Mean cisternal protein was 2.56 g/L ($\pm$ 9.8), and mean lumbar protein was 1.63 g/L ($\pm$ 2.5) (Bailey, 1986a). In nine dogs, cisternal CSF cell counts ranged from 0 to 11,000 $\times$ 10^6/L with predominantly macrophages and lymphocytes in each case (Thomas, 1989). There were low numbers of nondegenerate neutrophils present in four cases (Thomas, 1989). The Pandy test was positive in 519 dogs.

Eosinophilic Steroid-Responsive Meningoencephalitis (Figs. 6-46 to 6-48)

CLINICAL AND CYTOLOGICAL DIAGNOSES
A syndrome of idiopathic eosinophilic meningoencephalitis was reported in six dogs ranging in age from 14 weeks to 5 years (Smith-Maxie, 1989). As well, two other dogs with protozoan meningoencephalitis had eosinophilic pleocytosis (Smith-Maxie, 1989). Each dog presented with signs of diffuse inflammation of the CNS (Smith-Maxie, 1989). The dogs had increased CSF nucleated cell counts caused mainly by eosinophils (Smith-Maxie, 1989). Three of the eight dogs were golden retrievers. The CSF nucleated cell counts ranged from 11 to 5550 cells $\times$ 10^6/L with 21% to 98% eosinophils, and protein concentrations from 1.43 to 2.0 g/L (Smith-Maxie, 1989).

Eosinophilic meningoencephalitis has been reported in one cat with a CSF white blood cell count of 14 $\times$ 10^6/L. No clear cause was determined (Schultz, 1986).

Steroid-Responsive Meningoencephalitis

CLINICAL AND CYTOLOGICAL DIAGNOSES
A steroid-responsive meningoencephalitis is reported in medium- to large-breed dogs less than 16 months of age (Irving, 1990; Meric, 1985; Meric, 1988). In five dogs with steroid-responsive meningomyelitis, nucleated cell counts varied from 22 to 6400 cells $\times$ 10^6/L with protein concentrations of 0.49 to 2.50 g/L. Neutrophils varied between 2% and 80% with lymphocytes and mononuclears making up the other cells (Irving, 1990). In 10 affected dogs, protein concentration ranged from 0.15 to 9.40 g/L with nucleated cell counts ranging from 4 to 3500 $\times$ 10^6/L and most exceeding 55 cells $\times$ 10^6/L (Meric, 1985). In all but one dog there were greater than 80% neutrophils (Meric, 1985).

24 Hours after Iopamidol and Metrizamide Myelography

CLINICAL AND CYTOLOGICAL DIAGNOSES
Several studies have examined the effects of myelographic contrast agents used in dogs. Intrathecal administration of metrizamide caused a pleocytosis at 24 hours of 520 $\pm$ 350 $\times$ 10^6/L (Johnson, 1985). At 5 days mean CSF cell counts had decreased to 7 $\times$ 10^6/L and by 10 days to 2.91 $\times$ 10^6/L. Cells were mainly mononuclear with variable numbers of neutrophils (Johnson, 1985). Approximately 90 minutes after myelography with metrizamide, a slight increase in CSF nucleated cells was detected with a mean of 9.4 $\times$ 10^6/L and a mean total protein concentration of 0.28 g/L (Widmer, 1992). Differential CSF counts revealed 30% neutrophils and 45% lymphocytes with the remainder being mononuclear cells (Widmer, 1992). Approximately 90 minutes after iopamidol, the mean CSF nucleated cell count was 16.9 $\times$ 10^6/L and mean total protein was 0.21g/L. Neutrophils were 16% and lymphocytes were 49% of the nucleated cells (Widmer, 1992). CSF obtained 90 minutes after postmyelographic withdrawal of metrizamide revealed a more severe irritation with a CSF nucleated cell count of

84.32 × 10⁶/L and a protein concentration of 1.14 g/L (Widmer, 1990). There were 45% neutrophils, 30% lymphocytes, 2% eosinophils, and 12% mononuclear cells (Widmer, 1990).

Degenerative Disk Disease, Spinal Cord Trauma, Caudal Cervical Spondylomyelopathy, and Diskospondylitis

CLINICAL DIAGNOSIS

Canine spinal cord disease is a multifaceted problem with many origins. Neoplasia, degenerative disease, infectious agents, and trauma can all contribute to the final diagnosis. Changes in the CSF may assist in differentiating primary causes, although many focal spinal cord neurological problems are associated with normal CSF analysis.

CYTOLOGICAL DIAGNOSIS

Degenerative disk disease is often associated with a mild increase in CSF cellularity (<10 × 10⁶/L), which is primarily mononuclear but can have a small neutrophilic component (Bichsel, 1984; Vandevelde, 1977). In 10 dogs, CSF nucleated cells ranged from 1 to 27 × 10⁶/L (Vandevelde, 1977). In another 11 dogs, nucleated cell counts were 0 or 1 in most dogs, with one dog at 8 × 10⁶/L (Bischel, 1984). In 9 of these 11 dogs there was a positive Pandy reaction (Bischel, 1984). In both groups of dogs, mononuclear cells predominated (Bischel, 1984; Vandevelde, 1977). In 21 dogs with intervertebral disk disease, lumbosacral taps were consistently abnormal for both protein concentration and nucleated cell counts (Thomson, 1989). The nucleated cell counts rarely exceeded 12 × 10⁶/L and were predominantly mononuclear (Thomson, 1989). Rarely, neutrophils were increased, indicating acute inflammation (Thomson, 1989). Dogs with acute signs for less than 5 days and/or clinically severe lesions had greater increases in protein and nucleated cells (Thomson, 1989). Protein was more consistently elevated than nucleated cell counts and ranged from 0.22 to 2.00 g/L (Thomson, 1989). With both cervical and thoracic compressive spinal cord disease, CSF protein concentration was more consistently elevated than nucleated cell count (Thomson, 1990). Protein concentration was most often increased in acute compressive lesions (Thomson, 1990). Cervical disease had abnormalities 42% and 71% of the time in cerebromedullary and lumbar taps (Thomson, 1990). This compares with 27.5% and 87.5% in cerebromedullary and lumbar taps in dogs with thoracolumbar lesions (Thomson, 1990). This suggests that CSF obtained caudal to the lesion is more likely to detect abnormalities (Thomson, 1990). In nine dogs with infectious diskospondylitis, three had mildly increased cell counts (6, 9, and 18 × 10⁶/L) and four had mildly increased protein concentrations from 0.20 to 2.00 g/L (Kornegay, 1980).

CNS Vascular Disorders

CLINICAL AND CYTOLOGICAL DIAGNOSES

In the dog, the response in CSF to vascular disease of the spinal cord and brain is poorly documented. In three dogs with fibrocartilaginous emboli, the CSF nucleated cell count was increased to 10 × 10⁶/L in one dog, whereas in two others it was normal. Cell distribution was primarily mononuclear. CSF protein was mildly increased (Bischel, 1984). Two dogs, one with a cerebral infarction and one with hematomyelia, had increased CSF nucleated cell counts of 57 and 195 cells × 10⁶/L, respectively (Bichsel, 1984). Both had increased protein concentration with a mixture of mononuclear and polymorphonuclear cells (Bichsel, 1984). In eight other dogs with cerebrovascular disease, all but two had significant increases in CSF cellularity ranging from 7 to 120 × 10⁶/L (Vandevelde, 1977). In five of the eight dogs there was an increased percentage of neutrophils (11%-55%) and in two dogs there was erythrophagocytosis (Vandevelde, 1977).

Feline cerebral vascular disease, or feline ischemic encephalopathy (FIE), is a neurological diagnosis in cats usually less than 4 years of age (Rand, 1994a). It is suggested that FIE is a result of aberrant *Cuterebra* larval migration (Williams, 1998). CSF from seven affected cats showed a mild increase in protein (0.15-1.05 g/L), and only one cat had a mild increase in CSF nucleated cells, at 6 × 10⁶/L (Shepherd, 1980). One affected cat had a CSF nucleated cell count of 9 × 10⁶/L and a protein concentration of 0.18 g/L (Kornegay, 1981). CSF protein concentration was increased in three of four affected cats with a mean of 0.43 g/L (Rand, 1994a). Two of these cats had a mild increase in CSF white blood cells of 6 and 10 cells × 10⁶/L (Rand, 1994a). Increased cellularity was due to neutrophils or foamy macrophages (Rand, 1994a). In a report documenting the relationship between *Cuterebra* larval migration and FIE, two CSF analysis were performed (Williams, 1998). One CSF had no significant abnormalities, and one had an increased nucleated cell count of 26 × 10⁶/L (Williams, 1998). Cells were a combination of lymphocytes and macrophages with rare neutrophils (Williams, 1998).

Globoid Cell Leukodystrophy

CLINICAL AND CYTOLOGICAL DIAGNOSES

Globoid cell leukodystrophy is a progressive neurological disorder involving the white matter of the central and peripheral nervous systems (Shull, 1984). It is reported in several breeds and is an autosomal recessive trait in cairn and west highland white terriers (Shull, 1984). There is an increase in CSF protein concentration with a normal nucleated cell count and distribution (Shull, 1984). This is called *albuminocytological dissociation.* PAS-positive material within the cytoplasm of macrophages is described (Shull, 1972).

NEOPLASTIC DISEASE

Meningioma (Figs. 6-49 and 6-50)

CLINICAL AND CYTOLOGICAL DIAGNOSES
Meningioma is the only primary brain tumor in the dog in which CSF nucleated cell counts routinely exceed 50 × 10⁶/L often with greater than 50% neutrophils. These observations correlate with necrosis or neutrophilic infiltration of the tumor (Bailey, 1986b).

One report of impression smears of a meningioma revealed moderate cellularity with large plump spindle cells "in loose sheets or dense disorganized bundles" (Altman, 1984). Some bundles showed whorling. Cells had a moderate N:C ratio and pale cytoplasm with indistinct nucleoli. Cells were embedded in amorphous eosinophilic material (Altman, 1984).

Other CNS Tumors

CLINICAL AND CYTOLOGICAL DIAGNOSES
In 56 dogs with CNS tumors other than meningioma, the main protein concentration varied from 0.38 g/L to 1.49 g/L (Bailey, 1986b). Cell counts ranged from 2.8 × 10⁶/L to 11.4 × 10⁶/L (Bailey, 1986b). No tumor cells were detected within the CSF. A sedimentation technique has been reported that may increase cytological detection of malignant cells (Grevel, 1990). Seven other dogs with intracranial tumors had median cisternal protein concentrations of 0.59 g/L and nucleated cell counts of 7 × 10⁶/L, as opposed to two dogs with lumbosacral taps that had median protein concentrations of 3.97 g/L with 25 × 10⁶/L nucleated cells (Thomson, 1990). In 14 dogs with thoracolumbar neoplasia, 7 had cisternal taps and 7 had thoracolumbar taps. The cisternal median protein concentration was 0.32 g/L and nucleated cell count was 0 cells × 10⁶/L, whereas lumbosacral values were 1.45 g/L and 5 cells × 10⁶/L, respectively (Thomson, 1990). Atypical lymphocytes may be present in dogs with lymphoma and CNS involvement.

In 34 cats with noninflammatory CNS disease, neoplasia accounted for 12 of the cases (Rand, 1994b). In the 10 cats with primary CNS tumors, five were astrocytomas, three were meningiomas, one was ependymoma, and one was sarcoma (Rand, 1994b). Total protein was increased in 8 of 12 cats (mean 0.4 g/L), but no cat exceeded 0.85 g/L (Rand, 1994a). Cell distribution was abnormal in five cats, with an increase in either neutrophils or lymphocytes (Rand, 1994a). In 9 of the 12 cats the CSF nucleated counts were normal. Two of three cats had nucleated cell counts greater than 50 cells × 10⁶/L (Rand, 1994a).

Feline Cerebral Astrocytoma

CLINICAL AND CYTOLOGICAL DIAGNOSES
There are few reports describing CSF observations in cats with intracranial neoplasia. Although brain tumors are more common in older animals, astrocytomas were observed in younger cats comparable with the relative age ranges for humans with neuroectodermal tumors (Sarfaty, 1987). Two cats diagnosed with cerebral astrocytoma had pleocytosis with nucleated cell counts of 30 and 19 cells × 10⁶/L (Sarfaty, 1987). Neutrophils predominated in one case and lymphocytes in the other (Sarfaty, 1987). CSF protein was increased in one cat to 1.40 g/L (Sarfaty, 1987).

Lymphoma (Figs. 6-51 to 6-53)

CLINICAL AND CYTOLOGICAL DIAGNOSES
As described in Chapter 5, a monomorphic population of lymphocytes in the CSF prompts further examination for the diagnosis of lymphoma. Often these lymphocytes are larger and may have cytological abnormalities associated with neoplasia.

References

Alleman, A.R., Christopher, M.M., Steiner, D.A., et al. Identification of intracytoplasmic inclusion bodies in mononuclear cells from the cerebrospinal fluid of a dog with canine distemper. *Vet Pathol* 29:84-85, 1992.

Allen, D.G. Special techniques. In *Small Animal Medicine.* D.G. Allen, S.E. Kruth, M.S. Garvey (eds). Philadelphia, JP Lippincott, 1991.

Altman, D., Bolon, B., Meyer, D.J., et al. Cytologic features of a meningioma in a dog. *Vet Clin Pathol* 18:98-101,1984.

Bagley, R.S., Kornegay, J.N., Wheeler, S.J., et al. Generalized tremors in Maltese: clinical findings in seven cases. *J Am Anim Hosp Assoc* 29:141-143, 1993.

Bailey, C.S. and Higgins, R.J. Comparison of total white blood cell count and total protein content of lumbar and cisternal cerebrospinal fluid of healthy dogs. *Am J Vet Res* 46:1162-1165, 1985.

Bailey, C.S. and Higgins, R.J. Characteristics of cerebrospinal fluid associated with canine granulomatous meningoencephalomyelitis: a retrospective study. *J Am Vet Med Assoc* 188:418-421, 1986a.

Bailey, C.S. and Higgins, R.J. Characteristics of cisternal cerebrospinal fluid associated with primary brain tumors in the dog: a retrospective study. *J Am Vet Med Assoc* 188:414-417, 1986b.

Bailey, C.S. and Vernau, W. Cerebrospinal fluid. In *Clinical Biochemistry of Domestic Animals.* ed 5. J.J. Kaneko, J.W. Harvey, and M.L. Bruss (eds). Academic Press, New York, 1997.

Baker, J.L., Craig, T.M., Barton, C.L., et al. *Hepatozoon canis* in a dog with oral pylogranulomas and neurological disease. *Cornell Vet* 78:179-183, 1988.

Bichsel, P., Vandevelde, M., Vandevelde, E., et al. Immunoelectrophoretic determination of albumin and IgG in serum and cerebrospinal fluid in dogs with neurological diseases. *Res Vet Sci* 37:101-107, 1984.

Bullmore, C.C. Canine meningoencephalitis. *J Am Anim Hosp Assoc* 14:387-394, 1978.

Chrisman, C.L. Cerebrospinal fluid analysis. *Vet Clin North Am Small Animal Pract* 22:781- 810, 1992.

Christopher, M.M. Bone marrow contamination of canine cerebrospinal fluid. *Vet Clin Pathol* 21:95-98, 1992.

Cook, J.R., Evinger, J.V., and Wagner, L.A. Successful combination chemotherapy for canine cryptococcal meningoencephalitis. *J Am Anim Hosp Assoc* 27:61-64, 1991.

Cordy, D.R. and Holliday, T.A. A necrotizing meningoencephalitis of pug dogs. *Vet Pathol* 26:191-194, 1989.

Dillberger, J.E., Homer, B., Daubert, D., et al. Protothecosis in two cats. *J Am Vet Med Assoc* 192:1557-1559, 1988.

Dow, S.W., LeCouter, R.A., Henik, R.A., et al. Central nervous system infection associated with anaerobic bacteria in two dogs and two cats. *J Vet Intern Med* 2:171-176, 1988.

Dubey, J.P. Infectivity and pathogenicity of *Toxoplasma gondii* oocysts for cats. *J Parasitol* 82:957-961, 1996.

Dubey, J.P., Greene, C.E., and Lappin, M.R. Toxoplasmosis and neosporosis. In *Infectious Diseases of the Dog and Cat.* C.E. Greene (ed). WB Saunders, Philadelphia, 1990.

Esh, J.B., Cunningham, J.G., and Wiltor, T.J. Vaccine-induced rabies in four cats. *J Am Vet Med Assoc* 180:1336-1339, 1982.

Fallin, C.W., Raskin, R.E., and Harvey, J.W. Cytologic identification of neural tissue in the cerebrospinal fluid of two dogs. *Vet Clin Pathol* 25:127-129, 1996.

Greene, C.E., Burgdorfer, W., Cavagnolo, R., et al. Rocky Mountain spotted fever in dogs and its differentiation from canine ehrlichiosis. *J Am Vet Med Assoc* 186:465-472, 1985.

Greene, C.E. Rocky Mountain spotted fever and ehrlichiosis In *Current Veterinary Therapy IX.* R.W. Kirk (ed). WB Saunders, Philadelphia, 1986.

Greig, B., Rossow, K.D., Collins, J.E., et al. *Neospora caninum* pneumonia in an adult dog. *J Am Vet Med Assoc* 206:1000-1001, 1995.

Grevel, V. and Machus, B. Diagnosing brain tumors with a CSF sedimentation technique. *Vet Med Report* 2:403-408, 1990.

Harcourt, R.A. Polyarteritis in a colony of beagles. *Vet Rec* 102:519-522, 1978.

Hochwald, G.M. and Wallenstein, M.C. Exchange of albumin between blood, cerebrospinal fluid, and brain in the cat. *Am J Physiol* 19:115-126, 1967.

Hurtt, A.E. and Smith, M.O. Effects of iatrogenic blood contamination on results of cerebrospinal fluid analysis in clinically normal dogs and dogs with neurologic disease. *J Am Vet Med Assoc* 211:866-867, 1997.

Irving, G. and Chrisman, C. Long-term outcome of five cases of corticosteroid-responsive meningomyelitis. *J Am Anim Hosp Assoc* 26:324-328, 1990.

Jacobs, R.M., Cochrane, S.M., Lumsden, J.H., et al. Relationship of cerebrospinal fluid protein concentration determined by dye-binding and urinary dipstick methodologies. *Can Vet J* 31:587-588, 1990.

Jamison, E.M. *A study of cerebrospinal fluid in dogs with central nervous system disease.* Thesis. University of Guelph, 1992.

Jamison, E.M. and Lumsden, J.H. Cerebrospinal fluid analysis in the dog: methodology and interpretation. *Semin Vet Med Surg (Small Anim)* 3:122-132, 1988.

Johnson, G.C., Fucie, D.M., Fenner, W.R., et al. Transient leakage across the blood-cerebrospinal fluid barrier after intrathecal metrizamide administration to dogs. *Am J Vet Res* 46:1303-1308, 1985.

Johnson, G.C., Krakowka, S., and Axthelm, M.K. Albumin leakage into cerebrospinal fluid of dogs lethally infected with R252 canine distemper virus. *J Neuroimmunol* 14:61-74, 1987.

Jull, B.A., Merryman, J.I., Thomas, W.B., et al. Necrotizing encephalitis in a Yorkshire terrier. *J Am Vet Med Assoc* 211:1005-1007, 1997.

Kipar, A., Baumgartner, W., Vogl, C., et al. Immunohistochemical characterization of inflammatory cells in brains of dogs with granulomatous meningoencephalitis. *Vet Pathol* 35:43-52, 1998.

Kornegay, J. N. and Barber, D.L. Diskospondylitis in dogs. *J Am Vet Med Assoc* 177:337-341, 1980.

Kornegay, J.N. Cerebrospinal fluid collection, examination, and interpretation in dogs and cats. *Compend Cont Ed Pract* 3:85-90, 1981a.

Kornegay, J.N., Lorenz, M., and Zenoble, R.D. Bacterial meningoencephalitis in two dogs. *J Am Vet Med Assoc* 173:1334-1336, 1978.

Kornegay, J.N. Feline neurology. *Compend Cont Ed Pract* 3:203-213, 1981b.

Macdonald, J.M., Delahunta, A., and Georgi, J. *Cuterebra* encephalitis in a dog. *Cornell Vet* 66:372-380, 1976.

Macintire, D.K., Vincent-Johnson, N., Dillon, A.R., et al. Hepatozoonosis in dogs: 22 cases (1989-1994). *J Am Vet Med Assoc* 210:916-922, 1997.

Medleau, L. Feline cryptococcosis. In *Current Veterinary Therapy X, Small Animal Practice.* R.W. Kirk and J.D. Bonagura (eds). WB Saunders, Philadelphia, 1989.

Meric, S.M., Chjild, G., and Higgins, R.J. Necrotizing vasculitis of the spinal pachyleptomeningeal arteries in three Bernese mountain dog littermates. *J Am Anim Hosp Assoc* 22:459-465, 1986.

Meric, S.M. Canine meningitis: a changing emphasis. *J Vet Intern Med* 2:26-35, 1988.

Meric, S.M., Perman, V., and Hardy, R.M. Corticosteroid-responsive meningitis in ten dogs. *J Am Anim Hosp Assoc* 21:677-684, 1985.

Mesher, C.I., Blue, J.T., Guffroy, M.R.G., et al. Intracellular myelin in cerebrospinal fluid from a dog with myelomalacia. *Vet Clin Pathol* 25:124-127, 1996.

Nafe, L.A., Turk, J.R., and Carter, J.D. Central nervous system involvement of blastomycosis in the dog. *J Am Anim Hosp Assoc* 19:933-936, 1983.

Rakich, P.M. and Latimer, K.S. Altered immune function in a dog with disseminated prototobecosis. *J Am Vet Med Assoc* 185:681-683, 1984.

Rand, J.S. The analysis of cerebrospinal fluid in cats. In *Current Veterinary Therapy XII, Small Animal Practice.* R.W. Kirk and J.D. Bonagura (eds). WB Saunders, Philadelphia, 1995.

Rand, J.S., Parent, J., Jacobs, R., et al. Clinical, cerebrospinal fluid, and histological data from 34 cats with primary non-inflammatory central nervous system disease. *Can Vet J* 35:103-110, 1994a.

Rand, J.S., Parent, J., Jacobs, R., et al. Clinical, cerebrospinal fluid, and histological data from 27 cats with primary inflammatory central nervous system disease. *Can Vet J* 35:74-181, 1994b.

Rand, J.S., Parent, J., Jacobs, R., et al. Reference intervals for feline cerebrospinal fluid: cell counts and cytologic features. *Am J Vet Res* 51:1044-1048, 1990a.

Rand, J.S., Parent, J., and Jacobs, R. Reference intervals for feline CSF. *American College of Veterinary Internal Medicine Forum Proceedings,* p 118, 1989 (abstract).

Rand, J.S., Parent, J., Jacobs, R., et al. Reference intervals for feline cerebrospinal fluid: biochemical and serologic variables, IgG concentration, and electrophoretic fractionation. *Am J Vet Res* 51:1049-1054, 1990b.

Sarfaty, D., Carrillo, J.M., and Greenlee, P.G. Differential diagnosis of granulomatous meningoencephalitis, distemper and suppurative meningoencephalitis in the dog. *J Am Vet Med Assoc* 188:387-399, 1986.

Sarfaty, D., Carrill, J.M., and Patnaik, A.K. Cerebral astrocytoma in four cats: clinical and pathologic findings. *J Am Vet Med Assoc* 191:976-978, 1987.

Schultz, A.E., Cribb, A.E., and Tvedten, H.W. Eosinophilic meningoencephalitis in a cat. *J Am Anim Hosp Assoc* 22:623-627, 1986.

Sellon, R.K. and Breitschwerdt, E.B. CVT update: Rocky Mountain spotted fever. In *Current Veterinary Therapy XII, Small Animal Practice.* J.D. Bonagura (ed). WB Saunders, Philadelphia, 1995.

Shepherd, D.E. and deLahunta, A. Central nervous system disease in the cat. *Compend Cont Ed Pract* 2:305-311, 1980.

Shull, R., Rozel, J.F., Steinberg, S.A., et al. Periodic-acid - Schiff-positive cells in cerebrospinal fluid of dogs with globoid leukodystrophy. *Neurology* 22:738-742, 1972.

Shull, R., Selcer, E., and Selcer, R.R. Globoid cell leukodystrophy in two west highland white terriers and one Pomeranian. *Compend Cont Ed Pract* 6:621-624, 1984.

Smith-Maxie, L.L., Parent, J.P., Rand, J., et al. Cerebrospinal fluid analysis and clinical outcome of eight dogs with eosinophilic meningoencephalomyelitis. *J Vet Intern Med* 3:167-174, 1989.

Sorjonen, D.C. Cerebrospinal fluid electrophoresis: use in canine granulomatous meningoencephalomyelitis. *Vet Med Report* 1:399-401, 1989a.

Sorjonen, D.C., Cox, N.R., and Swango, L.J. Electrophoretic determination of albumin and gamma globulin concentrations in the cerebrospinal fluid of dogs with encephalomyelitis attributable to canine distemper virus infection: 13 cases (1980-1987). *J Am Vet Med Assoc* 195:977-980, 1989b.

Sorjonen, J.C. Total protein, albumin quota, and electrophoretic patterns in cerebrospinal fluid of dogs with central nervous system disorders. *Am J Vet Res* 48:301-305, 1987.

Sorjonen, D.C. Clinical and histopathological features of granulomatous meningoencephalomyelitis in dogs. *J Am Anim Hosp Assoc* 26:141-147, 1990.

Sornas, R. The cytology of the normal cerebrospinal fluid. *Acta Neurol Scand* 48:313-320, 1972.

Stalis, I.H., Chadwick, B., Dayrell-Hart, B.D., et al. Necrotizing meningoencephalitis of Maltese dogs. *Vet Pathol* 32:230-235, 1995.

Thomas, J.B. and Eger, C. Granulomatous meningoencephalomyelitis in 21 dogs. *J Small Anim Pract* 30:287-293, 1989.

Thomson, C.E., Kornegay, J.N., and Stevens, J.B Canine intervertebral disc disease: changes in the cerebrospinal fluid. *J Small Anim Pract* 30:685-688, 1989.

Thomson, C.E., Kornegay, J.N., and Stevens, J.B. Analysis of cerebrospinal fluid from the cerebellomedullary and lumbar cisterns of dogs with focal neurologic disease: 145 cases (1985-1987). *J Am Vet Med Assoc* 196:1841-1844, 1990.

Tipold, A., Fatzer, R., Jaggy, A., et al. Necrotizing encephalitis in Yorkshire terriers. *J Small Anim Pract* 34:623-628, 1993.

Tipold, A. Diagnosis of inflammatory and infectious diseases of the central nervous system in dogs: a retrospective study. *J Vet Intern Med* 9:304-314, 1995.

Tyler, D.E. Prototothecosis. In *Infectious Diseases of the Dog and Cat.* C.E. Greene (ed). WB Saunders, Philadelphia, 1990.

Tyler, D.E., Lorenz, M.D., Blue, J.L., et al. Disseminated protothecosis with central nervous involvement in a dog. *J Am Vet Med Assoc* 176:987-993, 1980.

Vandevelde, E. and Spano, J.S. Cerebrospinal fluid cytology in canine neurologic disease. *Am J Vet Res* 38:1827-1832, 1977.

Vincent-Johnson, N., Macintire, D.K., and Baneth, G. Canine hepatozoonosis: pathophysiology, diagnosis, and treatment. *Compend Cont Ed Pract* 19:51-63, 1997.

Widmer, W.R., DeNicola, D.B., Blevins, W.E., et al. Cerebrospinal fluid changes after iopamidol and metrizamide myelography in clinically normal dogs. *Am J Vet Res* 53:396-401, 1992.

Widmer, W.R., Blevins, W.E., Cantwell, H.D., et al. Cerebrospinal fluid response following metrizamide myelography in normal dogs: effects of routine myelography and postmyelographic removal of contrast medium. *Vet Clin Pathol* 19:66-76, 1990.

Williams, K.J., Summers, B.A., and De Lahunta, A. Cerebrospinal cuterebriasis in cats and its association with feline ischemic encephalopathy. *Vet Pathol* 35:330-343, 1998.

Wilson, J.W. and Stevens, JB. Effects of blood contamination on cerebrospinal fluid analysis. *J Am Vet Med Assoc* 171:256-258, 1977.

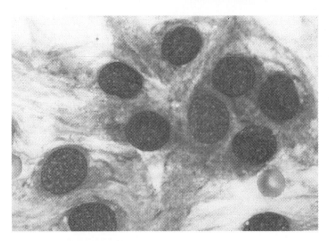

FIG. 6-1. Canine. Scraping. Normal brain. Spindle-shaped cells with abundant cytoplasm and indistinct adjoining borders. The nuclei have a distinct chromatin pattern with occasional small, single nucleoli. The cytoplasm is mildly basophilic, has a fibrillar pattern, and contains light pink granulation. (×400.)

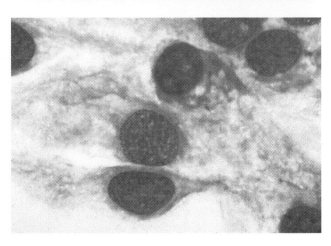

FIG. 6-2. Canine. Scraping. Normal brain. Greater spreading of cells described in Fig. 6-1 illustrate additional nuclear and cytoplasmic details, including angularity of cells. (×400.)

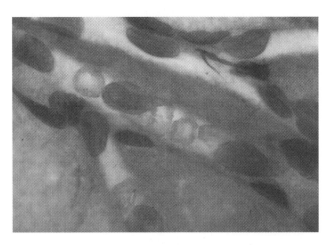

FIG. 6-3. Canine. Scraping. Normal Brain. Red blood cells within capillaries lined by endothelial cells may be observed in most tissues, especially after scraping techniques are used. (×400.)

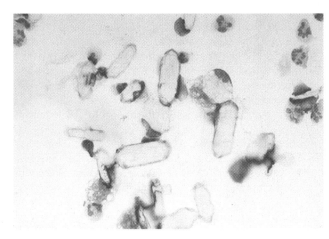

FIG. 6-4. Canine. Cerebrospinal fluid. Normal dog. Crystals occasionally found in cytocentrifuge preparations. Their origin is uncertain, but they are assumed to be an artifact of preparation. (×100.)

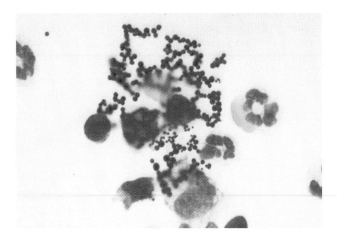

FIG. 6-5. Canine. Cerebrospinal fluid. The dark stain precipitate should not be mistaken for bacteria. (×500.)

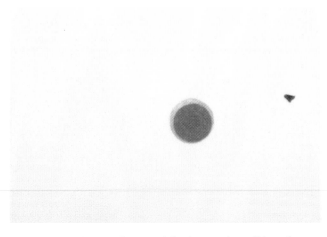

FIG. 6-6. Canine. Cerebrospinal fluid. Typical small lymphocyte with minimal cytoplasm. (×630.)

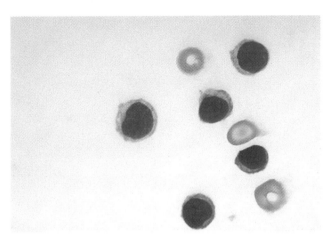

FIG. 6-7. Canine Cerebrospinal fluid. These cells would be classified as four small mononuclear cells and one small lymphocyte. (×500.)

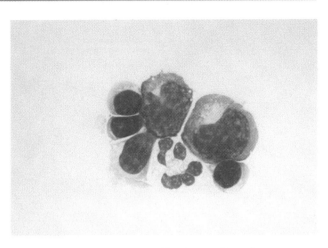

FIG. 6-8. Canine. Cerebrospinal fluid. A small lymphocyte, a neutrophil, three small and two large mononuclear cells. (×400.)

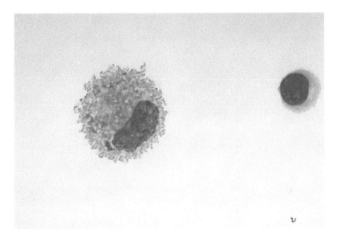

FIG. 6-9. Canine. Cerebrospinal fluid. A small mononuclear cell and a large mononuclear cell that borders on being a large foamy macrophage. (×400.)

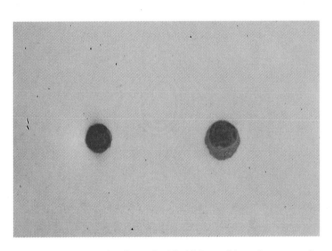

FIG. 6-10. Canine. Cerebrospinal fluid. A small lymphocyte and a small mononuclear cell. (×450.)

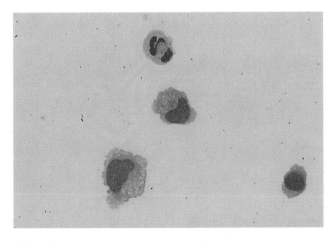

FIG. 6-11. Canine. Cerebrospinal fluid. One neutrophil, one small mononuclear cell, and two large mononuclear cells. (×450.)

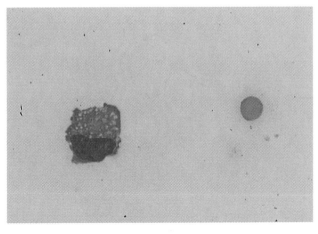

FIG. 6-12. Canine. Cerebrospinal fluid. One large mononuclear cell. (×450.)

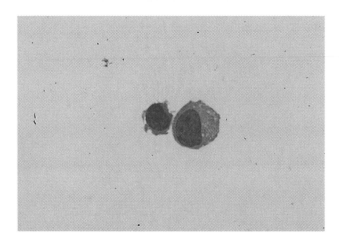

FIG. 6-13. Canine. Cerebrospinal fluid. One small mononuclear cell and one large mononuclear cell. (×450.)

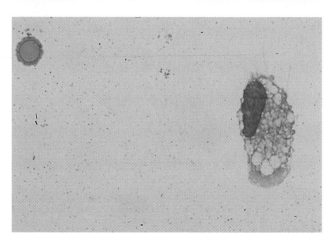

FIG. 6-14. Canine. Cerebrospinal fluid. One large, foamy macrophage. (×450.)

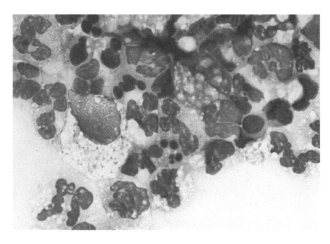

FIG. 6-15. Canine. Cerebrospinal fluid. Septic meningitis. Nucleated cell count was 300 × 10⁶/L. Many neutrophils with nuclear degeneration, indicating likely sepsis. Nuclear debris should not be misinterpreted as bacteria. (×400.)

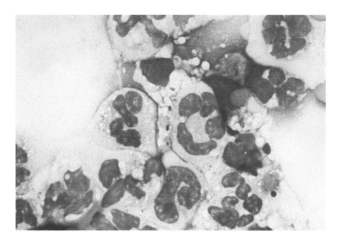

FIG. 6-16. Canine. Cerebrospinal fluid. Septic meningitis. (Same case as Fig. 6-15.) Neutrophil nuclear chromatolysis indicative of probable sepsis as confirmed by a few intracytoplasmic bacterial coccobacillio. (×500.)

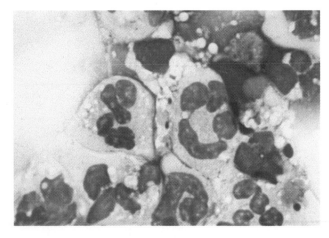

FIG. 6-17. Canine. Cerebrospinal fluid. Septic meningitis. Increased magnification of Fig. 6-16. Bacteria are frequently visible within the neutrophil cytoplasmic phagolysosomes. (×630.)

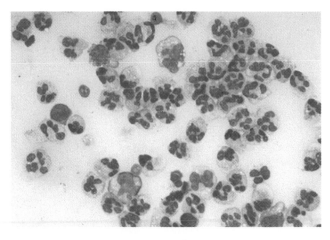

FIG. 6-18. Canine. Cerebrospinal fluid. Suppurative inflammation. Increased nondegenerate neutrophils and a few mononuclear phagocytic cells. This cytological observation may indicate an infectious or immune-mediated cause. (×200.)

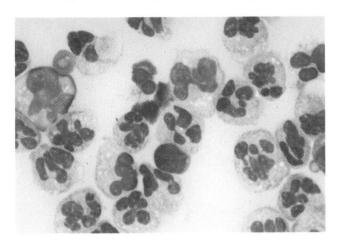

FIG. 6-19. Canine. Cerebrospinal fluid. Suppurative inflammation. (Same case as Fig. 6-18.) Many well-preserved neutrophils, intermixed with mononuclear cells, including monocytes and a small lymphocyte. Neutrophil nuclear morphology is suggestive of aging, in contrast to the karyolytic changes associated with bacterial toxins. (×400.)

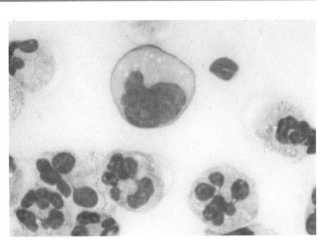

FIG. 6-20. Canine. Cerebrospinal fluid. Suppurative inflammation. (Same case as Fig. 6-18.) Background of nondegenerate neutrophils is contrasted with a single large mononuclear cell, likely of monocyte origin. (×500.)

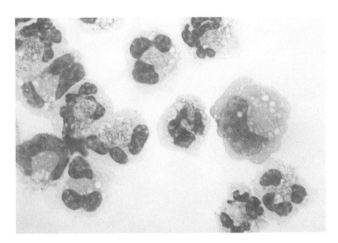

FIG. 6-21. Canine. Cerebrospinal fluid. Bernese mountain dog. Suppurative inflammation. Nondegenerate neutrophils and a large mononuclear cell. This cytological presentation is consistent with immune-mediated disease, but an infectious cause should not be excluded. (×400.)

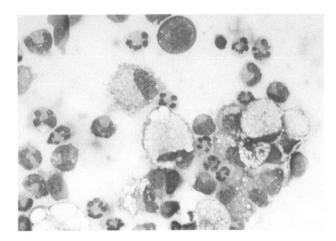

FIG. 6-22. Canine. Cerebrospinal fluid. Mixed inflammation. Macrophages, large and small mononuclear cells, and well-preserved neutrophils are present. It is not easy to differentiate whether the large mononuclear cell with basophilic cytoplasm is a lymphocyte or monocyte. (×200.)

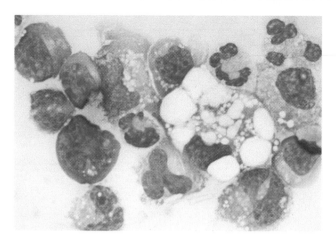

FIG. 6-23. Canine. Cerebrospinal fluid. Mixed inflammation. (Same case as Fig. 6-22.) The majority of cells are large mononuclear cells with a variable amount of cytoplasmic vacuolation. There is one large, foamy macrophage and two well-preserved neutrophils. Lymphoid origin is suggested for some cells by the basophilic cytoplasm and perinuclear clearing, whereas other cells appear to be monocytic in origin. (×400.)

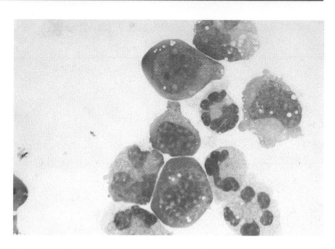

FIG. 6-24. Canine. Cerebrospinal fluid. Mixed inflammation. (Same case as Fig. 6-22.) This mixed population of cells would be identified as: four neutrophils, one small mononuclear, and five large mononuclear cells. Of the five large mononuclear cells, two appear to be lymphocytic and three monocytic in origin. Special stains are required for classification. (×400.)

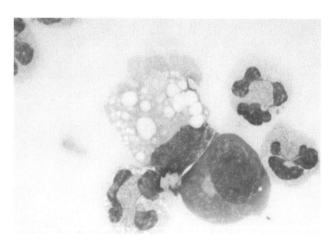

FIG. 6-25. Canine. Cerebrospinal fluid. Mixed inflammation. There is a foamy macrophage and a large mononuclear cell with markedly basophilic cytoplasm and perinuclear clearing. Nondegenerate neutrophils are also observed. The basophilic mononuclear cell may represent a large, "reactive" lymphocyte. (×500.)

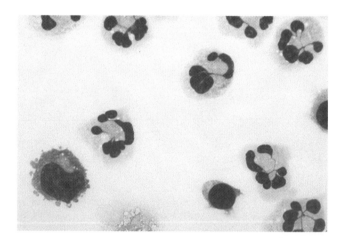

FIG. 6-26. Canine. Cerebrospinal fluid. Mixed inflammation. The predominance of neutrophils with distinct filaments separating lobules suggests nonseptic cause or low virulence of bacteria. (×400.)

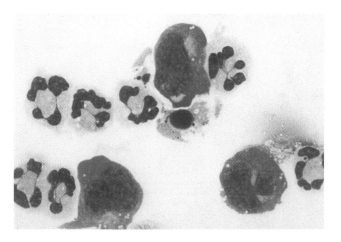

FIG. 6-27. Canine. Cerebrospinal fluid. Mixed inflammation. (Same case as Fig. 6-26.) Nondegenerate neutrophils and three large mononuclear cells with slightly convoluted nuclei and moderate to marked basophilic cytoplasm. These mononuclear cells illustrate the overlapping morphological appearance of the lymphocytic and monocytic cell populations. (×400.)

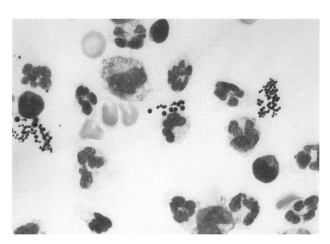

FIG. 6-28. Canine. Cerebrospinal fluid. Mixed inflammation. Moderately preserved neutrophils and a few large and small mononuclear cells. The dark basophilic stain precipitate should not be confused with bacteria. (×250.)

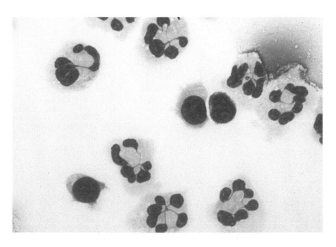

FIG. 6-29. Canine. Cerebrospinal fluid. Mixed inflammation. Nondegenerate neutrophils that appear hypersegmented. There is one typical small lymphocyte and two cells that are either small lymphocytes or small mononuclear cells. (×400.)

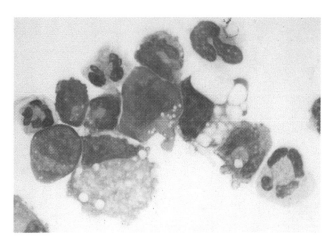

FIG. 6-30. Canine. Cerebrospinal fluid. Mixed inflammation. There are nondegenerate neutrophils, large mononuclear cells, and vacuolated macrophages. (×400.)

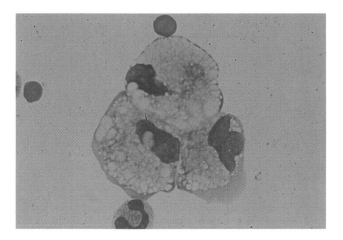

FIG. 6-31. Canine. Cytocentrifuge sediment. Cerebrospinal fluid. Foamy macrophages. Large cells of monocyte origin with abundant foamy cytoplasm indicate response to chronic inflammation. The close aggregation of the cells may be due to the physical forces established during the concentration procedure. (×380.)

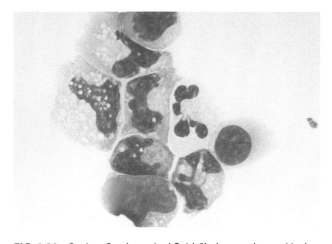

FIG. 6-32. Canine. Cerebrospinal fluid. Shaker syndrome. Moderate to large mononuclear cells and one neutrophil. An increase in lymphocytes may be the only change associated with this syndrome observed in small breeds such as West Highland white terriers. (×250.)

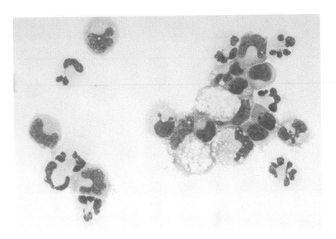

FIG. 6-33. Canine. Cerebrospinal fluid. Granulomatous meningoencephalitis. Mixed inflammatory cells consisting of nonlytic neutrophils, large and small mononuclear cells, and macrophages. The cytological presentation for GME is typically mixed inflammatory cells with large mononuclear cells, lymphocytes, and variable numbers of nonlytic neutrophils. (×100.)

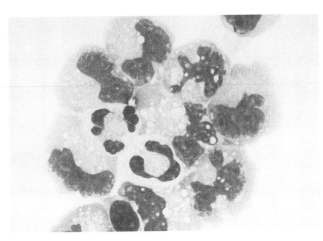

FIG. 6-34. Canine. Cerebrospinal fluid. Granulomatous meningoencephalitis. (Same case as Fig. 6-33.) Two neutrophils and eight large mononuclear cells likely of monocytic origin. (×400.)

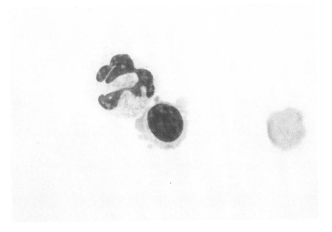

FIG. 6-35. Canine. Cerebrospinal fluid. Granulomatous meningoencephalitis. Neutrophil and a small mononuclear cell. Although the nuclear diameter is similar to small lymphocytes, there is more cytoplasm than expected. (×500.)

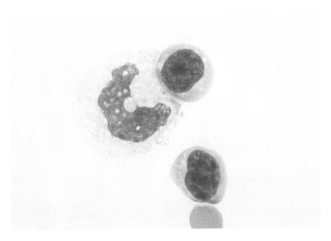

FIG. 6-36. Canine. Cerebrospinal fluid. Granulomatous meningoencephalitis. (Same case as Fig. 6-35.) Large mononuclear cell with indented nucleus and vacuolated cytoplasm with two small mononuclear cells, likely lymphoid in origin. (×500.)

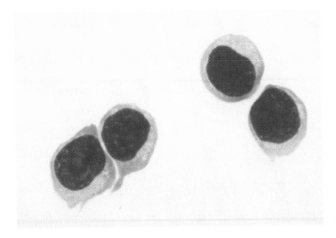

FIG. 6-37. Canine. Cerebrospinal fluid. Granulomatous meningoencephalitis. (Same case as Fig. 6-35.) Small mononuclear cells that appear lymphoid in origin with lightly basophilic cytoplasm and occasional perinuclear clear area. Lymphoid cells are often prominent in GME. (×630.)

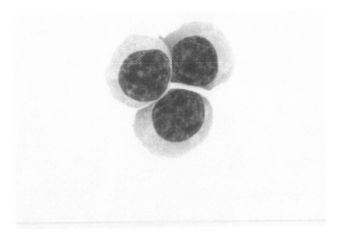

FIG. 6-38. Canine. Cerebrospinal fluid. Granulomatous meningoencephalitis. (Same case as Fig. 6-35.) Three small mononuclear cells with prominent heterochromatin clumping, suggesting lymphoid origin. (×630.)

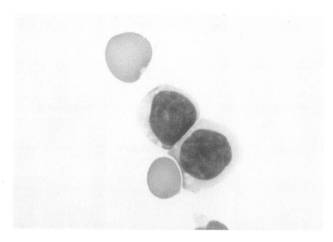

FIG. 6-39. Canine. Cerebrospinal fluid. Granulomatous meningoencephalitis. Total nucleated cell count was 23×10^6/L. There are two small mononuclear cells the diameter of $1^1/_2$ red cells that appear lymphoid in origin. ($\times$630.)

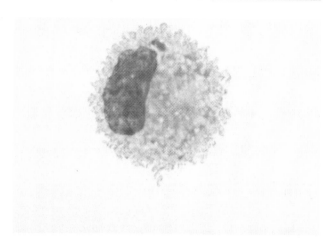

FIG. 6-40. Canine. Cerebrospinal fluid. Granulomatous meningoencephalitis. (Same case as Fig. 6-39.) Large mononuclear cell with slightly indented, eccentrically located nucleus and light basophilic granular cytoplasm. ($\times$400.)

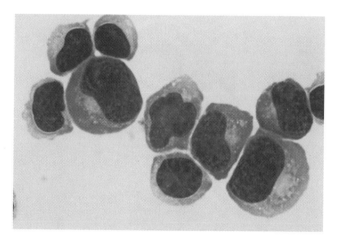

FIG. 6-41. Canine. Cerebrospinal fluid. Granulomatous meningoencephalitis. Small lymphocytes and small mononuclear cells that appear lymphoid in origin. ($\times$500.)

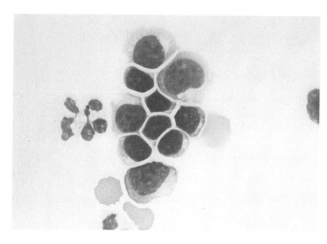

FIG. 6-42. Canine. Cerebrospinal fluid. Granulomatous meningoencephalitis. Mixed inflammatory response, including one neutrophil and large mononuclear cells. ($\times$500.)

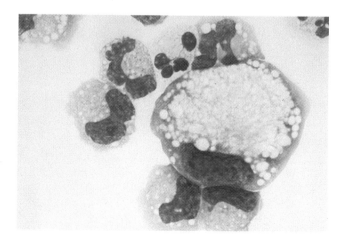

FIG. 6-43. Canine. Cerebrospinal fluid.. Granulomatous meningoencephalitis. (Same case as Fig. 6-42.) One neutrophil, large mononuclear cells, and one large, foamy macrophage. The appearance of "activation" of macrophages can be created during cytocentrifugation. ($\times$500.)

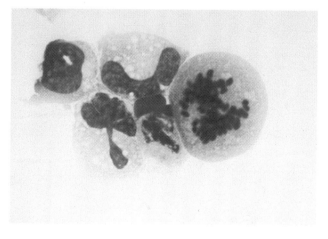

FIG. 6-44. Canine. Cerebrospinal fluid. Granulomatous meningoencephalitis. (Same case as Fig. 6-42.) Large mononuclear cells with round to convoluted nuclei. Mitotic figure is indicative of cell proliferation. ($\times$500.)

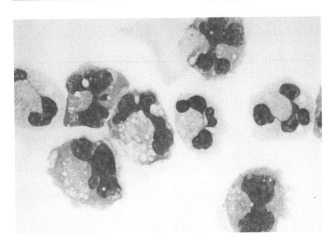

FIG. 6-45. Canine. Cerebrospinal fluid. Granulomatous meningoencephalitis. Large mononuclear cells adjacent to three neutrophils. Mononuclear cells usually predominate in GME. (×400.)

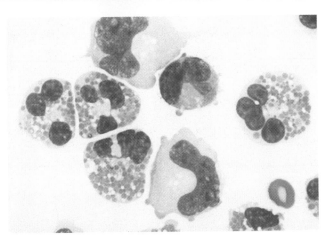

FIG. 6-46. Canine. Cerebrospinal fluid. Eosinophilic meningitis. Nucleated cell count was 893 × 10⁶/L. Three large mononuclear cells and four eosinophils. Note size comparison to the red blood cell. No etiologic agent was cultured. (×500.)

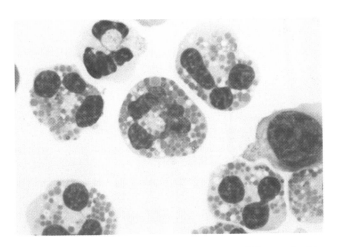

FIG. 6-47. Canine. Cerebrospinal fluid. Eosinophilic meningitis. (Same case as Fig. 6-46.) One large mononuclear cell and a neutrophil with several eosinophils. (×630.)

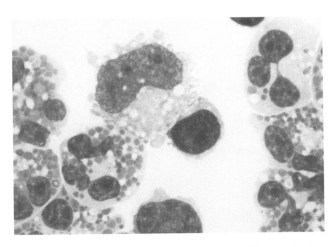

FIG. 6-48. Canine. Cerebrospinal fluid. Eosinophilic meningitis. (Same case as Fig. 6-46.) Three large mononuclear cells accompanied by eosinophils. Canine eosinophil granules can be mistaken for inclusions or erythrophagocytosis. (×630.)

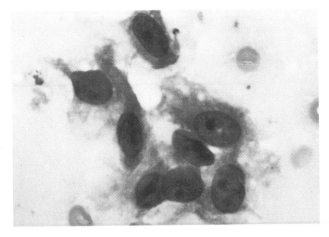

FIG. 6-49. Canine. Imprint. Meningioma. A cluster of loosely cohesive spindle-shaped cells with basophilic cytoplasm, hyperchromatic oval nuclei with prominent nucleoli, and a high N:C ratio. Diff-Quick stain. (×400.)

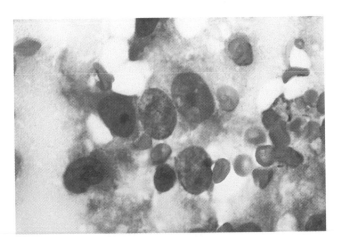

FIG. 6-50. Canine. Imprint. Meningioma. (Same case as Fig. 6-49.) Plump fusiform cells with one or two prominent nucleoli. Cytoplasm is lightly basophilic with indistinct cytoplasmic boundaries. (×400.)

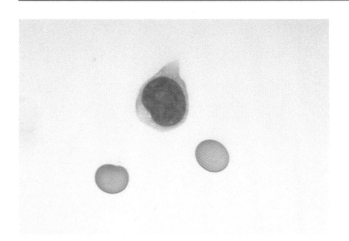

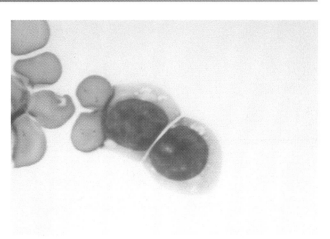

FIG. 6-51. Canine. Cerebrospinal fluid. Lymphoma. Small mononuclear cell consistent with lymphocyte. Nuclear diameter is 1 to $1\frac{1}{2}$ times the erythrocyte diameter. Nucleoli are prominent. ($\times$500.)

FIG. 6-52. Canine. Cerebrospinal fluid. Lymphoma. (Same case as Fig. 6-51.) Two lymphocytes with moderate light basophilic cytoplasm and nuclei with multiple nucleoli. ($\times$630.)

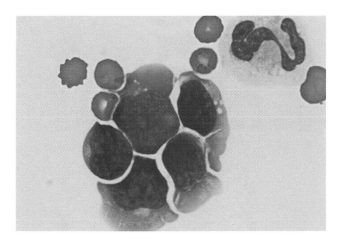

FIG. 6-53. Canine. Cerebrospinal fluid. Lymphoma. Closely aggregated lymphocytes, approximately two red blood cells in nuclear diameter. High N:C ratio and prominent nucleoli suggest a diagnosis of lymphoma. ($\times$500.)

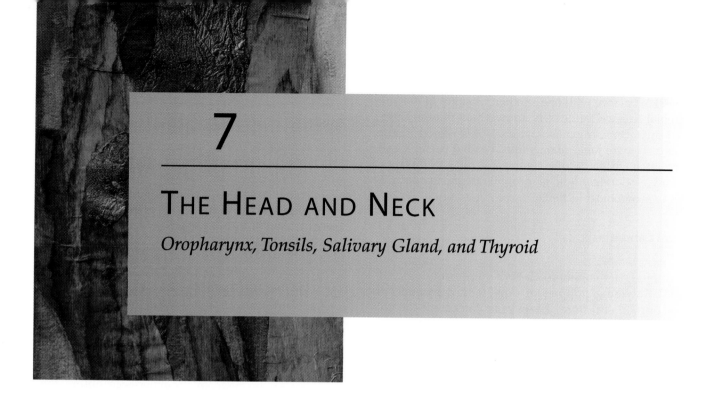

7

THE HEAD AND NECK

Oropharynx, Tonsils, Salivary Gland, and Thyroid

Diseases of the oropharyngeal cavity are common in the dog and cat. Presenting clinical signs vary widely, depending on the inciting lesion. Whereas inflammatory lesions are often treated before cytological investigation, intraoral masses may be aspirated before therapy and may assist in giving prognostic indicators to owners before expensive therapy begins. This chapter includes diseases of the oral cavity, including disorders of the tonsil and salivary gland. Diseases of the oropharyngeal lymph nodes other than the tonsil are discussed in Chapter 5.

TECHNIQUE

Lesions visible in the oral cavity are easily swabbed or scraped. The material is gently smeared onto a glass slide and stained as previously described. FNA is preferred for intraoral or tonsillar lesions, but sedation is often required. Techniques are described in Chapter 2. The cellular yield from periodontal masses is often minimal as a result of the stromal nature of many of the epulides. If aspiration biopsy fails to yield significant cells, a scraping of a tissue biopsy will often assist the diagnosis.

■ *OROPHARYNX*

NORMAL OROPHARYNX (Figs. 7-1 to 7-3)

A scraping of normal oropharynx contains many pleomorphic bacteria. The bacteria are free and adherent to the surface of mature, partially keratinized squamous epithelial cells. The squamous cells vary in maturity.

The oldest cells have blue-green cytoplasm and a condensed, small nucleus. Younger squames have larger nuclei and blue cytoplasm. Characteristic oral bacteria, such as *Simonsiella* spp., are usually present. Their palisading appearance is due to the parallel apposition of the bacteria.

NONNEOPLASTIC DISEASE

Several diseases of the oral cavity can be diagnosed using cytological techniques. The ease of sample collection, especially for superficial lesions, allows for ready examination, thus assisting final clinical decisions or demonstrating the need for additional investigative procedures. In some circumstances, for example, thrush, a final diagnosis can be made.

Pharyngitis, Gingivitis, Stomatitis, and Glossitis

CLINICAL DIAGNOSIS
Inflammation of the oral cavity usually presents with signs of excessive drooling, halitosis, and reluctance to chew or swallow. The inciting cause may be obvious (dental abnormalities) or may not lend itself to cytological evaluation (neuromuscular or autoimmune disorders). Oral inflammation associated with bacterial or fungal elements can be diagnosed from a simple smear preparation.

CYTOLOGICAL DIAGNOSIS
Bacterial Inflammation
Smears prepared from the oral cavity contain large numbers of pleomorphic bacteria. A monomorphic population of bacteria should alert the examiner to problems. *Actinomyces* spp., *Fusobacterium* spp., and

spirochetes normally inhabit the oral cavity (Tyler, 1999) in balance with one another. Changes in this microbial balance can lead to an overgrowth of individual organisms. *Nocardia* spp. may be involved. These anaerobes are long, filamentous, beaded bacteria and are often visible within neutrophil phagolysosomes. Many moderately lytic neutrophils frequently accompany anaerobic infections.

Oral Candidiasis

CLINICAL DIAGNOSIS
Although not common, *Candida* can infect dogs, especially young puppies or dogs with disruption of the normal oral flora. These yeast infect and inhabit the superficial layers of the epithelium (Barker, 1993).

CYTOLOGICAL DIAGNOSIS
Candida organisms have a characteristic appearance. They are thin-walled budding yeast, 2 to 6 μm in diameter, which form short tubular septate pseudohyphae (See Fig. 13-19).

Eosinophilic Granuloma Complex

CLINICAL DIAGNOSIS
Eosinophilic ulcers, linear granuloma, and eosinophilic plaque are grouped historically within the eosinophilic granuloma complex. Although these entities are not likely related, precedence continues to link them together (Barker, 1993). Eosinophilic ulcer is a superficial ulcerative condition typically found at the mucocutaneous junction of the lips but can also locate in the oral mucosa and skin (Barker, 1993). Linear granuloma, although commonly found on the skin, can also be seen on the tongue, gingiva, or palate (Barker, 1993). Eosinophilic plaque is a cutaneous lesion of cats that occasionally affects the oral cavity and is considered to be related to a hypersensitivity disorder. Recurrence after various therapies is common (Barker, 1993; Tyler, 1999).

CYTOLOGICAL DIAGNOSIS
Despite the name, eosinophilic ulcer is histologically associated with a neutrophilic and/or plasmacytic/mast cell inflammatory reaction (Barker, 1993). In both linear granuloma and eosinophilic plaque, eosinophils and mast cells predominate in histological sections. Large epithelioid macrophages, plump fibroblasts, and giant cells present in histological sections of linear granulomas would be expected in cytological preparations. The cytological picture of this complex has not been adequately studied, although large, reactive fibroblasts and eosinophils have been noted (Tyler, 1999).

NEOPLASTIC DISEASE

Epulis

CLINICAL DIAGNOSIS
Any tumorlike mass on the gingiva is classified as an epulis. Many hyperplastic, inflammatory, and neoplastic-like lesions are included within this umbrella diagnosis. Examples are giant cell epulis, fibrous hyperplasia, fibromatous epulis, and acanthomatous epulis (Barker, 1993). These lesions can be differentiated readily by histological but not cytological examination. Acanthomatous epulides tend to recur locally and may invade alveolar bone, whereas surgical excision is effective with the other lesions.

CYTOLOGICAL DIAGNOSIS
Although cytological reports are limited, some generalizations can be made. In our experience, fibromatous epulides yield poorly cellular samples containing rare, benign-appearing stromal cells. Many samples are nondiagnostic. In contrast, acanthomatous epulis yields benign squamous epithelial cells in various stages of maturation (Tyler, 1999).

NEOPLASTIC DISEASES OF THE ORAL CAVITY (Fig. 7-4)

In the dog and cat, malignant oral tumors account for 6% and 7%, respectively, of all neoplasms (Tyler, 1999). Oral tumors are more common in animals older than 7 years of age (Barker, 1993). Presenting clinical signs include excessive salivation, halitosis, dysphagia, and signs specific to tumor location (Barker, 1993). The oral mucosa is the fourth most common site of malignant tumors in the dog (Barker, 1993). The prognosis is poor for all oral malignant tumors in the dog and cat because the tumors usually follow a rapid clinical course (Barker, 1993).

Squamous Cell Carcinoma

CLINICAL DIAGNOSIS
In the dog, squamous cell carcinomas are second to melanomas in frequency, with the tonsil being the most common site. In the cat, squamous cell carcinoma is the most common oral malignancy, with the frenulum of the tongue the most common site (Barker, 1993; Stebbins, 1989). The gingivae are the next most common site for squamous cell carcinoma in dogs and cats (Barker, 1993).

CYTOLOGICAL DIAGNOSIS
The appearance of squamous cell carcinoma is described in Chapter 4.

Melanoma

CLINICAL DIAGNOSIS

Melanomas are the most common neoplasm of the canine oral cavity (Barker, 1993). Most oral melanomas are malignant and have a very poor prognosis. The majority have metastasized at the time of diagnosis, often to the submandibular lymph node (Barker, 1993). Oral melanomas are rare in cats (Barker, 1993).

CYTOLOGICAL DIAGNOSIS

The cytological appearance of melanomas is described in Chapter 4.

Fibrosarcoma

CLINICAL AND CYTOLOGICAL DIAGNOSES

Fibrosarcoma, unlike other oral neoplasms, is commonly reported in younger dogs (Barker, 1993). Fibrosarcoma is the third most common intraoral neoplasm of dogs (Barker, 1993), locating most frequently in the gingivae of the upper molars and the anterior lower mandible. Metastasis to regional nodes and recurrence after surgical resection occur frequently (Barker, 1993). Bone invasion is commonly observed in dogs (Barker, 1993). Fibrosarcoma is the second most common oral neoplasm of cats (Barker, 1993). The cytological description of fibrosarcoma is included in Chapter 4.

■ TONSIL

NORMAL TONSIL (Figs. 7-5 to 7-7)

The cytological harvest from a normal tonsil is somewhat confusing. The lymphoid component is a pleomorphic mixture of small to large lymphocytes, with small lymphocytes predominating. Many plasma cells may be present, especially if there is intraoral inflammation. Large squamous epithelial cells are interspersed with lymphocytes. These squamous cells can be misinterpreted as squamous cell carcinoma. Many of the tonsillar squames have large nuclei with an irregular chromatin pattern. The normal tonsillar cytological appearance must be considered when squamous cell carcinoma is suspected in a clinical case.

NONNEOPLASTIC DISEASE

CLINICAL AND CYTOLOGICAL DIAGNOSES

Benign tonsillar lesions are seldom examined in dogs and cats. The tonsil is aspirated if there is suspicion of neoplasia. The appearance of normal tonsillar cells must be known. Benign enlargement of the tonsil may

result from inflammatory conditions within the oral cavity, causing reactive change in the lymphatic tissue within the tonsil. Reactive hyperplasia of the nodal tissue is described in Chapter 5. Increased neutrophils are expected in inflammatory conditions involving the tonsil.

NEOPLASTIC DISEASE

CLINICAL AND CYTOLOGICAL DIAGNOSES

Squamous cell carcinoma is the primary consideration when neoplasia of the tonsil is suspected clinically. Next to melanoma, tonsillar squamous carcinoma is the most frequent oral cavity tumor in dogs (Barker, 1993). Tonsillar squamous cell carcinomas are locally invasive and may metastasize to regional nodes or distant organs, such as the lung (Barker, 1993).

Malignant squamous epithelial cells must be differentiated from benign squamous cells aspirated from the normal tonsil. With malignancy there is pronounced anisocytosis and variability in nuclear size. Nuclear cytoplasmic dissociation and nucleoli are often prominent. Remnants of a benign population of lymphocytes may be seen. A reactive hyperplasia with an associated increase in plasma cells may be present if the tumor is ulcerated and infected. The appearance of squamous cell carcinoma is also described in Chapter 4.

■ SALIVARY GLAND

NORMAL SALIVARY GLAND (Figs. 7-8 to 7-12)

The salivary gland is often aspirated inadvertently when investigating lesions in the neck and throat region. Aspiration smears from normal salivary gland contain pale blue epithelial cells arranged singly or in tight clusters, suggesting papillary or acinar origin. These cells have small, regular, eccentric nuclei with an even chromatin pattern. The cytoplasm is pale blue and granular to foamy, suggestive of secretory activity. Characteristic intercellular blue matrix is occasionally seen. Red blood cells may be arranged linearly because of the mucin content. Small clumps or sheets of dark cells may be ductular epithelial cells.

NONNEOPLASTIC DISEASE

Sialoadenitis

CLINICAL AND CYTOLOGICAL DIAGNOSES

Inflammation of the salivary gland is seldom diagnosed antemortem but is reported during postmortem examinations (Carberry, 1988; Spangler, 1991). The cytological presentation of sialoadenitis includes neutrophils, macrophages, and lymphocytes. Bacteria may be seen. Rabies and distemper are associated with sialoadenitis, but no documentation of the aspiration appearance is available (Carberry, 1988), although lymphocytes would be expected.

Mucocoele (Figs. 7-13 to 7-16)

CLINICAL DIAGNOSIS

Salivary mucoceles are the most common salivary disorder in the dog (Barker, 1993). Mucoceles locate most commonly in the cranial cervical area or on the floor of the mouth (ranulae) (Carberrry, 1988; Tyler, 1999). Mucoceles usually develop after blunt trauma but also occur secondary to inflammatory conditions that cause blockage of the ductal system. Mucoceles are uncommon in the cat.

CYTOLOGICAL DIAGNOSIS

Fluid aspirated from a mucocele is sticky and tenacious. Resulting smears are thick with a light blue mucinous background. The thickness of the smear reduces cell spreading and slows drying, resulting in dark pyknotic cells that provide limited morphological details. Large, foamy macrophages can be difficult to differentiate from epithelial cells. Moderate numbers of nonlytic neutrophils may be present. With secondary infection, neutrophils predominate and bacteria may be seen. Recognition of the characteristic blue mucin becomes critical for identification of the primary disorder.

NEOPLASTIC DISEASE

Salivary Carcinoma (Figs. 7-17 to 7-19)

CLINICAL DIAGNOSIS

Salivary carcinomas are the most common tumor of the salivary gland in the dog and cat, occurring more frequently in animals older than 10 years. Salivary carcinomas account for less than 0.2% of all tumors (Carberry, 1988). Salivary carcinomas may be slightly more common in cats (Spangler, 1991). Of the neoplastic salivary glands, 84% were malignant in dogs and cats (Carberry, 1988). Both the parotid and the mandibular salivary glands are cited as the most commonly affected gland (Carberry, 1988; Spangler, 1991). Of 85 cat salivary glands submitted for biopsy or examined during necropsy, 36 were diagnosed with neoplasia, the most common salivary disorder diagnosed in these cats (Spangler, 1991). In dogs, 41 of 160 salivary glands examined were neoplastic. It was the second most common diagnosis (Spangler, 1991). In dogs and cats, 75% to 85% of salivary tumors are adenocarcinomas (Carberry, 1988), frequently acinar cell in ori-

gin. Salivary carcinomas tend to recur after surgical excision and often metastasize to regional nodes and lungs (Barker, 1993; Carberry, 1988).

CYTOLOGICAL DIAGNOSIS

Adenocarcinomas of the salivary gland can be difficult to diagnose using cytological techniques. Cellularity is usually high, but in many tumors there is minimal cell pleomorphism. Cells are obviously epithelial and arranged in clusters or acinar formations. Cytoplasmic vacuolation may be prominent and with signet ring cells reflects the secretory nature. Anaplastic variants of these tumors occur and are diagnosed using the usual criteria of malignancy.

■ THYROID

Thyroid, salivary, and lymph node lesions are common palpable masses in the neck region of dogs and cats. FNA biopsies provide ready differentiation of thyroid origin. In the dog, carcinomas predominate, whereas in the cat, benign hyperplasia is more frequently diagnosed.

TECHNIQUE

Standard techniques are used to aspirate palpable neck masses. The vascularity of thyroid tissue may require modification of the aspiration technique to prevent dilution of cells. Use of decreased vacuum and cessation of aspiration immediately upon the observation of blood entering the tip of the syringe reduces dilutional effects. The aspirate is ejected onto a glass slide. The slide is tilted to allow blood to flow onto a gauze sponge, leaving visible clumps of tissue on the glass slide. The tissue clumps are transferred and spread, or gently squashed over a clean glass slide as for marrow granules. Alternatively, a needle may be inserted into the thyroid tissue and withdrawn. A syringe with plunger withdrawn is attached and used to eject needle contents onto a glass slide. Repeated aspirations may be required before obtaining representative cellular samples. In one study, 33% of the specimens contained only blood (Thompson, 1980).

NORMAL THYROID GLAND (Figs. 7-20 TO 7-22)

Thyroid epithelial cells are round to cuboidal with obvious cell borders. Acinar arrangements may be present. The cells have a low N:C ratio with little nuclear variability. Gray-blue amorphous colloid is often present as background material and less frequently within intact acinar structures. Perinuclear blue-black granulation is helpful in identifying the thyroid origin of the epithelial cells. These intracytoplasmic granules appear to represent tyrosine accumulation, but similar-appearing blood origin pigments may be seen free and within macrophages (Perman, 1979).

NONNEOPLASTIC DISEASE

CLINICAL AND CYTOLOGICAL DIAGNOSES

Nonneoplastic or hyperplastic conditions of the thyroid are rarely encountered in the dog. Feline hyperplastic and adenomatous changes are described under neoplastic conditions.

NEOPLASTIC DISEASE

Canine Thyroid Adenoma/Carcinoma (Figs. 7-23 to 7-28)

CLINICAL DIAGNOSIS

In dogs, thyroid gland tumors account for 1% to 4% of all canine neoplasms (Birchard, 1981; Capen, 1993; Leav, 1976; Leblanc, 1991). Thyroid adenomas may be palpably enlarged, but most are detected as an incidental finding during necropsy. Dogs with thyroid carcinomas frequently present with a palpable enlargement in the laryngeal region. Pressure on surrounding tissues or invasion of local vessels may create clinical signs resulting from interference with gastrointestinal, respiratory, or laryngeal function. If the tumor is functional, up to 10% of dogs may present with clinical signs associated with hyperthyroidism (Peterson, 1995) or occasionally hypothyroidism (Haley, 1989). Thyroid carcinomas in the dog grow rapidly, are very invasive, and frequently metastasize to the lungs (Bentley, 1990; Harari, 1986; Leblanc, 1991). Most thyroid carcinomas are tumors of follicular cells. Medullary carcinomas derived from parafollicular C cells are rare in dogs and cats (Patnaik, 1991).

In a series of 141 thyroid tumors in dogs, 44 adenomas and 97 carcinomas were diagnosed (Leav, 1976). Adenomas were usually small solid or cystic masses without well-defined capsules, but the largest were several centimeters in diameter (Leav, 1976). The cystic fluid was clear amber or blood-tinged, containing necrotic debris and red cells. A follicular pattern was observed in 43 of these adenomas (Leav, 1976). The cellular pattern varied within the carcinomas, with follicular and solid architecture observed less frequently than mixed follicular-solid cellularity (Leav, 1976). Other cell types were observed, including secondary tumors. In a study involving 17 dogs with clinically detectable masses, all were carcinomas (Sullivan, 1987). In a report including 26 thyroid tumors, 23 carcinomas were detected clinically and 3 adenomas were detected incidentally at necropsy (Harari, 1986). In 16 cases of canine thyroid tumors, 14 were malignant and 2 were benign (Birchard, 1981). Four of the 14 had

metastasis to the lung and 1 had metastasis to the local lymph node (Birchard, 1981). Average age at the time of diagnosis was 6.6 years (Birchard, 1981).

In 17 surgically treated dogs with carcinoma, the median survival time was 7 months (Harari, 1986). The size of tumor at diagnosis correlated well with prognosis and the probability of metastasis (Bentley, 1990). Beagles, boxers, and golden retrievers may have a higher risk than other breeds (Leav, 1976). In a series of beagles, increasing development of neoplasia late in life did not affect average life span even though 12% of tumor-bearing dogs died as a result of the neoplasm (Haley, 1989).

CYTOLOGICAL DIAGNOSIS

Aspirates are usually quite cellular with a heavy background of red blood cells. Cells may be present singly, in sheets or clusters, and occasionally with typical follicular cell clusters or acini. The usual cytological criteria of malignancy apply to thyroid carcinomas: increased N:C ratio, anisokaryosis, and multiple prominent nucleoli. Because cellular atypia is limited in well-differentiated carcinomas, differentiation from adenomas on the basis of cytology can be difficult. Thyroid cells normally have very little anisokaryosis, so when variation is present, it is a useful differentiating feature. Intracellular or extracellular blue-green pigment may be present in both benign and malignant lesions. From 11 dogs with thyroid carcinomas, based on histopathology, a positive or suspicious diagnosis was made for 10 cytology aspirates with one false negative (Thompson, 1980). In another study, a correct cytological diagnosis was made in 8 of 17 cases (Harari, 1986). Nondiagnostic specimens had too few epithelial cells or were too contaminated with blood to permit an accurate assessment (Harari, 1986).

Feline Adenomatous Hyperplasia (Figs. 7-29 to 7-34)

CLINICAL DIAGNOSIS

Hyperthyroid syndrome in cats is due primarily to benign adenomatous hyperplasia of the thyroid gland (Ferguson, 1991), with only 1% to 2% caused by thyroid carcinomas (Thoday, 1992). The severe and progressive clinical signs in hyperthyroid cats necessitates treatment. Choices include thyroid ablation using radioactive iodine, surgery, or the administration of antithyroid drugs.

CYTOLOGICAL DIAGNOSIS

In many cats with suspected hyperthyroidism the thyroid gland may not be enlarged, making aspiration difficult if not impossible. No reports describe cytological differentiation for benign hyperplasia, adenomas, and carcinomas in cats. In our experience, benign adenomatous hyperplasia has minimal cellular atypia, similar to that observed from normal thyroid cells in dogs. Many intracellular and extracellular pigmented granules may correlate with cellular activity and the clinical signs of hyperthyroidism. Cystic central cavities associated with an adenoma may yield pigment-laden macrophages, red blood cells, and cholesterol crystals (Maddux, 1999).

References

Barker, I.K., Van Dreumel, A.A., and Palmer, N. The alimentary system. In *Pathology of Domestic Animals, vol 2*. ed 4.. K.V.F. Jubb, P.C. Kennedy, and N. Palmer (eds). Academic Press, San Diego, 1993.

Bentley, J.F., Simpson, S.T., Hathcock, J.T., et al. Metastatic thyroid solid-follicular carcinoma in the cervical portion of the spine of a dog. *J Am Vet Med Assoc* 197:1498-1500, 1990.

Birchard, S.J. and Roesel, O.F. Neoplasia of the thyroid gland in the dog: a retrospective study of 16 cases. *Am Anim Hosp Assoc* 17:369-375, 1981.

Capen, C.C. The endocrine glands. In *Pathology of Domestic Animals, vol 2*. ed 4. K.V.F. Jubb, P.C. Kennedy. and N. Palmer (eds). Academic Press, San Diego, 1993.

Carberry, C.A., Flanders, J.A., Harvey, H.J., et al. Salivary gland tumors in dogs and cats: a literature and case review. *Am Anim Hosp Assoc* 24:561-567, 1988.

Ferguson, D.C. and Hoenig, M. Feline hyperthyroidism. In *Small Animal Medicine*. D.G. Allen (ed). JB Lippincott, Philadelphia, 1991.

Haley, P.J., Hahn, F.F., Muggenburg, B.A., et al. Thyroid neoplasms in a colony of beagle dogs. *Vet Pathol* 26:438-441, 1989.

Harari, J., Patterson, J.S., and Rosenthal, R.C. Clinical and pathologic features of thyroid tumors in 26 dogs. *J Am Vet Med Assoc* 188:1160-1163, 1986.

Leav, I., Schiller, A.L., Rijnberk, A., et al. Adenomas and carcinomas of the canine and feline thyroid. *Am J Pathol* 83: 61-93, 1976.

Leblanc, B., Parodi, A.L., Lagadic, M., et al. Immunocytochemistry of canine thyroid tumors. *Vet Pathol* 28:370-380, 1991.

Maddux, J.M. and Shull, R.M. Subcutaneous glandular tissue: mammary, salivary, thyroid and parathyroid. In *Diagnostic Cytology of the Dog and Cat*. ed 2. R.L. Cowell and R.D. Tyler (eds). Mosby, St Louis, 1999.

Patnaik, A.K. and Lieberman, P.H. Gross, histologic, cytochemical, and immunocytochemical study of medullary thyroid carcinoma in sixteen dogs. *Vet Pathol* 28:223-233, 1991.

Perman, V., Alsaker, R.D., and Riis, R.C. *Cytology of the Dog and Cat*. American Animal Hospital Association, South Bend, Ind, 1979.

Peterson, M. Hyperthyroid diseases. In *Textbook of Veterinary Internal Medicine*. ed 4. S.J. Ettinger and EC Feldman (eds). WB Saunders, Philadelphia, 1995.

Spangler, W.L. and Culbertson, M.R. Salivary gland disease in dogs and cats: 245 cases (1985-1988). *J Am Vet Med Assoc* 198:465-469, 1991.

Stebbins, K.E., Morse, C.C., and Goldschmidt, M.H. Feline oral neoplasia: a ten-year survey. *Vet Pathol* 26:121-128, 1989.

Sullivan, M., Cox, F., Pead, M.J., et al. Thyroid tumors in the dog. *J Small Anim Pract* 28:505-512, 1987.

Thoday, K.L. and Mooney, C.T. Medical management of feline hyperthyroidism. In *Current Veterinary Therapy XI*. R.W. Kirk and J.D. Bonagura (eds). WB Saunders, Philadelphia, 1992.

Thompson, E.J., Stirtzinger, T., Lumsden, J.H., et al. Fine needle aspiration cytology in the diagnosis of canine thyroid carcinoma. *Can Vet J* 21:186-188, 1980.

Tyler, R.D., Cowell, R.L., and Meinkoth, J.H. The oropharynx and tonsils. In *Diagnostic Cytology and Hematology of the Dog and Cat*. ed 2. R.L. Cowell, R.D. Tyler, and J.H. Meinkoth (eds). Mosby, St Louis, 1999.

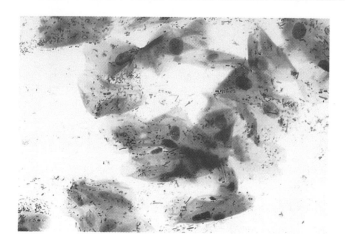

FIG. 7-1. Canine. Scraping. Normal gingiva. Intermediate to superficial squamous epithelial cells with typical lightly basophilic cytoplasm and round to angular borders. Adherent and free bacteria are visible. (×100.)

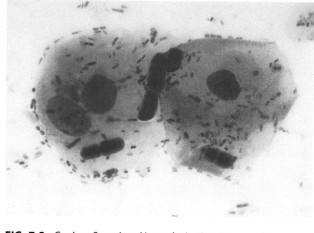

FIG. 7-2. Canine. Scraping. Normal gingiva. Intermediate squamous epithelial cells with adherent oral bacterial flora. The large *Simonsiella* sp. organisms are small rod-shaped bacteria arranged in parallel fashion. (×400.)

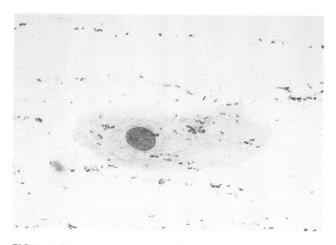

FIG. 7-3. Canine. Scraping. Normal gingiva. One large intermediate squamous epithelial cell with abundant pink cytoplasm and adherent oral bacterial flora. (×250.)

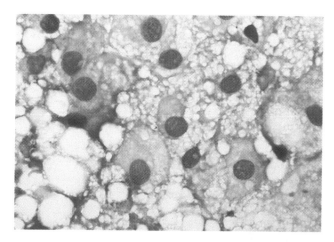

FIG. 7-4. Canine. Fine needle. Tongue mass. Oncocytoma. Loosely arranged cells with uniform central, round nuclei and abundant, pale, amorphous to finely granular cytoplasm. The significance of the vacuolation is uncertain but may indicate secretory function of some cells. Oncocytomas are rare, slow-growing adenomas of parotid and other small glands. Differentiation from other benign and malignant tumors may require histological examination. (×250.)

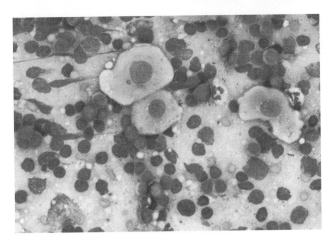

FIG. 7-5. Canine. Fine needle. Normal tonsil of young dog. There is a heterogeneous population of intact and ruptured lymphocytes and three epithelial cells with intermediate squamous differentiation. (×100.)

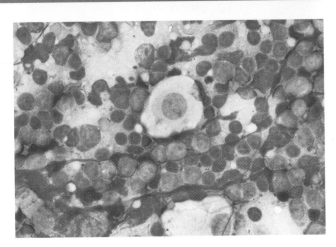

FIG. 7-6. Canine. Fine needle. Normal tonsil. (Same case as Fig. 7-5.) Many intact lymphocytes. The intermediate squamous epithelial cells have indistinct basophilic cytoplasmic aggregates common in any differentiating squamous epithelial population. (×200.)

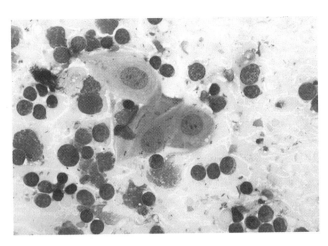

FIG. 7-7. Canine. Fine needle. Normal tonsil. Mixed population of lymphocytes, bare nuclei, and squamous epithelial cells with cytoplasmic basophilia and angular borders. (×200.)

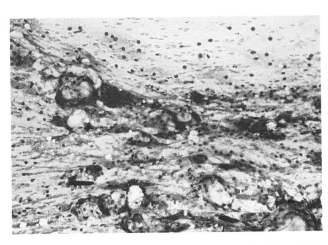

FIG. 7-8. Canine. Fine needle. Normal salivary gland. Basophilic mucin creates a "streaming" effect of the cellular elements when spread on a glass slide. Occasional acinar formations. (×50.)

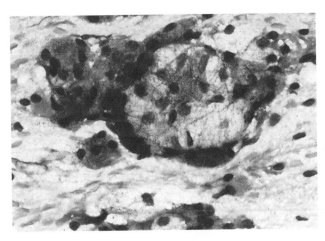

FIG. 7-9. Canine. Fine needle. Normal salivary gland. Acinar origin is suggested by the arrangement of secretory epithelial cells. Note low N:C ratio. (×200.)

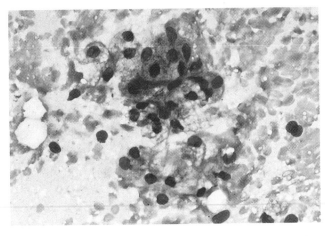

FIG. 7-10. Canine. Fine needle. Normal salivary gland. Cytoplasmic vacuolation, basophilia, and cellular arrangement consistent with acinar secretory cells. (×100.)

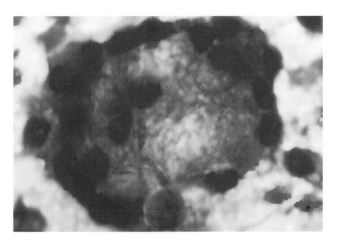

FIG. 7-11. Canine. Fine needle. Normal salivary gland. Typical acinar arrangement with peripheral nuclei and basophilic staining consistent with mucin. (×400.)

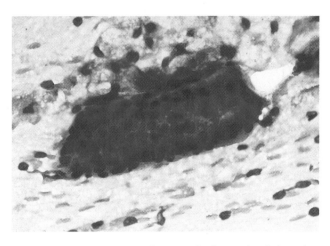

FIG. 7-12. Canine. Fine needle. Normal salivary gland. The tubular arrangement of the large sheet of epithelial cells suggests ductal rather than acinar origin. (×100.)

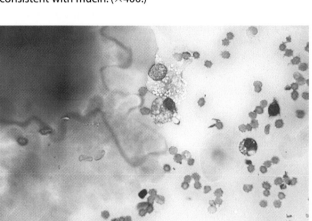

FIG. 7-13. Canine. Fine needle. Salivary mucocele. Basophilic light to dense amorphous background material is consistent with mucin. Cellularity is often low, especially in the absence of inflammation. (×100.)

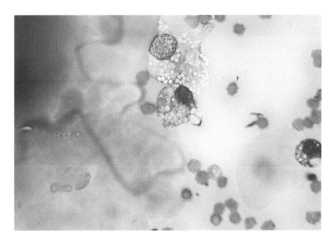

FIG. 7-14. Canine. Fine needle. Salivary mucocele. (Same case as Fig. 7-13.) Increased magnification of Fig. 7-13. Basophilic mucin, a few vacuolated mononuclear cells, and erythrocytes. The typical vacuolated mononuclear cells have been called mucinophages. Red blood cells are frequently observed within mucocele aspirates, possibly associated with trauma to the mass. (×250.)

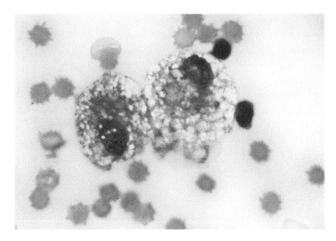

FIG. 7-15. Canine. Fine needle. Salivary mucocele. (Same case as Fig. 7-13.) Background of erythrocytes and macrophages with erythrophagocytosis indicates hemorrhage. The mucin slows cell drying, resulting in nuclear condensation and decreased ability to identify cells. (×400.)

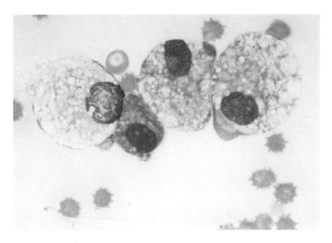

FIG. 7-16. Canine. Fine needle. Salivary mucocele. (Same case as Fig. 7-13.) Macrophages or mucinophages, with abundant vacuolated cytoplasm and a background of erythrocytes. (×400.)

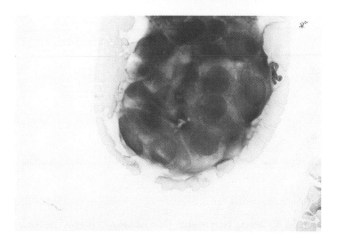

FIG. 7-17. Feline. Fine needle. Salivary carcinoma. A dense cluster of epithelial cells with some anisokaryosis and a moderate amount of basophilic cytoplasm. The cell arrangement suggests glandular origin without limitation to salivary tissue. The nuclear details visible within this illustration are insufficient to diagnose malignancy. (×200.)

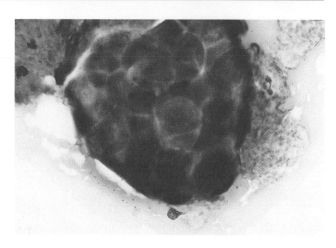

FIG. 7-18. Feline. Fine needle. Salivary carcinoma. (Same case as Fig. 7-17.) A cluster of epithelial cells that appear to have a high N:C ratio, anisokaryosis, and prominent nucleoli. The cytological details suggest a carcinoma; however, evidence of salivary differentiation is lacking. (×200.)

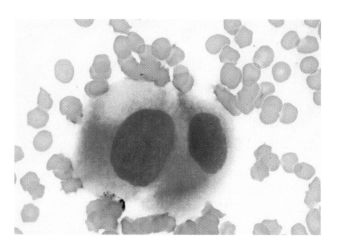

FIG. 7-19. Feline. Fine needle. Salivary carcinoma. (Same case as Fig. 7-17.) Two cells with amorphous basophilic cytoplasm, marked anisokaryosis, and large hyperchromatic nuclei. Nuclear details are consistent with neoplasia, but there is insufficient cytoplasmic differentiation to confirm salivary origin. (×400.)

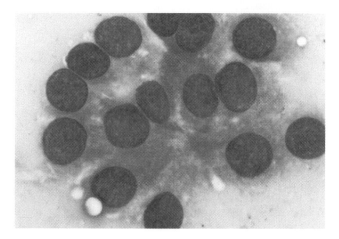

FIG. 7-20. Canine. Imprint. Normal thyroid gland. Uniform-appearing cells with abundant cytoplasm and some variation in nuclear size. There is a fine chromatin pattern and small, indistinct nucleoli. The cytoplasm is diffusely blue-gray, with some variation in density. Cellular pattern suggestive of acinar origin. (×400.)

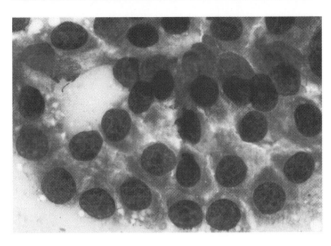

FIG. 7-21. Canine. Imprint. Normal thyroid gland. Sheet of thyroid epithelial cells with evidence of adjoining borders. There is abundant blue-gray cytoplasm, with some variation in density. These cytoplasmic tinctorial properties are typical of thyroid epithelial cells. (×400.)

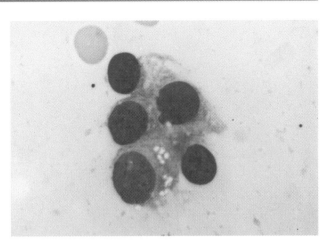

FIG. 7-22. Canine. Imprint. Normal thyroid gland. Epithelial cells with moderate N:C ratio, mild anisokaryosis, and amorphous chromatin pattern. The cytoplasm contains some small vacuoles and aggregated ribonucleic acid (RNA), suggestive of colloid precursors. (×500.)

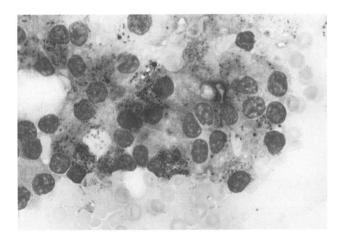

FIG. 7-23. Canine. Fine needle. Thyroid adenoma. Cohesive epithelial cells with indistinct cytoplasmic borders and moderately basophilic cytoplasm. There is minimal cellular atypia observed. Without adequate morphological criteria of malignancy or an anaplasia, it can be very difficult to distinguish between benign and malignant thyroid tumors. (×250.)

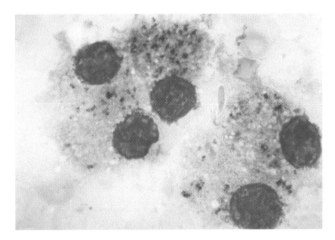

FIG. 7-24. Canine. Fine needle. Thyroid adenoma.(Same case as Fig. 7-23.) Epithelial cells with intracytoplasmic blue to black granular material that likely represents glandular secretory product (thyroglobulin). (×500.)

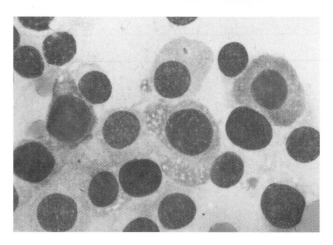

FIG. 7-25. Canine. Fine needle. Thyroid carcinoma. Moderately cohesive epithelial cells with round nuclei and a moderate amount of light basophilic cytoplasm. There is moderate anisokaryosis and mild cytoplasmic vacuolation. There are several free nuclei as often observed in aspirates from endocrine tumors. (×400.)

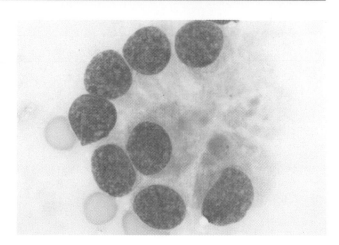

FIG. 7-26. Canine. Fine needle. Thyroid carcinoma. (Same case as Fig. 7-25.) Acinar arrangement of epithelial cells with a moderate amount of light basophilic granular cytoplasm and common adjoining borders. Lightly basophilic intracytoplasmic material may represent secretory product. (×500.)

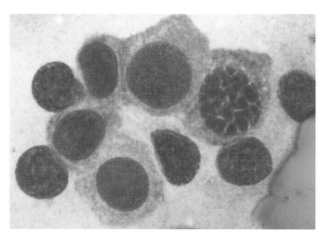

FIG. 7-27. Canine. Fine needle. Thyroid carcinoma. (Same case as Fig. 7-25.) Epithelial cells with marked anisocytosis, anisokaryosis, and one mitotic figure. Fine gray-blue cytoplasmic stippling and vacuolation is consistent with thyroid epithelial cells and aids the cytologist in confirming adequacy of sampling. (×630.)

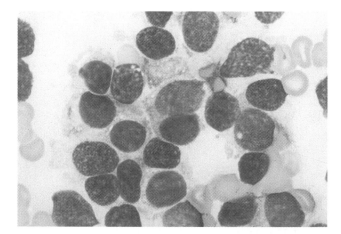

FIG. 7-28. Canine. Fine needle. Thyroid carcinoma. Moderately cohesive epithelial cells with mild anisocytosis and anisokaryosis and lightly basophilic granular cytoplasm. Free nuclei are also observed in the preparation. Red blood cells are present and are frequently observed because thyroid tumors can be highly vascular. (×400.)

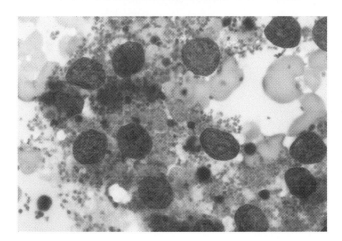

FIG. 7-29. Feline. Fine needle. Hyperthyroidism. Adenomatous hyperplasia. Epithelial cells have indistinct cytoplasmic borders and abundant moderate to marked basophilic granular material. Differentiation of feline adenomatous hyperplasia and carcinoma may be impossible from a cytological examination and requires close correlation with clinical information. (×400.)

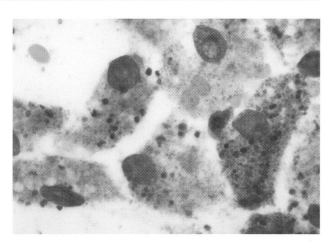

FIG. 7-30. Feline. Fine needle. Hyperthyroidism. (Same case as Fig. 7-29.) Adenomatous hyperplasia. Cells have a marked accumulation of deep basophilic granular material that represents increased production of glandular secretory product (thyroglobulin). Prominent cytoplasmic granulation appears to be characteristic of adenomatous hyperplasia, likely correlating with the hyperthyroid status of the cat. (×400.)

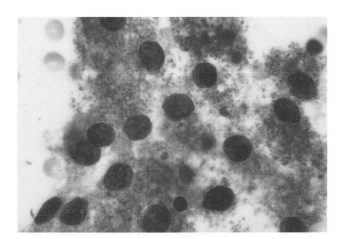

FIG. 7-31. Feline. Fine needle. Hyperthyroidism. Adenomatous hyperplasia. (Same case as Fig. 7-29.) Prominent cytoplasmic granulation, some of which has aggregated into larger globules. Note low N:C ratio of cells. (×400.)

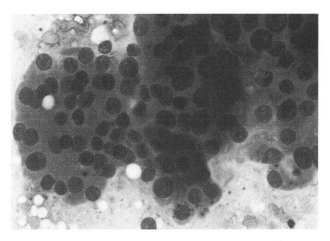

FIG. 7-32. Feline. Imprint. Thyroid adenocarcinoma. Large, cohesive sheet of epithelial cells with moderate to marked anisokaryosis and indistinct cytoplasmic borders. Blue-black cytoplasmic granules are present. (×200.) (Courtesy R. Gossett, 1991.)

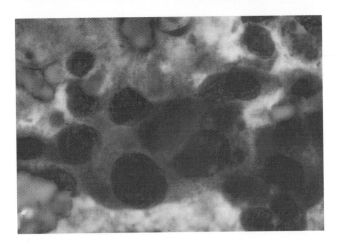

FIG. 7-33. Feline. Imprint. Thyroid adenocarcinoma. (Same case as Fig. 7-32.) Epithelial cells with marked anisokaryosis and blue-black cytoplasmic granulation. (×400.) (Courtesy R. Gossett, 1991.)

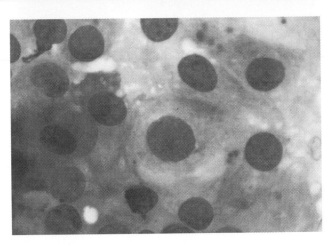

FIG. 7-34. Feline. Imprint. Thyroid adenocarcinoma. Thyroid epithelial cells with small aggregates of secretory product. Large nuclei, in comparison with the erythrocyte, and marked anisokaryosis are evident. (×400.)

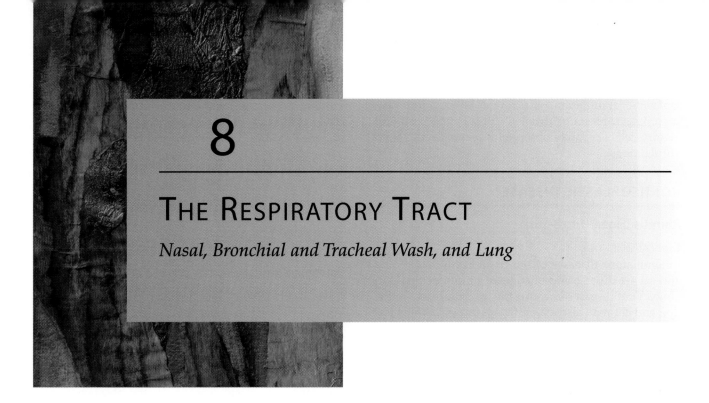

8

THE RESPIRATORY TRACT

Nasal, Bronchial and Tracheal Wash, and Lung

■ *NASAL*

Nasal cytological evaluation can be used as a rapid, noninvasive screening procedure of nasal lesions. Cytological examination of the nasal passage is most helpful when a definitive cause is found. A negative result may be due to the limitations of the blind biopsy techniques described for this location (French, 1987).

TECHNIQUE

In the dog or cat a chronic nasal discharge or sneezing may initiate cytological investigation of suspect lesions. Radiographic imaging should be used for guidance where lesions are discernible. Several techniques are described. Nasal swabs are the easiest but also the least useful. A cotton-tipped swab is inserted into the nasal cavity through the external nares and vigorously rubbed against the wall. The swab is gently rolled over the surface of a glass slide that is air dried and stained with Wright's stain.

A nasal wash technique is described. General anesthesia is induced in the patient. An endotracheal tube is inserted before passage of a polyethylene catheter into the nasal passageway. Between 5 and 10 ml of nonbacteriostatic sterile saline is flushed into the nose and then vigorously reaspirated. Multiple aspirates with repeated intermittent vigorous positive and negative pressure are applied to the syringe to dislodge fragments of tissue (Rakich, 1989; Rudd, 1985). Cells aspirated in the fluid are concentrated by centrifugation, and a smear is made of the sediment. Imprints are made of solid tissue fragments observed in the fluid or on the end of the catheter. Larger fragments are fixed

in formalin. In one study using this procedure, neoplastic cells were identified in 50% of the animals with histologically confirmed malignancy (MacEwen, 1977).

If a mass is apparent either radiographically or via rhinoscopy, the mass can be aspirated directly using a long, small-gauge needle. An alternative procedure is described using a tomcat catheter (Sherwood Medical). The tip is cut on a 45-degree angle to provide a cutting surface. The catheter is moved into and through the intranasal mass while gentle suction is applied using an attached large syringe (Rakich, 1989). Impression smears are made of the tissue samples, which can then be placed in formalin fixative for histopathology.

The vascularity of the nasal area leads to marked hemorrhage in many patients. Severe hemorrhage is a problem for the patient and clinician but also interferes with the quality of cytological samples, especially if coagulation is initiated. There is a strong suspicion that success rates would be higher if FNA were used routinely, especially where imaging could be used to improve accuracy in sampling lesion sites.

NORMAL NASAL CAVITY

A nasal swab or imprint made from healthy nasal tissue contains mature squamous epithelial cells and free or adherent mixed bacteria, including *Simonsiella*, as part of the normal flora. Basilar epithelial cells, some with cilia, may be included if vigorous swabbing techniques are used. Pseudostratified columnar epithelial cells line the nasal turbinates and are present in most nasal washes. Deeper into the nasal cavity, squamous epithelial cells are reduced and the proportion of columnar cells is increased (Rebar, 1988). Occasional goblet cells are observed containing metachromatic cytoplasmic granulation or a single, large, lightly basophilic cytoplasmic "droplet" (Rebar, 1988). Inflammatory cells are rarely observed in a nasal wash from normal dogs.

NONNEOPLASTIC DISEASE

Rhinitis (Figs. 8-1 to 8-10)

CLINICAL DIAGNOSIS

Inflammatory diseases of the nasal cavity in the dog and cat are diverse and often have a multifactorial etiology. Viral diseases infecting the upper airways in the dog and cat may also affect the nasal cavity. The nasal cavity is susceptible to opportunistic infection by bacteria and many fungal agents. Several specific infectious agents are associated with rhinitis. Cryptococcosis is the most frequent cause of granulomatous rhinitis in cats (Birchard, 1995; Dungworth, 1993), whereas *Aspergillus fumigatus* is the most common cause in dogs (Dungworth, 1993). Although *Aspergillus* spp. and *Penicillium* spp. are found in the nasal passage of healthy dogs, the organisms can cause nasal and sinus infections, often secondary to trauma, neoplasia, or immunosuppression (Rudd, 1985). Dolichocephalic breeds are predisposed.

CYTOLOGICAL DIAGNOSIS

Rhinitis is classified as purulent (neutrophils predominate), mixed (mixed neutrophils and monocyte/macrophages), mononuclear (mixed monocyte/macrophages and lymphocytes), or eosinophilic.

Epithelial hyperplasia is observed in response to inflammation or neoplasia. The epithelial cells have an increased N:C ratio and mild to moderate anisocytosis. Increased numbers of cuboidal cell rafts may be present. Epithelial hyperplasia (proplasia) can be very difficult to distinguish from a well-differentiated nasal carcinoma. Goblet cell hyperplasia develops in response to many irritations involving the nasal cavity.

If fungi are suspected, careful searching is required because the numbers are often low and the organisms stain poorly. A slow review of the slide, especially at the edges of necrotic clumps of cell debris, may be required to find the organisms. *Aspergillus* and *Penicillium* hyphae are septate, branching, and 4 to 6 μ wide (Rakich, 1989).

Rhinosporidiosis (Figs. 8-11 and 8-12)

CLINICAL AND CYTOLOGICAL DIAGNOSES

Rhinosporidium seeberi is a fungal organism responsible for canine polypoid intranasal masses detectable on rhinoscopy. With *Rhinosporidium* infection, spores may be numerous or rare. The spores are 5 to 10 μ in diameter and have a refractile, reddish-pink capsule when using Wright's stain. Spores contain many small, spherical bodies. Large sporangia are rarely seen but can exceed 100 μ. The spores stain magenta, which helps distinguish the large sporangia from *Coccidiomycosis* spores, which can appear similar but stain blue (Rakich, 1989). The inflammatory response is variable, with macrophages, lymphocytes, plasma cells, and neutrophils all present.

Allergic Rhinitis (Figs. 8-13 and 8-14)

CLINICAL AND CYTOLOGICAL DIAGNOSES

Allergic rhinitis is observed in dogs and cats. Lymphoplasmacytic rhinitis is uncommon but is also believed to have an immune-mediated cause (Gartrell, 1995). In the dog and cat, allergic rhinitis is characterized by the presence of increased neutrophils and/or eosinophils in nasal washes, in the absence of any causal agent, but before the institution of antibiotics. Lymphoplasmacytic rhinitis is characterized histologically by an infiltration of lymphocytes and plasma cells (Gartrell, 1995).

NEOPLASIA (Figs. 8-15 TO 8-22)

Nasal Neoplasia

CLINICAL DIAGNOSIS

Bloody nasal discharge, sneezing, and nasal swelling are clinical signs common to bacterial and fungal rhinitis, as well as nasal tumors. In the dog, tumors of the nose and paranasal sinuses are responsible for approximately 1% of all tumors (Norris, 1979; Rakich, 1989). In the cat, nasal tumors are responsible for 1% (Legendre, 1981) to 5.9% when tumors of the nasal planum are included (Cox, 1991). Of these tumors, 80% in the dog and 91% in the cat are malignant (Legendre, 1981; MacEwen, 1977). In dogs, dolichocephalic breeds and middle-aged to older dogs appear to be predisposed (Rudd, 1985; Theisen, 1996). Adenocarcinomas account for 68% to 75% of canine nasal tumors (Cox, 1991; Legendre, 1983; Norris, 1979), whereas in cats, squamous cell carcinomas are the most frequent (Cox, 1991; MacEwen, 1977). The prognosis for intranasal tumors of all types is generally poor. Death is due to local invasion rather than metastasis (Cox, 1991; MacEwen, 1977; Norris, 1979). Radiotherapy of the nasal planum in 16 cats with squamous cell carcinomas resulted in a 62% 1-year survival rate (Cox, 1991).

In a group of canine sinonasal neoplasms, 16% were soft-tissue tumors (Patnaik, 1989). Histological types included lymphoma (26.6%), fibrosarcoma (22%), and hemangiosarcoma (16%) (Patnaik, 1989). As with carcinomas, the prognosis is poor because of local invasion (Patnaik, 1989).

CYTOLOGICAL DIAGNOSIS

Cytological diagnosis of intranasal neoplasia can be a diagnostic challenge to the cytologist. Bacterial invasion, tissue necrosis, and inflammation are frequently associated with hyperplastic and dysplastic changes in epithelial cells. Caution should be exercised in diagnosing neoplasia when inflammation is present. Histological confirmation may be required.

In one study in dogs, five of eight samples were diagnostic for cancer using a nasal swab technique (Norris, 1979). Two submissions were required from four cases to confirm neoplasia using nasal flushes, whereas each of the three cases sampled using FNA were diagnosed correctly (Norris, 1979). Overall, 77% of the cases were correctly diagnosed as having cancer in the nasal cavity by cytological methods (Norris, 1979).

Diagnosis of nasal carcinoma is based on the usual features of malignancy: anisokaryosis, hyperchromasia, and a high N:C ratio. The changes in morphology are often subtle and can resemble those observed with hyperplastic or dysplastic epithelium. A pink, amorphous background is often observed that appears to be due to mucus production. Individual cells may contain large, intracellular vacuoles suggestive of secretory product. Cells may be arranged singly or in acinar arrangements. If the tumor is well vascularized, hemorrhage may be a prominent feature. Squamous cell carcinomas are described cytologically in Chapter 4.

Round cell tumors observed in the nasal cavity include lymphosarcoma (see Chapter 5), transmissible venereal cell tumors (see Chapter 4), and mast cell tumors (see Chapter 4).

Stromal tumors can develop in the nasal region. Their cytological appearance is reported elsewhere (see Chapter 11). Stromal masses, especially chondrosarcoma, frequently secrete a pink, amorphous ground substance that can be so plentiful that it obscures cellular details.

■ *BRONCHIAL AND TRACHEAL WASH*

Cytological examination of respiratory airways using wash, brush, or aspiration biopsy provides information regarding the presence and type of inflammation, infectious agents, and neoplasia. The clinical differential diagnosis predetermines the expected usefulness of cytological examinations. In addition, the representativeness of the sample also influences the reliability of the cytological interpretation.

METHODS

Tracheal Wash (Figs. 8-23 to 8-30)

CANINE

A transtracheal wash may be performed using manual restraint in most dogs. Sedation, if required, should not abolish the cough reflex. The area over the cricothyroid membrane, or the trachea at the thoracic inlet, is surgically prepared and infiltrated with lidocaine. With the dog in sternal recumbency and the neck extended, an intravenous catheter needle is inserted into the trachea at a 45-degree angle (Allen, 1991). A 14- to 16-gauge, 12- to 18-inch catheter with stylet is inserted through the needle into the trachea. The needle and stylet are removed. Between 3 and 10 ml of nonbacteriostatic saline is infused and aspirated as soon as a cough is elicited. Approximately 20% of infused fluid is usually recovered. The procedure is repeated 3 to 4 times to ensure adequate sample recovery. A pressure bandage is applied after removal of the catheter, and the animal is monitored closely for 2 to 3 hours (Allen, 1991).

FELINE

Tracheal washes are performed under general anesthesia. A 22-gauge catheter can be passed directly, or a polypropylene urinary catheter can be passed through an endotracheal tube to limit oropharyngeal contamination (Hawkins, 1994). The catheter is passed down the trachea to the thoracic inlet and 0.5 ml/kg of warm sterile nonbacteriostatic saline is infused and gently reaspirated (Padrid, 1990). Alternatively, 3 ml of sterile saline is infused and aspirated, then repeated at least once (Hawkins, 1994).

Bronchoalveolar Lavage

CANINE

In bronchoalveolar lavage (BAL), a sterile endotracheal tube is inserted into the airway of the anesthetized dog. A sterile fiberoptic bronchoscope is passed through the endotracheal tube and wedged in a distant bronchus. A 25-ml aliquot of warm sterile nonbacteriostatic saline is flushed through the bronchoscope into the bronchus and immediately aspirated through the bronchoscope attachment (Brown, 1983; Hawkins, 1990a). Repeated infusion and aspiration may be required (Hawkins, 1990a).

FELINE

In the anesthetized cat the tip of an endotracheal tube is passed just rostral to the carina and the cuff is inflated. Between 3 and 5 ml/kg aliquots of warmed sterile saline are infused and aspirated. Mild suction is applied using a 35-ml syringe attached to the endotracheal tube with a syringe adapter (Hawkins, 1989; Hawkins, 1990b; Hawkins, 1995a). The large volume of fluid is assumed to collect cells exfoliating from the bronchial surface (Rebar, 1988). Another procedure is described in which a sterile 14-gauge catheter with metal stylet is passed to the end of the endotracheal tube. The stylet is removed. The catheter is advanced a further 2 to 4 cm. After infusing 2 to 3 ml of sterile saline, the fluid is aspirated with a 12-ml syringe attached to the catheter (Moise, 1983).

Optimally, feline BAL is performed through a fiberoptic bronchoscope as in the dog. The end of the endoscope is wedged into the bronchus of one lung lobe and 2 ml/kg of sterile saline is instilled (Hawkins, 1991; Padrid, 1991b). Availability of equipment limits use of this preferred technique.

Bronchial Brush Biopsy

Bronchial brush biopsies provide excellent cytological preparations and selective sampling of bronchial lesions. The brush is passed through the biopsy port of the bronchoscope, rotated several times within the airway, and retracted into the bronchoscope. The brush is removed and gently agitated in 5 ml of sterile physiological saline to collect adherent cells (Rebar, 1980). Aliquots of fluid may be cultured and processed for cytological examination. Cells may be gently transferred directly from the brush to a glass slide for staining and microscopic examination.

PROCESSING OF SAMPLES

Cells adherent to biopsy brush or catheter tips can be transferred immediately onto glass slides for staining and microscopic examination. Fluid samples must be processed as soon after collection as possible to preserve cell details. Cells may be counted, but the interpretative value is limited unless reference values have been developed that consider animal size, volume of fluid instilled and aspirated, and disease process being investigated. Cells are concentrated, using a centrifuge, onto glass slides for staining and examination.

NORMAL TRACHEAL WASH IN THE DOG (Figs. 8-23 TO 8-31)

Tracheal wash specimens from healthy dogs contain limited numbers of columnar and cuboidal respiratory epithelial cells, many of which are ciliated. Occasional neutrophils and macrophages are present. Mucous strands can be seen in the background. Oropharyngeal bacteria are regarded as contaminants. Frequency of bacteria and the cellular inflammatory response aid in determining the significance of bacteria present on the smear. Tracheal wash cultures are usually negative (Hawkins, 1995a).

NORMAL BAL IN THE DOG

There is wide variation in BAL cell reference values reported from clinically healthy dogs. The variation appears to be due to within-animal variation and the influence of BAL fluid collection procedures and sample processing. Cell counts of 400 to 500×10^6/L are reported in BAL fluid from normal dogs (Hawkins, 1990a; Rebar, 1980).

The average percentage of nucleated cells observed in the BAL fluid from 10 healthy dogs, collected using 140-ml infusions, was 50.5% macrophages, 46% lymphocytes, and 3.5% neutrophils (Brown, 1983). Another study reported 80% to 95% macrophages, 1% epithelial cells, and less than 5% neutrophils (Rebar, 1980). In a study of 14 healthy purpose-bred dogs, BAL fluid contained 87% macrophages, 5% lymphocytes, 5% neutrophils, and 3% eosinophils (Baudendistel, 1992). In 18 random-source dogs, there were 69% macrophages, 3% lymphocytes, 3% neutrophils, and 24% eosinophils (Baudendistel, 1992). The high percentage of eosinophils was attributed to earlier parasite burdens in "mongrel" dogs (Baudendistel, 1992). In 18 beagles aged 2.5 to 10 years, with epithelial cells included in the differential, cell distribution was 35% lymphocytes, 42% macrophages, 1% to 2% neutrophils, and 15% epithelial cells (Mayer, 1990). Cell distribution was not affected by age (Mayer, 1990). In six dogs with histologically normal lungs, mean percentages of cells were 78% macrophages, 7% lymphocytes, 5% neutrophils, 6% eosinophils, 1% mast cells, and 1% epithelial cells (Hawkins, 1991).

NORMAL BAL IN THE CAT

There is controversy concerning the influence of technique and animal source on BAL reference values in the cat (Hawkins, 1991; Padrid, 1991a). Cell distribution from eight adult specific pathogen free (SPF) cats lavaged with 20 ml of saline through a blind catheter was 87% pulmonary alveolar macrophages and 10% eosinophils, whereas in eight conventional adult cats the mean cell distribution was 61% pulmonary macrophages and 29% eosinophils (McCarthy, 1989). Eosinophils were rare in young kittens, and neutrophils and lymphocytes accounted only for 1% to 3% of the total cells in adult cats (McCarthy, 1989). The BAL fluid collected through an endotracheal tube from 34 SPF cats contained total nucleated cells of 169 to 456 cells/μl with 78% macrophages, 5% neutrophils, 16% eosinophils, and 0.4% lymphocytes (Hawkins, 1994). Sequential aliquots were examined to determine the effects of combining aliquots (Hawkins, 1994). Differences were found between the cell distribution in the second and third aliquots compared with the combined three aliquots, but the differences were not considered of clinical significance (Hawkins, 1994).

In 11 clinically normal cats, BAL cell distribution was 7% neutrophils, 71% macrophages, 5% lymphocytes, and 16% eosinophils (King, 1989). The BAL mean nucleated cell count was 241 × 10^6/L (King, 1989). In seven cats with allergic or parasitic pulmonary disease there were 63% to 90% eosinophils in the BAL (King, 1989). These cats usually had BAL nucleated cell counts greater than 1000 × 10^6/L (King, 1989). Cats with BAL nucleated cell counts greater than 1000 × 10^6/L may help distinguish healthy cats with high eosinophil counts from cats with disease-associated increased eosinophils (King, 1989).

In another study, BAL fluid was collected from 14 pet cats, 6 random-source cats, and 4 SPF cats lavaged with 5 infusions of 10 ml through a bronchoscope (Padrid, 1991b). The average nucleated cell count for all 24 cats was 301 × 10^6/L (SD = 126) with an average of 25% (SD = 21%) eosinophils. Eosinophils were the predominant cell in the BAL from five cats, including one cat from the SPF colony (Padrid, 1991b). In eight cats lavaged through a bronchoscope, mean cell distribution was as follows: macrophages 60%, neutrophils 24%, eosinophils 11%, and lymphocytes 5%. The mean cell count was 280 × 10^6/L (Lecuyer, 1995). A wide range of eosinophil counts in BAL fluid of cats appears to be normal. Also, with sequential sampling it appears that eosinophil counts vary greatly within and between healthy cats (McCarthy, 1986; Padrid, 1991b). In another study, bronchial brush biopsy and endotracheal tube bronchial washes were performed on 15 healthy cats (Dye, 1992). The bronchial wash fluid contained 16% to 100% epithelial cells, and 25% to 30% macrophages with no fluid containing greater than 9% eosinophils (Dye, 1992). Bronchial brush biopsy on these cats contained a high percentage of epithelial cells, often up to 100% (Dye, 1992).

BAL CELL MORPHOLOGY (Figs. 8-32 TO 8-36)

Nucleated cells in BAL fluid include neutrophils, eosinophils, lymphocytes, goblet cells, macrophages, and epithelial cells. The ciliated epithelial cells vary from cuboidal to tall columnar. Apical terminal plates with extending cilia are prominent within some cells. The nuclei usually have a basilar location, just above a narrow tail of cytoplasm. There is often a small, clear zone above the nucleus. With hyperplasia in response to inflammation or increased cell turnover the cells have increased basophilic cytoplasm, larger nuclei, and possibly prominent nucleoli.

Alveolar macrophages are large (10-15 μ) and round. Cytoplasm is variably vacuolated and may contain blue to black particulate matter representing phagocytized inhaled contaminants or heme pigments. Other cell types include neutrophils, eosinophils, lymphocytes, plasma cells, and mast cells.

Squamous epithelial cells are routinely observed in tracheal wash fluids because these cells readily exfoliate from the oral mucosa onto the catheter or bronchoscope. Squamous epithelial cells are large with abundant blue-gray cytoplasm and a central pyknotic nucleus and often have adherent bacteria. If squamous cells are present in the tracheal or BAL fluid, caution should be used when interpreting results from bacterial culture because the bacteria may be normal oropharyngeal flora.

The BAL fluid from clinically healthy dogs contains low numbers of goblet cells, which are columnar with basilar, lightly staining nuclei. The cytoplasm contains round mucin granules that frequently distend the borders of the cell. Small concentrations of mucus are also found in the normal tracheal or bronchial wash. With air-dried slides and Romanowsky's stains the mucus is usually pink and homogenous. It may have a fibrillar appearance and occur in strands. Cells trapped within mucus dry more slowly and tend to round up, making identification difficult. Inspissated mucus can form casts within small bronchioles. The spiral casts of basophilic mucus, called Curschmann's spirals, are seen in association with excessive mucus production and are not restricted to respiratory tract origin.

NONNEOPLASTIC DISEASE

General Interpretation of Tracheal Wash (Figs. 8-37 to 8-43)

Diseases that affect the large airways and trachea are reflected in tracheal wash samples (Hawkins, 1995a). When there is coughing and mucus regurgitation, diseases of the lung parenchyma can be evaluated in tracheal wash specimens (Hawkins, 1995a).

Tracheal washes were performed in 42 dogs with bacterial bronchopneumonia. A septic purulent exudate was seen in 20 dogs and a mucopurulent exudate in 11 dogs. In 11 dogs, cytological examination did not suggest an inflammatory process (Thayer, 1984). Both BAL and tracheal washes were performed on dogs with respiratory tract disease for comparative purposes (Hawkins, 1995a). Tracheal washes and BAL cell harvest were different in 45 of 66 dogs (68%) for one or more of the following categories: inflammation, hemorrhage, infectious agents, and criteria of malignancy (Hawkins, 1995a). Although tracheal wash techniques are more readily accessible to clinicians, the limitations for diagnosis must be recognized.

General Interpretation of the BAL (Figs. 8-44 to 8-51)

Cytological examination of bronchoalveolar fluid can predict many histological changes in lungs. The histologic/cytologic correlation is best when the disease process is diffuse. The cytological response, based on

BAL nucleated cells, can be divided into six categories: neutrophilic, eosinophilic, mixed (chronic-active inflammation), hemorrhagic, lymphoid, and neoplastic. Increased mucus or goblet cell hyperplasia can be seen as a nonspecific response to any of the above categories. In one study, increased BAL goblet cells were associated with histological evidence of mucous metaplasia (Greenlee, 1984). BAL cytology is frequently not diagnostic for a specific type of lesion because most disorders involving the respiratory tract can present with any one or combination of the above cellular responses. When combined with physical examination, complete blood count (CBC), radiographs, and, where indicated, culture, cytological examination can make a significant contribution to the final clinical diagnosis. In a study involving 66 dogs with respiratory disease, BAL provided a definitive diagnosis in 25% and a supportive diagnosis in 50%, and was not helpful in 25% of the cases (Hawkins, 1995b). BAL was most helpful in diagnosing disease of the alveolar or bronchial tree or in pulmonary masses (Hawkins, 1995b). Lavage of multiple lung lobes improves the chances of identifying the primary disease process (Hawkins, 1995b).

In dogs with pulmonary mycosis, organisms were seen in six of nine dogs (Hawkins, 1990b). However, only three dogs had organisms present in every lobe lavaged (Hawkins, 1990b).

Neutrophilic inflammation is associated with bacterial infection but can be observed with parasites, neoplasia, allergic bronchitis, chronic bronchitis, mycoplasma, protozoa, aspiration pneumonia, and inhaled toxins (Hawkins, 1995a). Eosinophilic inflammation is most commonly associated with allergic bronchitis and less frequently with pulmonary parasites and heartworm (Hawkins, 1995a). A mixed inflammatory reaction containing a predominance of macrophages was called chronic, or chronic-active inflammation in the earlier veterinary cytology literature. Use of this terminology for cytological description is discouraged because of the different definitions for these terms used by histopathologists, cytologists, and clinicians. A mix of neutrophils and macrophages is nonspecific as to etiology (Greenlee, 1984). A mixed inflammatory response is observed in response to hemorrhage as indicated by hemosiderin-laden macrophages, erythrocytophagy, and erythrocyte concentration.

A pure population of lymphocytes is occasionally observed, suggesting a nonspecific immune response. Depending on morphology, a monotonous population of lymphocytes suggests that lymphoma be included in the differential diagnosis.

Neoplasia can be diagnosed with BAL and is superior to tracheal washes. Neoplastic cells must be carefully differentiated from hyperplastic epithelial cells. As in any tissue, if large numbers of inflammatory cells are present, caution must be exercised in the diagnosis of malignancy.

The respiratory syndromes with documented characteristic cytological descriptions are presented.

Canine Chronic Bronchitis (Figs. 8-52 to 8-58)

CLINICAL DIAGNOSIS
Chronic cough of obscure origin is one of the most common respiratory problems in the dog. Chronic airway inflammation and excess mucus production are hallmarks of chronic bronchitis (Padrid, 1992). Other causes of chronic cough must be excluded before making the diagnosis of chronic bronchitis. Underlying conditions and chronic bronchitis can coexist (Padrid, 1992).

CYTOLOGICAL DIAGNOSIS
Many neutrophils intermixed with mucus are routinely seen in tracheal wash specimens from dogs with chronic bronchitis. Increased alveolar macrophages are harvested using a bronchial wash. Intracellular bacteria may or may not be present (Padrid, 1992). Increased eosinophils are often present, which suggests an "allergic" component to the syndrome (Padrid, 1992). A clinical response after glucocorticoid therapy supports this conclusion.

Feline Bronchial Disease

CLINICAL DIAGNOSIS
Cats with bronchial disease present with a history of coughing, wheezing, or dyspnea. Typically there is no evidence of upper airway disease or radiographic evidence of irregular bronchial walls (Moise, 1989). In 65 affected cats, older female and Siamese cats were overrepresented (Moise, 1989). In another study, Siamese cats were overrepresented, accounting for 17% of 24 cats with bronchopulmonary disease (Dye, 1996).

CYTOLOGICAL DIAGNOSIS
In cats with bronchial disease the BAL fluid cytology frequently contains increased inflammatory cells intermixed with abundant mucus (Dye, 1992). The inflammatory response is categorized according to the predominant cell type. Bacteria were isolated from 25% to 40% of all cats with bronchial disease (Dye, 1992). *Pasteurella multocida* and *Moraxella* spp. are the usual etiologic agents. (Dye, 1992). However, the presence of inflammatory cells in the BAL wash did not correlate with a positive bronchial culture (Dye, 1996).

When used alone, BAL cytology was inadequate for evaluating disease in an individual cat (Moise, 1989). In 58 exudative bronchial washes, eosinophils were predominant in 24%, neutrophils in 33%, macrophages in 22%, and a mixed cell population in 21% (Moise, 1989). Mast cells were observed in all types of exudates (Moise, 1989). Peripheral blood eosinophilia did not predict the predominant cell type in bronchial exudates, although it did correlate with moderate to severe clinical disease (Dye 1992; Dye, 1996). In 24 cats with bronchopulmonary disease the BAL fluid contained decreased epithelial cells (Dye, 1996). The severely affected cats (based on pulmonary function tests and clinical and radiographic scoring) generally had an increase of eosinophils and/or neutrophils (Dye, 1996). In 17 of 22 affected cats, bronchial brush cytology did not reflect the inflammatory component seen in the wash cytology (Dye, 1996). Perhaps wash samples are more representative of intraluminal inflammatory cells than brush biopsies; however, further comparison studies are needed (Dye, 1996). Cats with bronchial disease frequently have abundant mucus (Dye, 1992).

Parastic Diseases (Figs. 8-59 to 8-68)

CLINICAL AND CYTOLOGICAL DIAGNOSES

Occasionally larva or parasitic eggs are found within tracheal or bronchial lavage samples. Dogs often present with a chronic, productive cough. Larvae that pass first larval stage in the sputum and feces are *Crenosoma vulpis, Oslerus osleri, Filaroides hirthi,* and *Filaroides milksi* (Andreasen, 1992; McConkey, 1997). Larva of *Filaroides osleri* can also be found on tracheal or bronchial washes because the adults are found in the submucosa of the tracheal bifurcation (Dungworth, 1993). *Aelurostrongylus abstrusus* is the most common lungworm of cats (Dungworth, 1993). Differentiation of the various parasitic lung infections is based on morphologic criteria using Baerman or zinc sulfate fecal flotation techniques (McConkey, 1997).

Cytologically, a highly cellular background with moderate to many eosinophils and a mix of neutrophils and macrophages is reported (McConkey, 1997). In one dog, a lung aspirate contained adult and larval nematodes (Andreasen, 1992). The smear contained many neutrophils, plasma cells, macrophages and a lower number of eosinophils (Andreasen, 1992). In our experience with intrapulmonary larvae the cytological response includes a mixed neutrophil/macrophage reaction with limited eosinophils. Further study is required.

Mycotic Infections (Figs. 8-69 and 8-70)

CLINICAL DIAGNOSIS

Organisms that cause systemic mycotic infections are found frequently in the respiratory tract as a result of their ubiquitous distribution and the airborne spread of the spores. The initial acute pulmonary infection is followed by either elimination of the infectious agents by the host or progression to a chronic pyogranulomatous pneumonia (Roudebush, 1992).

CYTOLOGICAL DIAGNOSIS

In tracheal wash and BAL cytology examined from seven dogs with pulmonary mycotic infections, five dogs had *Blastomyces* organisms in the BAL fluid and

three of five had the organisms in the tracheal wash (Hawkins, 1990b). Organisms were generally seen in greater numbers in the BAL than in the tracheal wash (Hawkins, 1990b). There was no typical cellular pattern because the inflammatory component varied from neutrophilic to eosinophilic to normal (Hawkins, 1990b). In one dog with coccidioidomycosis infection, no organisms were detected in either the tracheal wash or BAL (Hawkins, 1990b).

Mycoplasma

CLINICAL DIAGNOSIS

Mycoplasma organisms are normal flora within the canine pharynx (Randolph, 1993). In dogs older than 1 year, tracheobronchial lavage mycoplasma recovery rates were similar between dogs with and without pulmonary diseases (Randolph, 1993). Young dogs (<1 year old) with pulmonary disease and dogs with concurrent bacterial pulmonary infections may have increased susceptibility to mycoplasma colonization of the lower airways (Randolph, 1993).

Mycoplasma was not isolated from lavage fluid of 24 clinically healthy cats (Padrid, 1989; Padrid, 1991b) and may not normally inhabit the respiratory tract of the cat. Mycoplasma culture of lavage fluid has been recommended in wheezing cats with chronic bronchial disease (Padrid, 1990). Although the role of mycoplasma is unknown, significant numbers of cats with clinical signs of chronic disease have positive mycoplasma cultures (Padrid, 1990).

CYTOLOGICAL DIAGNOSIS

The typical cellular response observed in synovial fluid associated with mycoplasma infection is a predominance of abundant nonlytic neutrophils. It is suggested that the chemotactic response in BAL fluid might be similar depending on the stage of the disease.

Viral Pneumonia

CLINICAL DIAGNOSIS

Canine distemper virus, canine adenovirus, and feline calicivirus are frequently implicated in upper and lower respiratory infections (Roudebush, 1992).

CYTOLOGICAL DIAGNOSIS

In 19 SPF beagle puppies infected with canine adenovirus type 2 (CAV2), the percentage of neutrophils in the BAL fluid correlated directly with bronchiolar histological inflammation (Grad, 1990).

Pulmonary Infiltration with Eosinophils

CLINICAL DIAGNOSIS

Pulmonary infiltration with eosinophils (PIE) describes a set of allergic diseases in which pulmonary infiltration of the lung with eosinophils is the predominant pathological finding. This increase is frequently but not always associated with an increase in eosinophils in the tracheobronchial lavage fluid (Calvert, 1992). PIE is an inclusive term that encompasses alveolitis, bronchitis, eosinophilic pneumonia, and pulmonary eosinophilic granuloma (Corcoran, 1991). It has been suggested that the use of the term PIE be restricted to conditions in which an underlying cause cannot be found (Kuehn, 1995). In dogs that were sensitized neonatally to ragweed, challenge with the antigen caused an increase in eosinophils and mast cells in the BAL (Baldwin, 1993).

Pulmonary eosinophilic granuloma appears to be associated with *Dirofilaria immitis* approximately 80% of the time (Calvert, 1992; Neer, 1986). Pulmonary eosinophilic granuloma was accompanied by peripheral eosinophilia and/or basophilia in 13 of 19 dogs (Calvert, 1992).

CYTOLOGICAL DIAGNOSIS

The cytological picture is characterized by eosinophils with variable numbers of plasma cells, neutrophils, macrophages, and lymphocytes (Calvert, 1992).

NEOPLASTIC DISEASE

Neoplasia involving the bronchial tree can be diagnosed using bronchial and occasionally tracheal washes. A description of cell types is included in the section for diseases of the lung.

■ LUNG

Many diseases of the lung can be diagnosed using bronchial wash techniques, especially when there is diffuse disease of the pulmonary tree. However, isolated solitary lesions may require image-guided FNA biopsy. The following text refers to disorders not readily diagnosed by BAL and not previously described.

TECHNIQUE

Aspiration biopsy of the lung is an easy, safe method for diagnosing lung lesions (Roudebush, 1981). FNA is performed as previously described. The needle should be inserted on the cranial aspect of the rib to avoid intercostal vessels on the caudal rib border. Any part of the lung field may be aspirated, but isolated solitary lesions identified by radiography or ultrasonography can be targeted. The dorsal portion of the right caudal lung lobe is the preferred aspiration site for diffuse lesions. The lung is thickest in this area and therefore most accessible, minimizing risk of damage to other vital organs. Sedation is not usually required. The biopsy may be performed with the animal standing, sternal, or in a lateral position. Multiple aspirations are often necessary to obtain representative samples. The quantity of cells aspirated from the lung is typically small and may be contained within the needle. Allow the plunger to advance within the syringe to eliminate the vacuum before gently removing the needle in order to prevent aspiration of the small sample into the needle hub or syringe tip. Expel aspirate gently onto slides before preparing the monolayer of cells.

Scrapings and impressions of surgical or postmortem samples can be used to assist identification of disease processes. During surgery an impression smear of diseased lung tissue may allow immediate identification of the primary disorder, leading to selection of the appropriate surgical procedure.

Postsampling pneumothorax is a possible complication. Animals should be monitored closely for 24 hours. Lung laceration and hemorrhage are potential risks but uncommonly encountered. FNAs are contraindicated in animals with uncontrollable coughing.

NORMAL LUNG (Figs. 8-71 TO 8-78)

Aspirates from normal lung have poor cellularity. The direct smear background contains primarily erythrocytes. There may be occasional stromal and endothelial cells, sometimes in capillary formation. Typical macrophages and pulmonary epithelial cells are sometimes indistinguishable. Macrophages frequently contain phagocytized material, including pigments. Large vacuolated macrophages are occasionally seen. Aspirate smears from normal lung may contain single epithelial cells or pneumocytes. Both type I and type II pneumocytes may be seen. Type I pneumocytes line 90% to 95% of the alveolus (DeMay, 1996). Type II pneumocytes account for the remaining 5% and are responsible for surfactant production (DeMay, 1996). A distinction between type I and type II pneumocytes is not usually made cytologically. These alveolar cells are generally round to cuboidal with a basally located round to oval nucleus (Cowell, 1999). With hyperplasia, in humans, it is primarily the type II pneumocyte that becomes hyperplastic. (DeMay, 1996). These reactive pneumocytes can mimic carcinoma, demonstrating increased N:C ratio, macronucleoli, and multinucleation (DeMay, 1996). Ciliated and nonciliated columnar and cuboidal epithelial cells, as well as goblet cells, may be present in low numbers. These cells are identical to those seen in BALs. Neutrophils, eosinophils, lymphocytes, plasma cells, and mast cells may all be seen occasionally in the normal lung aspirate.

NONNEOPLASTIC CONDITIONS (Figs. 8-79 AND 8-80)

Most nonneoplastic conditions of the lung are readily diagnosed using BAL, and these have been described above. Occasionally, organisms such as blastomyces, not detected within BAL fluid, may be identified using a fine-needle aspirate. Aspirates from lungs with inflammatory disorders can be expected to contain similar cells as collected in a BAL. Hyperplastic and dysplastic epithelial changes are frequently observed in association with inflammation. Aspirates containing epithelial cells arranged in large aggregates, with increased N:C ratio, hyperchromasia, and moderate anisokaryosis, indicate epithelial response to inflammation. Caution should be exercised when diagnosing malignancies in these circumstances. As within other tissues, pneumonic inflammatory conditions are categorized according to the predominant cell type (see Chapter 2). Increased epithelial cells in the absence of severe inflammation may indicate pulmonary atelectasis (Larkin, 1994). Phagocytized erythrocyte breakdown products, such as hemosiderin and hematoidin, observed within pulmonary macrophages indicate previous intrapulmonary hemorrhage.

In one study including 41 dogs and 2 cats with widespread interstitial or multinodular lung disease, use of needle lung biopsy allowed diagnosis of malignancy in 24 cases (Teske, 1991). Cytological diagnosis under these conditions was accurate in 83% of the cases (Teske, 1991). In 22 of these cases, diagnosis was confirmed using histology. The 11 cases with inflammatory lesions were diagnosed correctly. The one false-positive cytological diagnosis of malignancy was found to be due to torsion of a middle lung lobe with resulting severe necrosis and fibroblastic proliferation. In our experience the marked inflammatory, fibroblastic, and mesothelial proliferation observed in lung lobe torsion can easily be mistaken for neoplasia. For the dogs in this study, although pneumothorax occurred in 31% of the cases, drainage was required in only 6% (Teske, 1991). The 18-gauge needle used in this study possibly increased the incidence of pneumothorax (Teske, 1991). In our experience a 22-gauge needle is found to be adequate and is associated with low risk.

Blind intrathoracic aspiration biopsies may result in aspiration from organs other than the lung. These ectopic tissues must be recognized to avoid misdiagnosis. In our experience, hepatic tissue is most frequently aspirated in error.

NEOPLASTIC DISEASE

Primary Lung Carcinoma (Figs. 8-81 to 8-84)

CLINICAL AND CYTOLOGICAL DIAGNOSES
Primary lung tumors of the dog and cat are rare. Affected dogs and cats are usually older, the average age being 10 to 12 years (Dungworth, 1993). In the dog, reported incidence is 4 to 5 per 100,000 animals (Dungworth, 1993; Ogilvie, 1989). The incidence of primary lung tumors in the cat is approximately half that of the dog (Dungworth, 1993). Most primary lung tumors are epithelial in origin (Dungworth, 1993). Ade-

nocarcinomas account for 77% and 72% of lung tumors in the dog and cat, respectively (Moulton, 1990). In 34 cats with primary pulmonary tumors, 83% were malignant (Wilson, 1997). The most common feline pulmonary tumor appears to originate from bronchial glands or airway epithelium and have a mixed basosecretory appearance (Wilson, 1997).

At the time of diagnosis, tumor development is often advanced, making the histogenetic tumor origin difficult to determine. Most tumors appear to be bronchogenic or bronchoalveolar in origin (Dungworth, 1993). Squamous differentiation is common. Bronchoalveolar carcinoma is the primary lung tumor found incidentally at necropsy. They typically appear as solitary tumors in the periphery of the lung lobe (Dungworth, 1993). The regular alveolar pattern of these tumors may be visible in the cytological preparation.

When examined cytologically, primary lung tumors resemble other epithelial tumors. On FNA, large clumps of epithelial cells may be accompanied by a heavy background of secretory product or mucus. Clusters and clumps of epithelial cells usually have prominent cell borders, marked hyperchromasia, frequent anisokaryosis, and cell crowding. An alveolar or papillary pattern may be prominent. The adenomatous cells may have single, large, secretory vacuoles (signet ring cells). An absence of cilia is a characteristic of malignant cells but is associated with dysplastic epithelial cells, as well. Accompanying severe inflammation is common. Epithelial changes secondary to inflammation can mimic neoplasia, and every effort must be made to differentiate this possibility. Well-differentiated carcinomas may be impossible to distinguish from severe dysplastic change. In one study the two most successful clinical methods of diagnosing pulmonary malignancy were radiography and cytology (Ogilvie, 1989). Fine-needle aspirates were helpful in diagnosing malignancy 24.8% of the time (Ogilvie, 1989).

Secondary Tumors of the Lung

CLINICAL AND CYTOLOGICAL DIAGNOSES
Multiple nodules scattered throughout the lung is the typical pattern for metastatic neoplasia. In dogs and cats, mammary and endocrine glands and skin are common origins for neoplastic lesions (Dungworth, 1993). Sarcomas may include osteosarcoma and hemangiosarcoma (Dungworth, 1993). The primary site may or may not be readily suggested during cytological examination of the metastatic lesion. However, combined with radiographic and other clinical data, it is frequently possible to differentiate metastatic epithelial from sarcomatous lesions. Aspiration of lung for confirmation of hemangiosarcoma is frequently requested. Cellularity is low for these stromal masses, and multiple attempts are frequently necessary. Care-

ful scanning of the slide for single aberrant stromal cells often supports or may confirm the diagnosis.

References

Allen, D.G. Special techniques. In *Small Animal Medicine*. D.G. Allen, S.A. Kruth, and M.S. Garvey (eds). JB Lippincott, Philadelphia, 1991.

Andreasen, C.B. and Carmichael, P. What is your diagnosis? *Vet Clin Pathol* 21:78,1992.

Baldwin, F. and Becker, A.B., Bronchoalveolar eosinophilic cells in a canine model of asthma: two distinctive populations. *Vet Pathol* 30:97-103, 1993.

Baudendistel, L.J., Vogler, G.A., Frank, P.A., et al. Bronchoalveolar eosinophilia in random-source versus purpose-bred dogs. *Lab Anim Sci* 42:491-496, 1992.

Birchard, S.J. Surgical diseases of the nasal cavity and paranasal sinuses. *Semin Vet Intern Med (Small Anim)* 10: 77-86, 1995.

Brown, N.O., Noone, K.E., and Kurzman, I.D. Alveolar lavage in dogs. *Am J Vet Res* 44:335-337, 1983.

Calvert, C.A. Eosinophilic pulmonary granulomatosis. In *Current Veterinary Therapy XI, Small Animal Practice*. R.W. Kirk and J.D. Bonagura (eds). WB Saunders, Philadelphia, 1992.

Corcoran, S.M., Thoday, K.L., Henfrey, J.I., et al. Pulmonary infiltration with eosinophils in 14 dogs. *J Small Anim Pract* 32:494-502, 1991.

Cowell, R.L., Tyler, R.D., and Baldwin, C.J. The lung parenchyma. In *Diagnostic Cytology of the Dog and Cat*. ed 2. R.L. Cowell and R.D. Tyler (eds). Mosby, St Louis, 1999.

Cox, N.R., Brawner, W.R., Powers, R.D., et al. Tumours of the nose and paranasal sinuses in cats: 32 cases with comparison to a national database (1977 through 1987). *J Am Anim Hosp Assoc* 27:339-347, 1991.

DeMay, R.M. Respiratory cytology. In *The Art and Science of Cytopathology, vol 1, Exfoliative Cytology*. R.M. DeMay (ed). American Society of Clinical Pathologists Press, Chicago, 1996.

Dungworth, D.L. The respiratory system. In *Pathology of Domestic Animals*. ed 4. K.V.F. Jubb, P.C. Kennedy, and N. Palmer (eds). Academic Press, San Diego, 1993.

Dye, J.A., McKiernan, C., Rozanski, E.A., et al. Bronchopulmonary disease in the cat: historical, physical, radiographic, clinicopathologic, and pulmonary functional evaluation of 24 affected and 15 healthy cats. *J Vet Intern Med* 10:385-400, 1996.

Dye, J.A. and Moise, N.S. Feline bronchial disease. In *Current Veterinary Therapy XI, Small Animal Practice*. R.W. Kirk and J.D. Bonagura (eds). WB Saunders, Philadelphia, 1992.

French, T.W. The use of cytology in the diagnosis of chronic nasal disorders. *Compend Cont Ed Pract* 9:115-121, 1987.

Gartrell, C.L., O'Handley, P.A., and Perry, R.L. Canine nasal disease—part 11. *Compend Cont Ed Pract* 17:539-546, 1995.

Grad, R., Sobonya, R.E., Witten, M.L., et al. Localization of inflammation and virions in canine adenovirus type 2 bronchiolitis. *Am Rev Respir Dis* 142:691-699, 1990.

Greenlee, P.G. and Roszel, J.F. Feline bronchial cytology: histologic/cytologic correlation in 22 cats. *Vet Pathol* 21: 308-315, 1984.

Hawkins, E.C. Tracheal wash and bronchoalveolar lavage in the management of respiratory disease. In *Current Veterinary Therapy XI*. R.W. Kirk and J.D. Bonagura (eds). WB Saunders, Philadelphia, 1995a.

Hawkins, E.C. and DeNicola, D.B. Collection of bronchoalveolar lavage fluid in cats, using an endotracheal tube. *Am J Vet Res* 50:855-859, 1989.

Hawkins, E.C. and DeNicola, D.B. Cytological analysis of tracheal wash specimens and bronchoalveolar lavage fluid in the diagnosis of mycotic infections in dogs. *J Am Vet Med Assoc* 197:79-83, 1990a.

Hawkins, E.C., DeNicola, D.B., and Kuehn, N.F. Bronchoalveolar lavage in the evaluation of pulmonary disease in the dog and cat. *J Vet Intern Med* 4:267-274, 1990b.

Hawkins, E.C., DeNicola, D.B., and Kuehn, N.F. Letter to the editor. *J Vet Intern Med* 5:53-55, 1991.

Hawkins, E.C., DeNicola, D.B., and Plier, L. Cytological analysis of bronchoalveolar lavage fluid in the diagnosis of spontaneous respiratory tract disease in dogs: a retrospective study. *J Vet Intern Med* 9:386-392, 1995b.

Hawkins, E.C., Kennedy-Stoskopf, S., Levy, J., et al. Cytologic characterization of bronchoalveolar lavage fluid collected through an endotracheal tube in cats. *Am J Vet Res* 55:795-802, 1994.

King, R.R. and Zeng, Q.Y. Further observation on the characterization of the alveolitis in cats with eosinophilic pneumonitis. *Am Coll Vet Intern Med Forum* 1044, 1989 (abstract).

Kuehn, N.F. Diagnostic methods for upper airway disease. *Semin Vet Med Surg (Small Animal)* 10: 70-76,1995.

Larkin, H.A. Veterinary cytology—cytological diagnosis of diseases of the respiratory tract in animals. *Irish Vet J* 47: 304-312, 1994.

Lecuyer, M., Dube, P.G, DiFruscia, R., Desnoyers, M., *et al*. Bronchoalveolar lavage in normal cats. *Can Vet J* 36: 771-773, 1995.

Legendre, A.M., Krahwinkel, D.J. and Spaulding, K.A. Feline nasal and paranasal sinus tumors. *J Am Anim Hosp Assoc* 17:1038-1039, 1981.

Legendre, A.M., Spaulding, K., and Krahwinkel, D.J. Canine nasal and paranasal sinus tumors. *J Am Anim Hosp Assoc* 19:115-123, 1983.

MacEwen, E.G., Withrow, S.J., and Patnaik, A.K. Nasal tumors in the dog: retrospective evaluation of diagnosis, prognosis and treatment. *J Am Vet Med Assoc* 170:45-48, 1977.

Mayer, P., Laber, G., and Walzl, H. Bronchoalveolar lavage in dogs. Analysis of proteins and respiratory cells. *Zendralbl Veterinarmed [A]* 37:392-399, 1990.

McCarthy, G. and Quinn, P.J. The development of lavage procedures for the upper and lower respiratory tract of the cat. *Irish Vet J* 40:6-9, 1986.

McCarthy, G.M. and Quinn, P.J. Bronchoalveolar lavage in the cat: cytological findings. *Can J Vet Res* 53:259-263, 1989.

McConkey, S., Horney, B., Conboy, G., et al. What is your diagnosis? *Vet Clin Pathol* 26:21,35, 1997.

Moise, N.S. and Blue, J. Bronchial washings in the cat: procedure and cytologic evaluation. *Compend Cont Ed Pract* 5:621-627, 1983.

Moise, N.S., Wiedenkeller, D., Yeager, A.E., et al. Clinical, radiographic, and bronchial cytologic features of cats with bronchial disease: 65 cases (1980-1986). *J Am Vet Med Assoc* 194:1467-1473, 1989.

Moulton, J. E. Tumors of the respiratory system. In *Tumors in Domestic Animals.* ed 3. J.E. Moulton (ed). University of California Press, Berkeley, Calif, 1990.

Neer, M. and Waldron, R. Eosinophilic pulmonary granulomatosis in two dogs and literature review. *J Am Anim Hosp Assoc* 22:595-599, 1986.

Norris, A.M. Intranasal neoplasms in the dog. *J Am Anim Hosp Assoc* 15:231-236, 1979.

Ogilvie, G.K., Haschekm, W.M., Withrow, S.J., et al. Classification of primary lung tumours in dogs: 210 cases (1975-1985). *J Am Vet Med Assoc* 195:106-108, 1989.

Padrid, P. Diagnosis and therapy of canine chronic bronchitis. In *Current Veterinary Therapy XI, Small Animal Practice.* R.W. Kirk and J.D. Bonagura (eds). WB Saunders, Philadelphia, 1992.

Padrid, P. Letter to the editor. *J Vet Intern Med* 5:52-53, 1991a.

Padrid, P., Feldman, B.F., Funk, K., et al. Cytologic, microbiologic, and biochemical analysis of bronchoalveolar lavage fluid obtained in 24 healthy cats. *Am J Vet Res* 52:1300-1307, 1991b.

Padrid, P., Feldman, B.F., Samitz, E., et al. Feline bronchoalveolar lavage. *Am Coll Vet Intern Med Forum* 1044, 1989 (abstract).

Padrid, P.A. and Koblik, P.D. The techniques used to diagnose feline respiratory disorders. *Vet Med* 85:956-985, 1990.

Patnaik, A.K. Canine sinonasal neoplasms: soft tissue tumours. *J Am Anim Hosp Assoc* 25:491-496, 1989.

Rakich, P.M. and Latimer, K.S. Cytology of the respiratory tract. *Vet Clin North Am Small Anim Pract* 19:823-850, 1989.

Randolph, J.F., Moise, N.S., Scarlett, J.M., et al. Prevalence of mycoplasmal and ureaplasmal recovery from tracheobronchial lavages and prevalence of mycoplasmal recovery from pharyngeal swab specimens in dogs with or without pulmonary disease. *Am J Vet Res* 54:387-391, 1993.

Rebar, A.H. and DeNicola, D.B. The cytological examination of the respiratory tract. *Semin Vet Med Surg (Small Anim)* 3:109-121, 1988.

Rebar, A.H., DeNicola, D.B., and Muggenburg, B.A. Bronchopulmonary lavage cytology in the dog: normal findings. *Vet Pathol* 17:294-304, 1980.

Roudebush, P. Infectious pneumonia. In *Current Veterinary Therapy XI, Small Animal Practice.* R.W. Kirk and J.D. Bonagura (eds). WB Saunders, Philadelphia, 1992.

Roudebush, P., Green, R.A., and Digilio, K.M. Percutaneous fine-needle aspiration biopsy of the lung in disseminated pulmonary disease. *J Am Anim Hosp Assoc* 17:109-116, 1981.

Rudd, G. and Richardson, D.C. A diagnostic and therapeutic approach to nasal disease in dogs. *Compend Cont Ed Pract* 7:103-111, 1985.

Teske, E., Stokhof, A.A., van den Ingh, T.S.G.A.M., et al. Transthoracic needle aspiration biopsy of the lung in dogs with pulmonic diseases. *J Am Anim Hosp Assoc* 27:291-294, 1991.

Thayer, G.W. and Robinson, S.K. Bacterial bronchopneumonia in the dog: a review of 42 cases. *J Am Anim Hosp Assoc* 20:731-736, 1984.

Theisen, S.K., Hosgood,G., and Lewis, D.D. Intranasal tumors in dogs: diagnosis and treatment. *Compend Cont Ed Pract* 18:131-138,1996

Wilson, D.W. Pulmonary neoplasia in cats. *Vet Pathol* 34: 485, 1997.

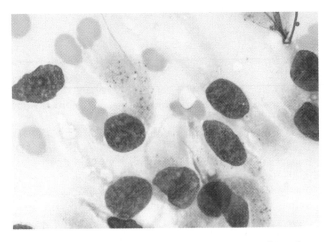

FIG. 8-1. Canine. Nasal flush. Nasal occlusion resulting from necrotizing rhinitis. Nasal columnar epithelial cells with basilar nuclei and indistinct metachromatic cytoplasmic granularity and cilia. Distortion and rupture of cells occurs readily within saline solutions. (×400.)

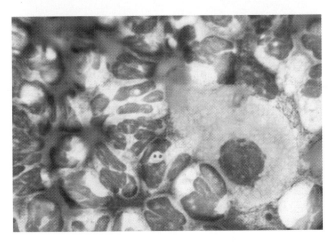

FIG. 8-2. Canine. Nasal flush. Septic suppurative inflammation. There are many neutrophils, a single epithelial cell, and a few phagocytized coccoid bacteria. (×500.)

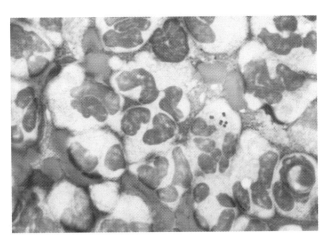

FIG. 8-3. Canine. Nasal flush. Septic suppurative inflammation. (Same case as Fig. 8-2.) Moderately degenerate neutrophils and intracellular bacteria. (×500.)

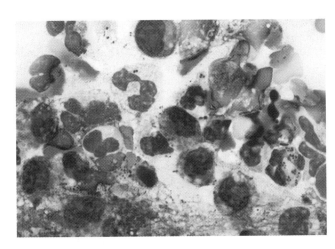

FIG. 8-4. Canine. Nasal flush. Septic inflammation. Mixed inflammatory response with mononuclear cells, neutrophils, and free and phagocytized bacteria. The azurophilic extracellular material may be mucin and/or nuclear debris. (×400.)

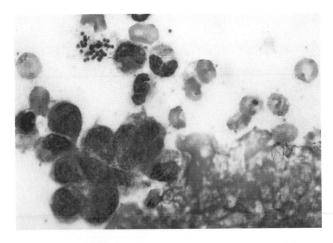

FIG. 8-5. Canine. Nasal flush. Septic inflammation. Basophilic epithelial cells are located adjacent to the mucinous material and a cluster of bacteria. Epithelial cell dysplasia is a common response to inflammation. (×400.)

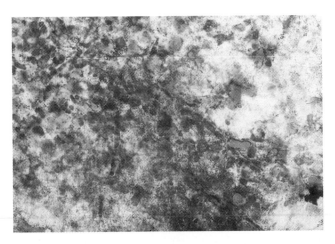

FIG. 8-6. Canine. Nasal flush. Mycotic rhinitis. There are numerous septate fungal hyphae visible within the cellular debris, erythrocytes, and mucus. Basophilic internal structures and the thin negative-staining wall help outline the hyphae. (×200.)

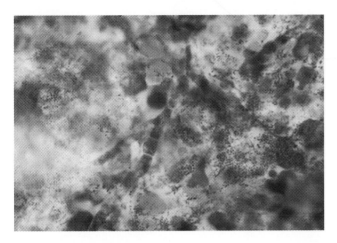

FIG. 8-7. Canine. Nasal flush. Mycotic rhinitis. Indistinct septate, branching, positively and negatively stained fungal hyphae are visible. The negative outlines of parallel walls may be the initial morphological indicator of fungal organisms. (×400.)

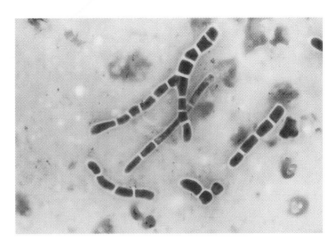

FIG. 8-8. Canine. Nasal flush. Mycotic rhinitis. Septate, branching hyphae and a few red blood cells. (×400.)

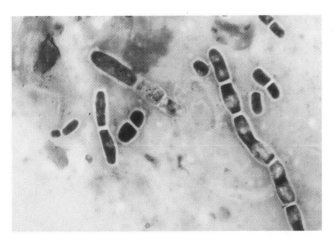

FIG. 8-9. Canine. Nasal flush. Mycotic rhinitis. Variably sized septate hyphae with amorphous background debris. Uptake of Romanowsky's stains by fungi is quite variable. (×400.)

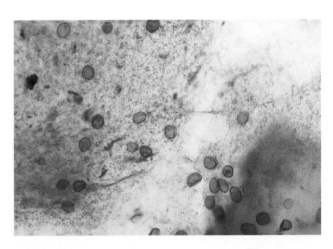

FIG. 8-10. Canine. Nasal flush. Mycotic rhinitis. Many round to oval, blue-green fungal spores are visible. The significance of fungal spores in nasal washes must be correlated with the presence of inflammatory cells and the holding environment of the animal. (×200.)

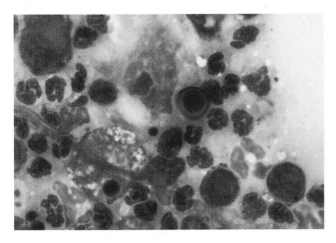

FIG. 8-11. Canine. Imprint. Nasal mass. Rhinosporidiosis. There is one round eosinophilic to pink *Rhinosporidium seeberi* endospore surrounded by mixed inflammatory cells. (×400.)

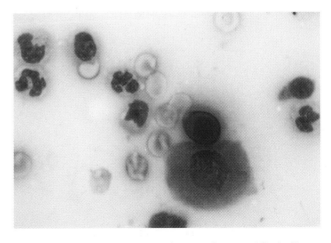

FIG. 8-12. Canine. Imprint. Nasal mass. Rhinosporidiosis. (Same case as Fig. 8-11.) A round *Rhinosporidium* endospore with a dark basophilic nucleus and magenta-staining limiting membrane is contrasted with the neutrophils and basophilic epithelial cell. (×500.)

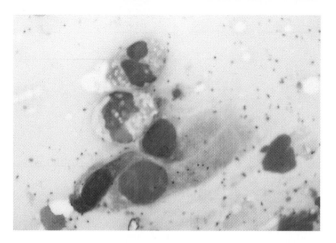

FIG. 8-13. Feline. Nasal wash. Allergic rhinitis. There are poorly preserved ciliated columnar epithelial cells, eosinophils with indistinct granulation and vacuolation, and a background of eosinophil granules. (×400.)

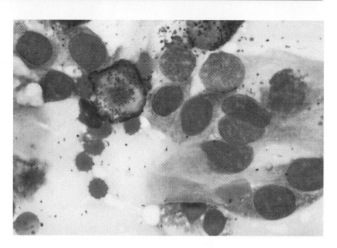

FIG. 8-14. Feline. Nasal wash. Allergic rhinitis. There are columnar and cuboidal epithelial cells. The eosinophil and two mast cells support, but do not confirm, a clinical diagnosis of hypersensitivity. (×400.)

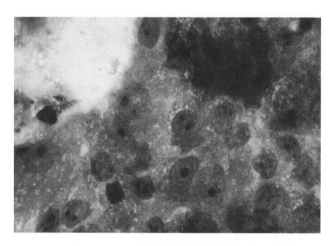

FIG. 8-15. Canine. Nasal flush. Epithelial cell dysplasia. Dysplasia is suggested within these epithelial cells, which have indistinct borders, basophilic lightly vacuolated cytoplasm, anisokaryosis, and prominent nucleoli. (×250.)

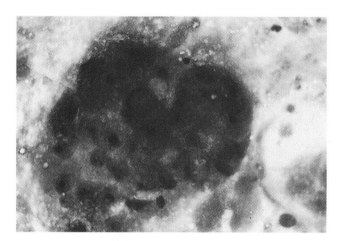

FIG. 8-16. Canine. Nasal flush. Epithelial cell dysplasia. (Same case as Fig. 8-15.) A cluster of dark, cohesive epithelial cells with increased cytoplasmic basophilia, mild cytoplasmic vacuolation, anisocytosis, and prominent nucleoli. Alternative staining methods would allow examination of nuclear details within such dense clusters. (×100.)

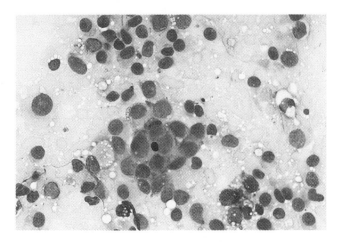

FIG. 8-17. Canine. Imprint. Nasal carcinoma. Epithelial cells with moderate anisokaryosis and slight cytoplasmic vacuolation. The morphological changes associated with malignant transformation may be very subtle and may closely resemble changes observed with hyperplasia or dysplasia. The central cells require closer examination. (×100.)

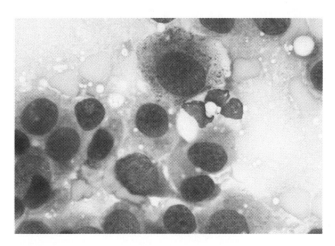

FIG. 8-18. Canine. Imprint. Nasal carcinoma. (Same case as Fig. 8-17.) Epithelial cells with moderate to marked anisokaryosis and a moderate amount of gray-blue cytoplasm. The prominent red cytoplasmic granules in one cell suggest mucin production. With a clinical signalment of tumor mass, the cytological details shown support malignancy rather than dysplasia. (×400.)

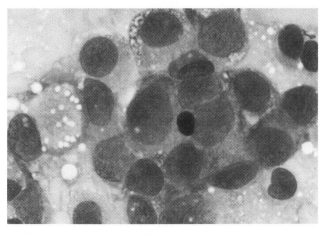

FIG. 8-19. Canine. Imprint. Nasal carcinoma. (Same case as Fig. 8-17.) Epithelial cells with multiple indistinct nucleoli and high N:C ratio. (×400.)

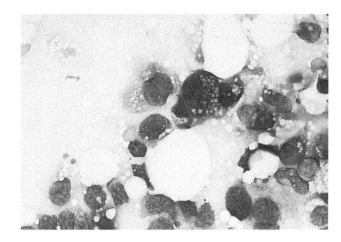

FIG. 8-20. Canine. Fine needle. Mandibular lymph node. Nasal carcinoma. Hyperchromatic epithelial cells, lymphocytes, and bare nuclei. Epithelial cells are not normally located within a lymph node and are consistent with metastasis. (×200.)

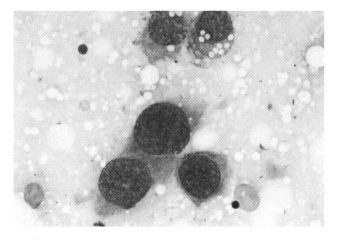

FIG. 8-21. Canine. Fine needle. Mandibular lymph node. Nasal carcinoma. Metastatic epithelial cells with moderate anisokaryosis, gray-blue cytoplasm, and slight cytoplasmic vacuolation. (×400.)

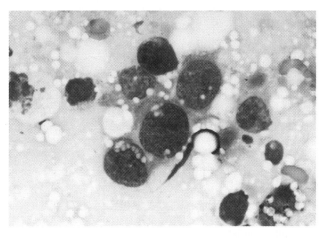

FIG. 8-22. Canine. Fine needle. Mandibular lymph node. Nasal carcinoma. Several large cells with high N:C ratio and cytoplasmic vacuolation. Their presence in the lymph node confirms malignancy. (×400.)

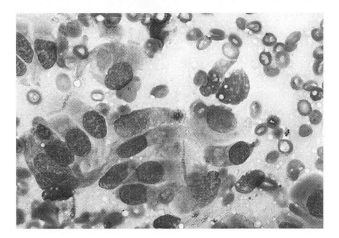

FIG. 8-23. Canine. Scraping. Normal trachea, mid-region. Cuboidal to columnar ciliated epithelial cells. (×250.)

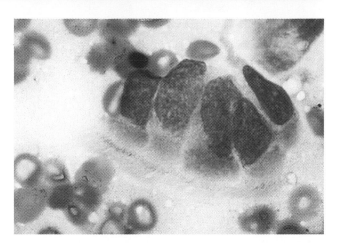

FIG. 8-24. Canine. Scraping. Normal trachea, mid-region. Basilar nuclei in columnar epithelial cells. Basophilic cytoplasm with apical terminal bar and cilia. (×500.)

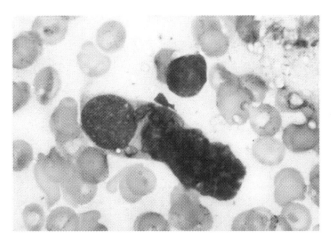

FIG. 8-25. Canine. Scraping. Normal trachea, mid-region. Goblet cell with metachromatic granulation. (×400.)

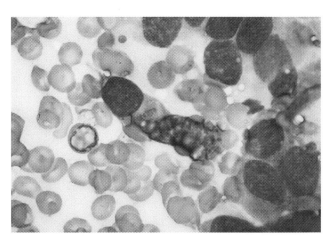

FIG. 8-26. Canine. Scraping. Normal trachea, mid-region. Cuboidal epithelial cells and goblet cell with metachromatic mucinous granules. (×400.)

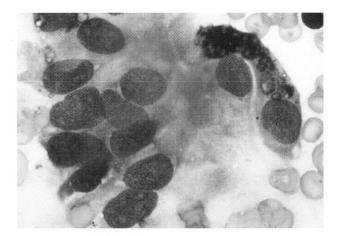

FIG. 8-27. Canine. Scraping. Normal trachea. Cluster of ciliated columnar epithelial cells. One goblet cell with intracytoplasmic mucin droplets. (×400.)

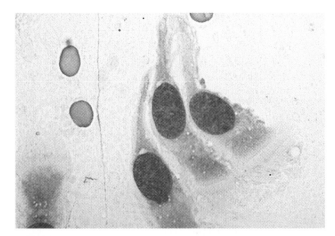

FIG. 8-28. Canine. Scraping. Normal trachea. Columnar epithelial cells with indistinct terminal bar and cilia. Basilar tags may be artifacts created during smear preparation. (×400.)

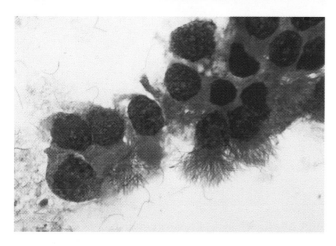

FIG. 8-29. Canine. Tracheal wash. Columnar epithelial cells with prominent cilia. Cuboidal appearance may be an artifact associated with collection and slide preparation or may indicate dysplasia in response to the *Filaroides osleri* infection subsequently diagnosed. (×400.)

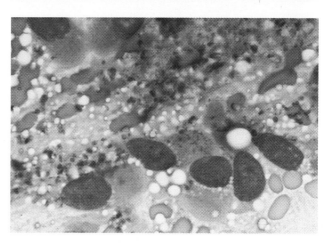

FIG. 8-30. Feline. Scraping. Normal trachea. Background of goblet cell secretory granules and a few columnar epithelial cells. (×400.)

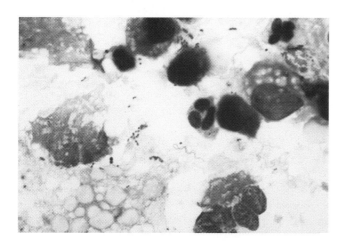

FIG. 8-31. Canine. Tracheal wash. The background of intact cells and debris surround a central indistinct spirochete. The significance is undetermined. (×500.)

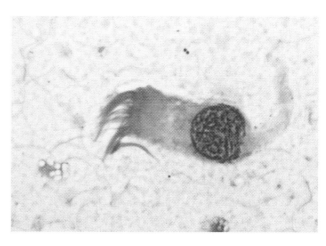

FIG. 8-32. Canine. Bronchial brushing. Normal bronchus. Ciliated columnar epithelial cell. Nuclear detail suggests retroplasia or early cell degeneration. (×630.)

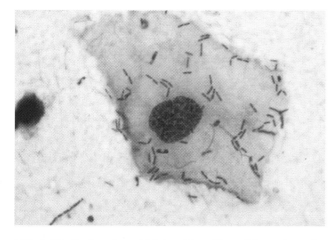

FIG. 8-33. Canine. Bronchial brushing. Normal bronchus. The presence of superficial squamous cells with bacteria indicates oropharyngeal contamination during the sampling procedure. (×500.)

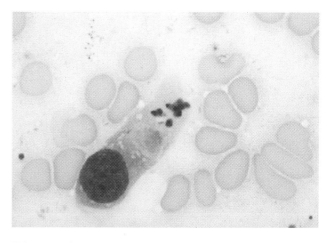

FIG. 8-34. Canine. Scraping. Normal bronchus. Goblet cell illustrating terminal location of purple mucin. (×500.)

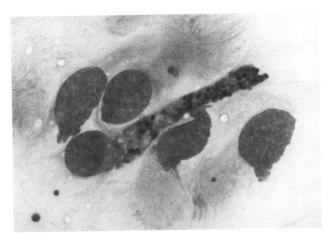

FIG. 8-35. Canine. Scraping. Normal bronchus. Ciliated columnar epithelial cells and an elongated goblet cell. Note indistinct terminal cilia. (×500.)

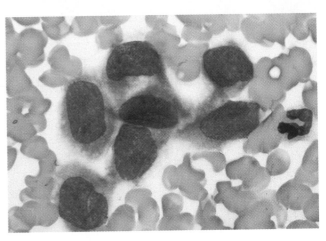

FIG. 8-36. Canine. Imprint. Normal bronchus. Several cuboidal to low columnar epithelial cells with uniform, large nuclei. (×400.)

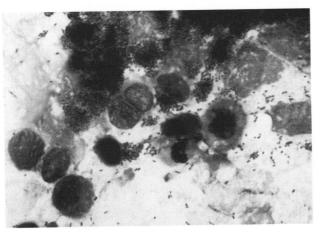

FIG. 8-37. Canine. Tracheal wash. Septic tracheitis. There are many bacteria, both singly and in clusters. The nucleated cells are mononuclear and appear to be poorly preserved epithelial cells. The observation of bacteria and inflammatory cells in tracheal washes, in contrast to BAL, does not confirm infection. Interpretation of tracheal wash cytology requires close correlation with clinical signs. (×400.)

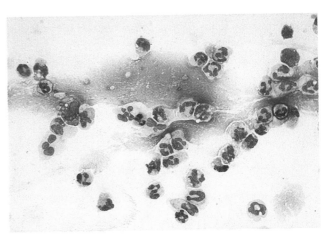

FIG. 8-38. Canine. Tracheal wash. Septic tracheitis. Many neutrophils with pink-staining mucinous material. Some neutrophils are expected within normal tracheal washes, but when increased, further investigation should be conducted for an infectious cause. (×100.)

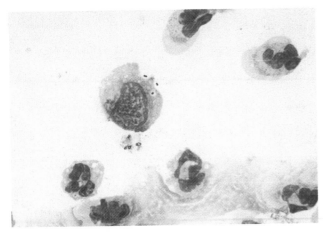

FIG. 8-39. Canine. Tracheal wash. Septic tracheitis. Several mildly degenerate neutrophils and a large macrophage containing a small bacterial rod within a phagolysosome. Extracellular bacteria are visible. A similar cellular response can be seen in dogs free of clinical signs. (×400.)

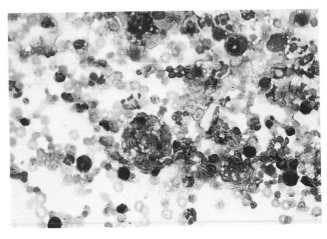

FIG. 8-40. Canine. Tracheal wash. Hemorrhage. Background of erythrocytes and mixed inflammatory cells. Several erythrocytes have been phagocytized by a large macrophage, indicating response to previous hemorrhage. (×100.)

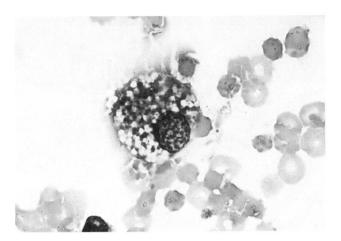

FIG. 8-41. Canine. Tracheal wash. Hemorrhage. (Same case as Fig. 8-40.) There are many erythrocytes in the background. The central vacuolated macrophage contains dark pigment consistent with hemosiderin and possibly erythrocytophagy. (×500.)

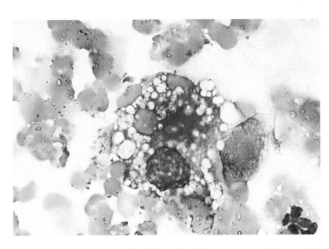

FIG. 8-42. Canine. Tracheal wash. A large macrophage with phagocytized red blood cells, indicating recent erythrocytophagy. (×400.)

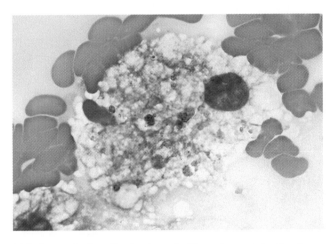

FIG. 8-43. Canine. Tracheal wash. The pigment in the large macrophage is consistent with hemosiderin and hematoidin pigment, indicating previous erythrocytophagy. (×100.)

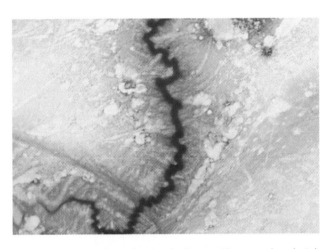

FIG. 8-44. Canine. Bronchoalveolar lavage. The convoluted pink structure, a Curschmann's spiral, can be created when mucin becomes inspissated within any gland. Curschmann's spirals are frequently observed when chronic pulmonary disorders are associated with increased mucin production. (×400.)

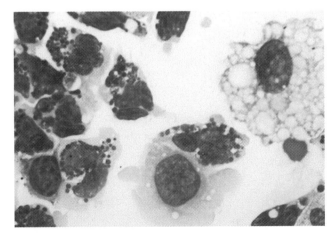

FIG. 8-45. Canine. Bronchoalveolar lavage. Eosinophilic bronchitis. Several eosinophils with dull orange to purple cytoplasmic granules and a larger foamy macrophage. Increased numbers of eosinophils within the respiratory tract may indicate allergic airway disease. (×500.)

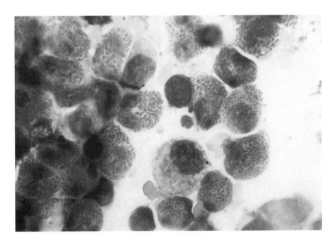

FIG. 8-46. Canine. Bronchoalveolar lavage. Eosinophilic bronchitis. The concentration of eosinophils suggests allergic airway disease. (×400.)

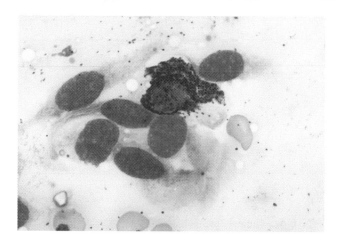

FIG. 8-47. Feline. Bronchial brushing. A mast cell and columnar ciliated epithelial cells. Some mast cells are present within normal respiratory epithelium. (×400.)

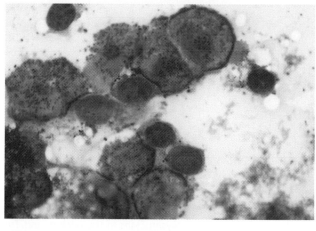

FIG. 8-48. Feline. Bronchial brushing. Several mast cells intermixed with small, round, basilar epithelial cells. Increased mast cells may be associated with an allergic response. Basilar epithelial cells may be seen in bronchial brush samples. (×400.)

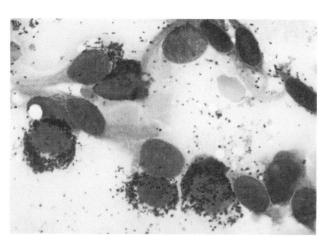

FIG. 8-49. Feline. Bronchial brushing. Mast cells and elongated columnar epithelial cells. (×400.)

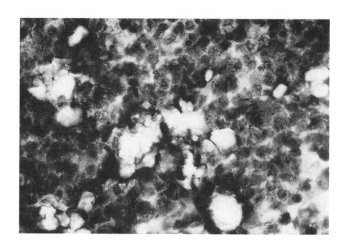

FIG. 8-50. Feline. Bronchoalveolar lavage. Microlithiasis. High cellularity consisting primarily of macrophages. Large, unstained crystalline material is consistent with aspirated substance of unknown origin. (×100.)

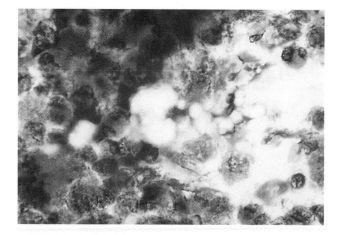

FIG. 8-51. Feline. Bronchoalveolar lavage. Microlithiasis. Increased magnification of Fig. 8-50. (×400.)

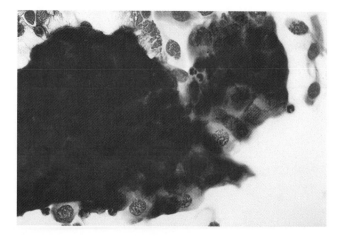

FIG. 8-52. Canine. Bronchoalveolar lavage. Chronic cough. The dense cluster of deeply basophilic epithelial cells with high N:C ratio is consistent with epithelial dysplasia. Romanowsky's stains only allow examination of single layers of cells when differentiating possible neoplasia. (×100.)

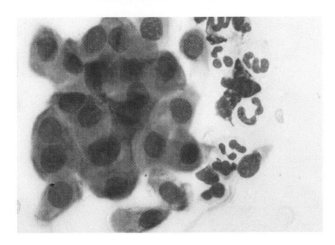

FIG. 8-53. Canine. Bronchoalveolar lavage. Chronic cough. (Same case as Fig. 8-52.) Irregular sheet of round to columnar epithelial cells with high N:C ratio, anisokaryosis, and increased cytoplasmic basophilia consistent with dysplasia. (×250.)

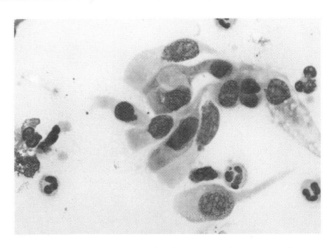

FIG. 8-54. Canine. Bronchoalveolar lavage. Chronic cough. Loss of cilia and cuboidal appearance of some columnar epithelial cells indicates proplastic or retroplastic changes. In vivo changes must be differentiated from the possibility of in vitro damage of cells during sampling procedure. Basilar cytoplasmic tags also suggest epithelial cell injury. (×250.)

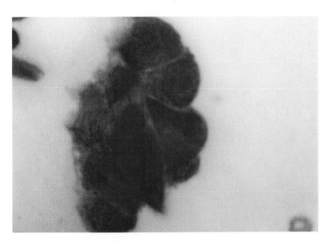

FIG. 8-55. Canine. Bronchoalveolar lavage. Chronic cough. (Same case as Fig. 8-54.) Although intracellular details are poorly visible because of dense basophilia, the cells appear to have a high N:C ratio and have cuboidal outlines consistent with epithelial dysplasia. Epithelial dysplasia resulting from chronic inflammation can mimic malignant transformation. (×400.)

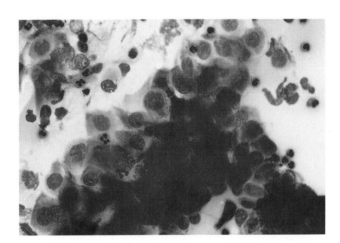

FIG. 8-56. Canine. Bronchoalveolar lavage. Chronic cough. (Same case as Fig. 8-54.) Large sheet of epithelial cells with increased N:C ratio and deeply basophilic cytoplasm, suggesting dysplastic change. Neutrophils are visible between the epithelial cells. (×100.)

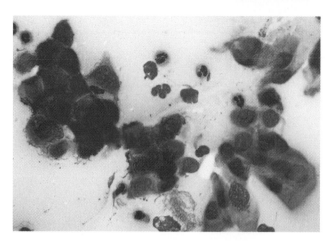

FIG. 8-57. Canine. Bronchoalveolar lavage. Epithelial dysplasia. Chronic cough. (Same case as Fig. 8-54.) Cluster of basophilic cuboidal epithelial cells with a high N:C ratio are contrasted with the more normal-appearing columnar epithelial cells and warrant further examination to confirm or rule out possible malignancy. (×200.)

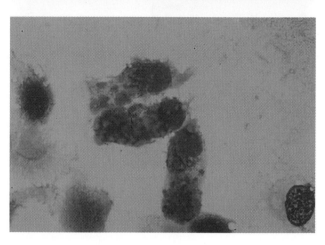

FIG. 8-58. Canine. Bronchoalveolar lavage. Lung. Goblet cell hyperplasia. Columnar cells with large metachromatic granules. Goblet cell hyperplasia develops in response to chronic stimulation. (×380.)

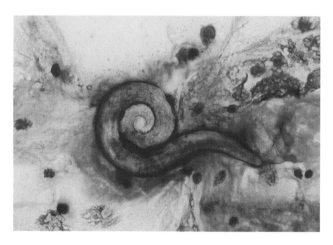

FIG. 8-59. Feline. Bronchoalveolar lavage fluid. *Aleurostrongylus* infection. There is a background of mucus containing poorly defined mononuclear cells and one large, curled organism compatible with *Aleurostrongylus* sp. (×100.)

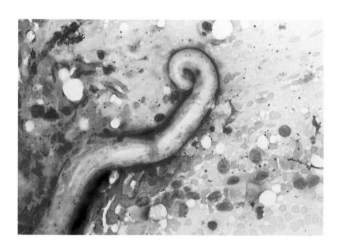

FIG. 8-60. Feline. Lung. Imprint. *Aleurostrongylus* sp. with macrophages. (×100.)

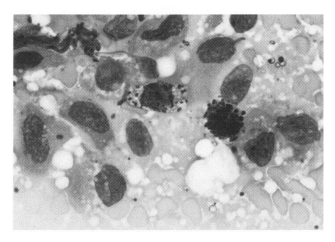

FIG. 8-61. Feline. Lung. Imprint. *Aleurostrongylus.* (Same case as Fig. 8-60.) Background of round to oval cells, which may be hyperplastic type II alveolar epithelial cells or alveolar macrophages. Cytological differentiation may be impossible without special markers. The two central mast cells reflect a hypersensitivity reaction to *Aleurostrongylus* sp. (×400.)

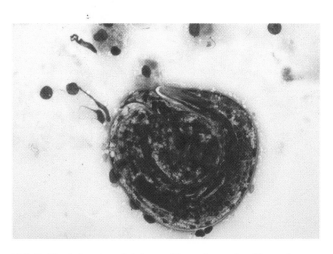

FIG. 8-62. Feline. Imprint. Lung. *Aleurostrongylus. Aleurostrongylus* sp. (×100.)

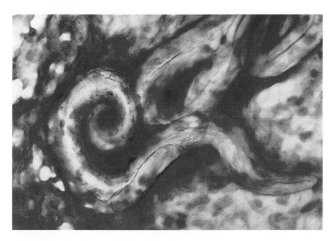

FIG. 8-63. Feline. Imprint. Lung. *Aleurostrongylus. Aleurostrongylus* sp. with a coiled appearance and light granular internal structures. (×100.)

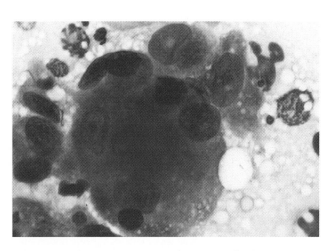

FIG. 8-64. Feline. Imprint. Lung. *Aleurostrongylus.* (Same case as Fig 8-63.) Mixed inflammatory response, including multinucleated giant cell. (×400.)

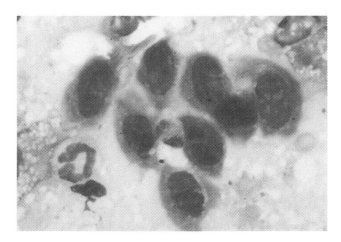

FIG. 8-65. Feline. Bronchoalveolar lavage. *Aleurostrongylus.* Epithelial dysplasia associated with *Aleurostrongylus* sp. Epithelial cells are elongated with round to oval large nuclei, have a high N:C ratio, and increased basophilia of the cytoplasm. (×400.)

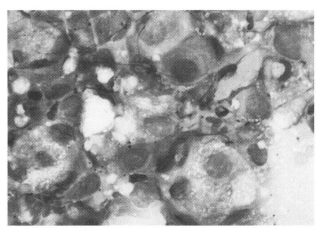

FIG. 8-66. Feline. Bronchoalveolar lavage. *Aleurostrongylus.* Background of epithelioid macrophages associated with the cellular response to *Aleurostrongylus* infection. (×250.)

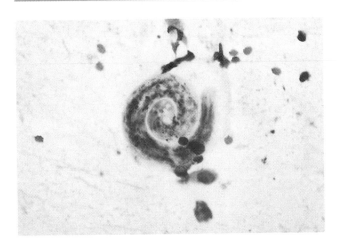

FIG. 8-67. Canine. Bronchoalveolar lavage. *Filaroides osleri* larva. (×100.)

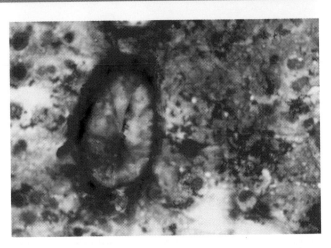

FIG. 8-68. Feline. Lung. Imprint. *Paragonimus* spp. *Paragonimus* spp. are large, ovoid structures with indistinct internal granularity. (×100.)

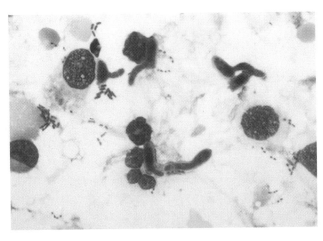

FIG. 8-69. Canine. Bronchoalveolar lavage. Mycotic pneumonia. Bare nuclei, bacteria, and septate fungal hyphae. (×400.) (Courtesy J. Andrews, 1991.)

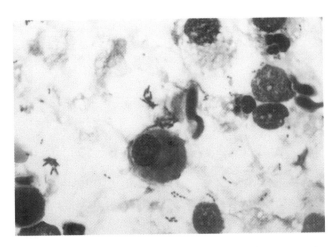

FIG. 8-70. Canine. Bronchoalveolar lavage. Mycotic pneumonia. (Same case as Fig. 8-69.) Hemosiderin-laden macrophage and two neutrophils. There are low numbers of free bacteria and fungal hyphae. (×400.) (Courtesy J. Andrews, 1991.)

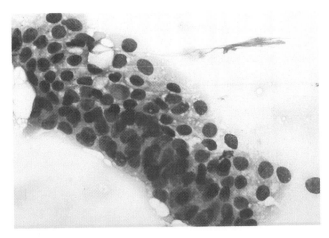

FIG. 8-71. Canine. Imprint prepared from cross section immediately after euthanasia. Normal lung. A sheet of round to cuboidal epithelial cells with dark round to oval nuclei and light basophilic cytoplasm. Cells appear to originate from lower bronchial tree. (×200.)

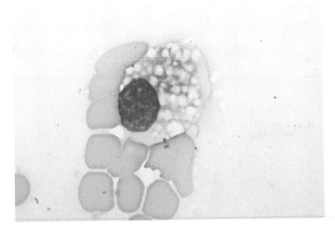

FIG. 8-72. Canine. Imprint. Normal lung. Alveolar macrophage with abundant vacuolated cytoplasm and a round nucleus with indistinct coarse heterochromatin. (×400.)

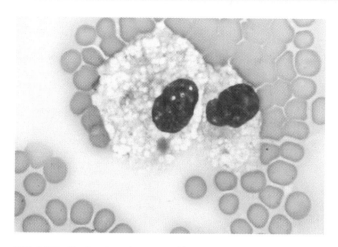

FIG. 8-73. Canine. Imprint. Normal lung. Two large macrophages with typical vacuolated cytoplasm and indistinct heterochromatin clumping. The indistinct basophilic cytoplasmic material may be RNA aggregation or remnants of phagocytized nuclear debris. (×400.)

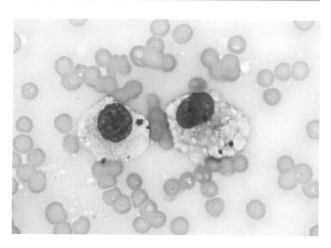

FIG. 8-74. Canine. Imprint. Normal lung. Large macrophages with abundant, slightly basophilic and indistinctly vacuolated cytoplasm. Intracytoplasmic basophilic pigment may be environmental carbon particles, hemosiderin, or cellular debris. (×400.)

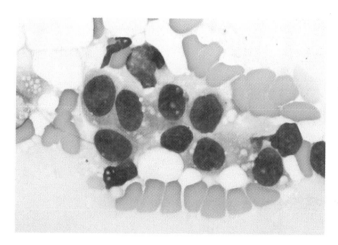

FIG. 8-75. Canine. Imprint. Normal lung. Sheet of round to cuboidal type I or type II epithelial cells with indistinct adherent adjoining borders. The nuclei contain a few large, indistinct chromocenters without apparent nucleoli. The cytoplasm is light in density. (×400.)

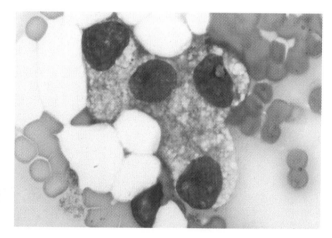

FIG. 8-76. Canine. Imprint. Normal lung. Closely adherent medium-sized cells without apparent connecting cytoplasmic borders. These cells have low N:C ratio, indistinct basophilic aggregation, and vacuolation. In normal lung type I alveolar epithelial cells predominate, but differentiation from alveolar macrophages is difficult. (×500.)

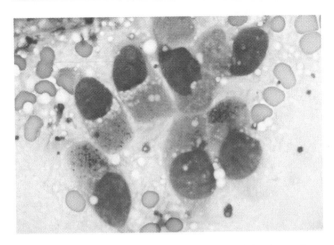

FIG. 8-77. Canine. Imprint. Normal lung. Cuboidal to low columnar epithelial cells with low N:C ratio and lightly basophilic cytoplasm. A few cells have fine and occasionally coarse metachromatic granulation suggestive of mucin formation. (×400.)

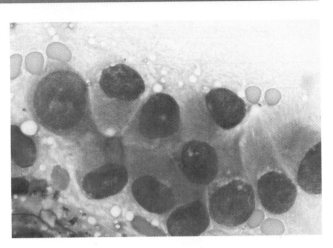

FIG. 8-78. Canine. Imprint. Normal lung. Cluster of cuboidal to columnar ciliated epithelial cells. There is mild variation in nuclear size, uniform nuclear density with indistinct chromatin. Ciliated columnar epithelial cells line the airways down to terminal bronchioles. (×400.)

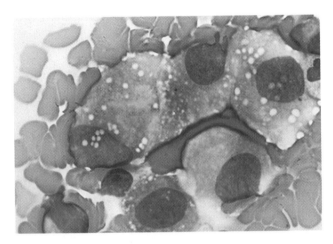

FIG. 8-79. Canine. Fine needle. Granulomatous pneumonia. Epithelioid macrophages with amorphous basophilic cytoplasm containing a few vacuoles. The morphology of the cytological aspirate is consistent with the histological diagnosis but would not allow independent confirmation. (×400.)

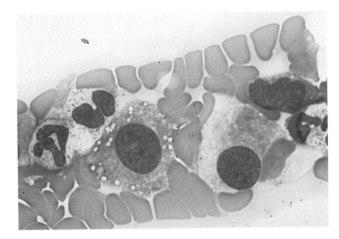

FIG. 8-80. Canine. Fine needle. Granulomatous pneumonia. (Same case as Fig. 8-79.) Macrophages and neutrophils. (×400.)

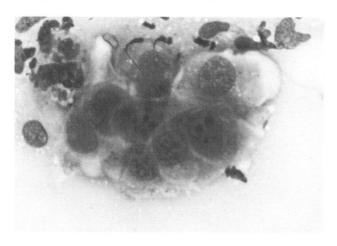

FIG. 8-81. Canine. Scraping. Lung mass. Bronchogenic carcinoma. Sheet of epithelial cells with large nuclei, anisokaryosis, high N:C ratio, and multiple prominent nucleoli consistent with malignant epithelial cells. (×400.) (Courtesy G.S. Elliott, 1991.)

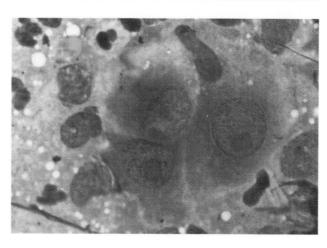

FIG. 8-82. Canine. Scraping. Lung mass. Bronchogenic carcinoma. (Same case as Fig. 8-81.) Epithelial cells with large nuclei, multiple prominent nucleoli consistent with exfoliating malignant epithelial cells (×400.) (Courtesy G.S. Elliott, 1991.)

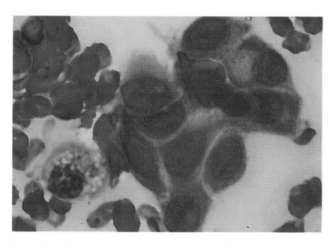

FIG. 8-83. Canine. Fine needle. Lung. Bronchogenic carcinoma. Large, cohesive cells with variable large round to oval hyperchromatic nuclei containing large, indistinct nucleoli and dense, uniform cytoplasm. The cell shape and common adjoining borders support epithelial differentiation. (×375.)

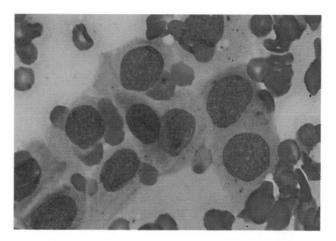

FIG. 8-84. Canine. Fine needle. Lung. Bronchogenic carcinoma. (Same case as Fig. 8-83.) Large cells with large round to oval nuclei, fine chromatin pattern, and multiple indistinct nucleoli. There is some indistinct cytoplasmic pigmentation and less distinctive adjoining cell borders. The variation in cell morphology may be due to phenotypic expression or increased spreading of cells on the glass surface. (×375.)

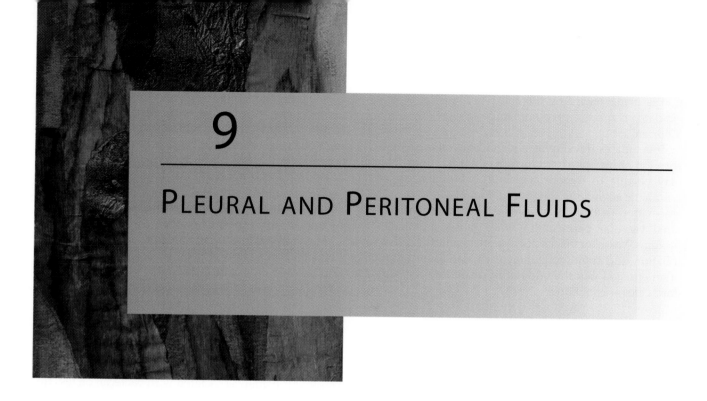

9

PLEURAL AND PERITONEAL FLUIDS

Effusions are observed frequently within pleural and peritoneal cavities in dogs and cats. Effusions develop for multiple reasons. Although the protein and cell changes are not specific for each cause, cytological analysis of these fluids is an integral part of the diagnostical workup. Disorders with specific cytological fluid abnormalities are described in detail.

TECHNIQUE

Cavity fluids are collected using aseptic technique. For abdominocentesis the needle is inserted 1 to 2 cm posterior to the umbilicus on the ventral midline (Cowell, 1999). For thoracocentesis the radiographic location of the fluid determines the site of aspiration. If effusion is generalized, the needle is inserted ventrally between the seventh or eighth intercostal space (Cowell, 1999). The needle is inserted along the cranial edge of the rib to prevent laceration of the larger vessels located on the rib's caudal surface. The fluid is collected into a vial containing EDTA. If desired, a small portion can be collected into a serum tube and observed for clotting as a crude test for the presence of fibrinogen found in exudative effusions. If sepsis is suspected, a sample is submitted for culture.

The total white blood cell count (WBC) is performed. If the cell count is high ($>10,000 \times 10^6/L$), the smears can be made directly. Otherwise the cells should be concentrated using a centrifuge at low rpm for 5 to 10 minutes before making cytological preparations from the sediment. The protein concentration is measured in the supernatant. Smears are made from the resuspended sediment in a manner similar to preparation of a blood smear. Smears are air dried and stained with a Romanowsky's stain as previously described.

NORMAL CAVITY FLUIDS

Protein Determination

The refractometer is a reliable method for measuring protein concentration greater than 25 g/L unless there is interference from chyle where light refraction by lipids is unrelated to protein concentration. High concentrations of bilirubin or hemoglobin also interfere with refractometer protein determination. In normal serous fluid, protein concentration is usually less than 25 g/L with a mode of 10 g/L (O'Brien, 1988).

Cell Counts

Nucleated cells are counted using a hemocytometer chamber or an electronic cell counter. Cell counts are normally less than $3000 \times 10^6/L$ with a mode less than $1000 \times 10^6/L$ (O'Brien, 1988). Erythrocytes can be counted or estimated from packed cell volume determination.

■ CLINICAL DIAGNOSIS OF EFFUSIONS

Traditionally, effusions are placed into three categories based on total protein, cell counts, and cell distribution. Effusions are called *transudates* when protein concentration and cell count are within the reference limits, *exudates* when protein and cell concentration are both increased, and *modified transudates* when either protein or cells are increased but not both. No distinction is made regarding the cell type, but the typical exudate contains predominantly phagocytic cells (O'Brien, 1988).

Transudates develop as a result of decreased reabsorption or increased production of normal fluid. This may be due to hypoproteinemia, overhydration, or lymphatic or venous congestion. Exudates develop in association with chemotaxis of inflammatory cells, altered vascular permeability, and leakage of plasma proteins. Vessel or viscus disruption, neoplastic cell exfoliation, and chylothorax may each lead to formation of an effusion, but they do not fit easily into the standard categories (O'Brien, 1988).

Alternative classification schemes have been proposed (O'Brien, 1988), such as:

A: Transudate

B: Exudate nonseptic

C: Exudate septic: caused by aerobic or anaerobic bacteria, fungi, mycoplasma

D: Hemorrhage

E: Viscus rupture (gallbladder, urinary bladder, intestine)

F: Neoplasia

SEPTIC EFFUSIONS (Figs. 9-1 to 9-6)

Exudate Septic

CLINICAL DIAGNOSIS

Septic effusions are characteristically exudative and due to bacterial agents. Septic effusions may develop subsequent to traumatic penetration, hematogenous spread, pneumonia, gastroenteritis, internal abscessation involving prostate or liver, or surgical entry. Septic effusions may develop secondary to repeat pleural aspirations while investigating suspected lung pathology. Fungi and mycoplasma may also initiate marked chemotaxis of phagocytic cells and exudative change. Bacterial agents isolated include *Bacteroides*, *Fusobacterium*, *Clostridium*, *Pasteurella*, and *Actinomyces* (Jonas, 1983; O'Brien, 1988). Nocardiosis is also reported, although less commonly than actinomycosis (Dow, 1987; Marino, 1993; O'Brien, 1988; Tyler, 1989).

Sepsis accounted for 20 of 178 cases of pleural effusions reported in cats and 18 of 59 dogs with pleural and peritoneal effusions (O'Brien, 1988).

CYTOLOGICAL DIAGNOSIS

Septic fluid characteristically contains increased neutrophils and macrophages with free or phagocytized bacteria, the latter more often within neutrophils. Fungal organisms are more frequently detected in the cytoplasm of macrophages. Neutrophil nuclear degeneration can be mild to marked depending on the amount and virulence of toxins present. Aerobic bacteria are

associated with a greater degree of neutrophil nuclear chromatin degeneration (lytic neutrophils) than anaerobic organisms. *Nocardia* and other members of the family Actinomycetaceae appear as branching filamentous rods (Marino, 1993). *Actinomyces* spp. tend to colonize in the fluid and may be overlooked during sampling and examination of the smear. The typical "sulfur granules" observed floating on the fluid surface represent colonies of bacteria as readily confirmed by microscopic examination.

The microscopic appearance of neutrophil nuclear degeneration within effusions, as well as concentration, is used as an indicator of likely sepsis. The combination of nuclear degeneration in the absence of bacteria indicates the need for more intensive microscopic examination and for bacterial culture, possibly including anaerobic collection and culture techniques. Neutrophil aging degeneration includes karyopyknosis and karyorrhexis but not the swelling and chromatolysis that is usually associated with bacterial or, less frequently, chemical toxins.

The cytoplasmic "toxic changes" reported in peripheral blood neutrophils may be observed in neutrophils within effusions. These cytoplasmic changes should be interpreted with caution because they have limited specificity. Vacuolation will appear in the cytoplasm of cells within a fluid because of exposure to EDTA and as an aging change.

Macrophages, lymphocytes, and plasma cells are present to varying degrees in both acute and chronic effusions. Plasma cells indicate a response to chronic antigenic stimulation.

In 17 cats with pyothorax, the mean nucleated cell count was $128,875 \times 10^6/L$ and in every case was greater than $10,000 \times 10^6/L$ (Jonas, 1983). Organisms were cultured from only half of the cases in which they were visible on cytological slides (Jonas, 1983).

NONSEPTIC EFFUSIONS (EXCLUDING CHYLOTHORAX)

Nonseptic effusions may be transudative or exudative in origin.

Exudate Nonseptic

CLINICAL DIAGNOSIS

Nonseptic exudative effusions develop in feline infectious peritonitis, steatitis, foreign bodies, immune-mediated disease, parasitic migration (O'Brien, 1988), and hemorrhage.

CYTOLOGICAL DIAGNOSIS

It is recommended that exudates be classified according to the predominant cell type present, that is, *purulent* or *suppurative* if predominantly neutrophils and *mononuclear* if predominantly monocytes, macrophages, or lymphocytes. In many cases, mixed inflammation is present. Eosinophilic exudates may be observed.

The traditional classification for effusions is *acute* if greater than 70% of cells are neutrophils, *chronic active* if 50% to 70% are neutrophils, and *chronic* if there are less than 30% neutrophils. As discussed in Chapter 2, this terminology has some merit if criteria are understood, but because different definitions apply to acute, subacute, and chronic for clinicians, histopathologists, and cytologists, miscommunication is common. Consequently, we encourage classification of exudates based on the predominant cell or mixture of cells.

Feline Infectious Peritonitis (Figs. 9-7 to 9-9)
CLINICAL AND CYTOLOGICAL DIAGNOSES
FIP is characterized by a nonseptic exudative effusion. The most consistent observation is a moderate to marked increase in protein concentration. The nucleated cells include a mixture of neutrophils, macrophages, lymphocytes, and occasionally plasma cells. Neutrophil nuclear degenerative changes may be minimal, and usually only age-related changes of pyknosis and karyorrhexis are seen. The background is dense, purple-blue, and often finely granular, suggesting the increased globular protein concentration. Lighter-staining crescent artifacts are often distinctive within the dense background. FIP accounted for 10% of 178 cats with pleural effusions (O'Brien, 1988).

Transudates/Modified Transudates

CLINICAL DIAGNOSIS
Congestive heart failure, liver failure, and hypoproteinemia are the most common syndromes associated with transudation (O'Brien, 1988). Venous congestion, decreased colloidal osmotic pressure, or extravascular compression are explanatory pathogenetic mechanisms. Modified transudates result from chronic transudation. Fluid transudation accounts for approximately 20% to 40% of body fluid accumulations when tumor cell exfoliation is excluded (O'Brien, 1988). Cardiac failure was diagnosed in 28% of 178 cats with effusions (O'Brien, 1988). In 59 dogs with pleural and peritoneal effusion, transudate formation was due to cardiac failure in 16% and hypoproteinemia in 25% (O'Brien, 1988).

CYTOLOGICAL DIAGNOSIS
Transudates have a protein concentration less than 25 g/L and a nucleated cell count less than 3000×10^6/L. Some authors suggest the cell count should be less than 1000×10^6/L (Forrester, 1988). Mononuclear cells, either macrophages or mesothelial cells, predominate. If cells are degenerate and vacuolated, differentiation may be difficult, but it is not usually of clinical importance.

Viscous Rupture

Bile Duct Rupture (Fig. 9-10)
CLINICAL AND CYTOLOGICAL DIAGNOSES
Bile duct or gallbladder rupture will initiate a modified transudate or in later stages an exudate. Release of bile into the cavity results in chemical peritonitis and chemotaxis of phagocytic cells, including neutrophils and monocytes/macrophages. It is not uncommon to have accompanying bacterial peritonitis. Tan to light brown to blue-green pigment is visible in the background or phagocytized within macrophages. Protein and cellularity increase with time.

Hemorrhage (Figs. 9-11 to 9-15)

CLINICAL DIAGNOSIS
Hemorrhage into a body cavity can result from trauma or, less frequently, neoplasia, splenic rupture, hemostatic defects, and heartworm.

CYTOLOGICAL DIAGNOSIS
In some cases it may be difficult to differentiate acute hemorrhage from an iatrogenic bloody tap. The presence of, or lack of, clinical signs associated with acute blood loss should help the clinician make this distinction at the time of sample collection. Comparison of effusion and blood-packed cell volume may be helpful. Platelets are likely to be present on the slide with iatrogenic contamination compared with chronic hemorrhage, in which platelets quickly degranulate and disappear. After hemorrhage into a body cavity, macrophages become activated and phagocytize erythrocytes. The absence of erythrophagocytosis and the presence of platelets would suggest peracute bleeding or a bloody tap, whereas the presence of erythrophagocytosis and the absence of platelets would suggest chronic hemorrhage (Cowell, 1999).

Neoplasia (Figs. 9-16 to 9-26)

CLINICAL DIAGNOSIS
Effusions associated with exfoliation of tumor cells do not fit readily into the transudate/exudate classification. Exfoliation of tumor cells into pleural or peritoneal fluid occurs most frequently with epithelial tumors and only rarely with stromal masses. In 42 dogs with pericardial effusions, 57% were neoplastic in origin (O'Brien, 1988). In cats, neoplastic effusion accounted for 37% of 178 pleural fluids, whereas in dogs it accounted for 11% of 59 dogs with pleural or peritoneal effusion (O'Brien, 1988).

CYTOLOGICAL DIAGNOSIS
The protein and nucleated cell concentrations may be low or increased. Initially tumor cells may not be exfoliating, and only hyperplastic mesothelial cells are

present. A mild inflammatory component may accompany the tumor cells or, subsequent to tissue invasion and exfoliation or necrosis, the inflammatory component may become very marked. Reactive mesothelial cells must be differentiated from exfoliating neoplastic epithelial cells. The differential diagnosis of the rare mesothelioma must also be considered. The anaplastic exfoliating cells may be poorly differentiated, limiting ability to deduce origin. A monomorphic population of nonmesothelial or hematopoietic cells within an effusion is likely of clinical significance regardless of the criteria of malignancy apparent. With adequate differentiation of cells, cytoplasmic criteria are most helpful in identifying cell origin, especially if there is evidence of secretory activity as expected for an adenocarcinoma. Cytoplasmic secretory product suggests adenocarcinoma. For many clinical cases, a diagnosis of malignancy may be all that is required.

Chylothorax (Figs. 9-27 to 9-37)

CLINICAL DIAGNOSIS

Milky white pleural fluids that do not clear with centrifugation are called *chylous effusions.* Chyle is an emulsion of chylomicrons and lymph. Chylomicrons are formed in the intestinal mucosa from dietary fats and are composed primarily of triglycerides. They traverse the thoracic duct and empty into the venous system. They are cleared within 4 to 6 hours after eating and are not found in fasting blood samples of normal dogs and cats (Meadows, 1994).

Although traumatic rupture of the thoracic duct is the most obvious cause of chylous effusion, it is probably the least common (Fossum 1986a; Meadows, 1994). Obstruction of thoracic duct flow is the major cause of chylothorax (Meadows, 1994). Obstruction leads to a combination of lymphatic hypertension, dilation of thoracic lymphatics, and obstruction of the flow of lymph into the venous system, leading to leakage (Fossum, 1986a; Fossum, 1989; Meadows, 1994).

Clearance of the fluid with ether, an often-quoted procedure, is a crude test for chylomicrons and does not always provide definitive results. The pleural fluid must first be alkalinized with several drops of sodium hydroxide. Equal volumes of ether and pleural fluid are mixed. Chylomicron solubility in ether should result in clearing of the sample. The unreliability of the test and the safety hazard as a result of ether suggests this test should be of historical interest only.

High levels of triglyceride are characteristic of chylous effusions, whereas pseudochylous effusions have increased cholesterol concentrations. Several ratios for serum and fluid cholesterol and triglyceride content have been proposed to help differentiate chylous effusions. Ratios of greater than 2 to 3:1 of fluid to serum triglycerides are reported characteristic for chylous effusions (Fossum, 1986a). A cholesterol to triglyceride

(C:T) ratio less than 1 supports an effusion as chylous (Fossum, 1986b). However, one study reported that 12% of dogs and 50% of cats with nonmilky effusions had C:T ratios less than 1 (Waddle, 1990). In these same animals, those with chylous effusions based on chylomicrons present on lipoprotein electrophoresis had triglyceride concentrations greater than 1.13 mmol/L (100mg/dl) and all those with nonchylous effusions had triglyceride concentrations less than 1.13 mmol/L (100 mg/dl) (Waddle, 1990). It was felt that measurement of the absolute value of triglycerides in the fluid was superior to the calculation of C:T ratios (Waddle, 1990). However, triglyceride concentrations have never been measured in true pseudochylous effusion because they are rare according to the veterinary literature. In humans there is increasing evidence that fluid triglyceride levels may also be increased in pseudochylous effusions (Hamm, 1991).

In general, chylous effusions have a C:T ratio less than 1, a ratio for fluid:serum triglycerides greater than 3:1, and fluid triglyceride concentrations greater than 1.13 mmol/L (100 mg/dl). Perhaps too much effort has been used to define rigid diagnostical criteria because the causes of chylous effusions are varied. Even after the physicochemical differentiation of chylous effusion has been determined, there are similar multiple clinical differential diagnoses to consider.

In one study involving 34 dogs with chylothorax, the cause was unknown in 24, 5 were associated with neoplasia, and 5 were associated with trauma (Fossum, 1986a). Abdominal chylous effusions also occur with lymphatic obstruction and with trauma to intestinal lymphatics (Fossum, 1992).

In cats, chylothorax has been associated with cardiomyopathy (Birchard, 1986; Fossum, 1993; Waddle, 1990), dirofilariasis (Birchard, 1990), thoracic and pulmonary neoplasia (Fossum, 1991; Fossum, 1986b), mediastinal lymphosarcoma (Forrester, 1988), lymphoma (Forrester, 1991), and mediastinal granuloma (Meadows, 1994). Many cases remain idiopathic.

CYTOLOGICAL DIAGNOSIS

The small lymphocyte, which is expected to predominate in chylous effusions, is smaller than a neutrophil and has a small oval nucleus, coarse nuclear chromatin, and no visible nucleoli. The cytoplasm is scant and clear to light blue. However, if the chylous effusion is long-standing, the chemotactic response to pleural irritation results in neutrophils and macrophages outnumbering the lymphocytes (Meadows, 1994). Refractile lipid droplets are outlined with NMB staining, whereas chylomicrons take up Sudan 3 stain.

When nucleated cell differentials were performed for 19 of the 34 dogs with chylothorax, 2 of the 19 cases had a preponderance of small lymphocytes, 13 had mostly neutrophils, and 4 had mostly macrophages (Fossum, 1986a). In 29 cats with opaque nonclearing effusions the mean nucleated cell count was 11,919 cells $\times$ 10^6/L (Fossum, 1991). When cells were differentiated for 26 of the 29 cats, lymphocytes predominated in 19 and neutrophils in 7 (Fossum, 1991). With subsequent pleural taps, neutrophil numbers increased (Fossum, 1991). C:T ratios in the pleural fluid were less than 0.15 in the 17 cats that were evaluated (Fossum, 1991).

Pseudochylous Effusions

By definition, chylous effusions contain chyle and pseudochylous effusions do not contain chyle, although they appear similar macroscopically (Meadows, 1994).

CLINICAL DIAGNOSIS

When the pleura become thickened and mineralized in response to chronic pleural effusions, a pseudochylous effusion can develop. Cholesterol accumulates in the pleural cavity as a result of decreased transfer of cholesterol out of the pleural space. Recently it has been hypothesized that low-density-lipoprotein (LDL) cholesterol becomes trapped in the pleural space (Meadows, 1994). Cholesterol then accumulates in complexes that contain triglyceride and proteins (Meadow, 1994). The high levels of triglycerides are not of dietary origin as proven by the associated apolipoprotein present (Meadows, 1993; Meadows, 1994).

CYTOLOGICAL DIAGNOSIS

A milky effusion that fails to clear with centrifugation and has an increased cholesterol concentration, independent of serum cholesterol concentration, is likely pseudochylous (Meadows, 1994). There is usually a history of chronic inflammatory disease and cholesterol crystals in the fluid.

Documented cases of true pseudochylous effusions in the dog and cat are rare. A combination of mononuclear cells and neutrophils can be expected depending on the initiating cause.

■ *MESOTHELIUM*

NORMAL (Fig. 9-38)

Mesothelial cells line the parietal and visceral surfaces of the pleural and peritoneal cavities. Nonstimulated, euplastic mesothelial cells are observed in flat sheets on aspirate smears or impressions of the serosal surface. The quiescent mesothelial cells have small basophilic nuclei with one or two nucleoli and light blue cytoplasm. They are often polygonal or elongate in shape.

NONNEOPLASTIC DISEASE (Figs. 9-39 to 9-50)

CYTOLOGICAL DIAGNOSIS

When fluid accumulates within cavities, the mesothelial cells become hyperplastic and exfoliate singly or as small to large clusters, or "balls." Hyperplastic mesothelial cells, that is, proplastic or "reactive," have large, round nuclei with one to three prominent nucleoli and dark basophilic cytoplasm. The cells often are multinucleated. Within the cell clusters, nuclei are of regular size and shape, helping distinguish them from adenocarcinomas. The cytoplasm may contain pink granulation and pseudopod-like projections of the cytoplasm. If the cells dry slowly, an eosinophilic to bright red fluffy halo (Prasse, 1976) appears to surround the edge of the cell when stained with Wright's stain. Reactive mesothelial cells often contain very large cytoplasmic vacuoles that may peripheralize the nuclei, giving a signet ring appearance to the cell and suggesting a secretory nature. Mitosis may be frequent. These properties mimic morphological changes expected in neoplastic cell clusters. In benign mesothelial effusions there is usually a continuum from single cells to syncytial sheets to large cell clusters. Histology may be required to differentiate benign mesothelial hyperplasia from neoplasia.

NEOPLASTIC DISEASE

Mesotheliomas (Figs. 9-51 to 9-56)

CLINICAL DIAGNOSIS

Mesotheliomas develop from the mesodermal origin cells that line the pleural, pericardial, and peritoneal cavities. Mesotheliomas are rare (Dubielzig, 1979; Harbison, 1983; McDonough, 1992; Morrison, 1984; Smith, 1989) and are considered malignant tumors primarily because of their propensity for implantation, but occasionally they metastasize to other locations (Morrison, 1984; Smith, 1989). Mesotheliomas usually present with extensive effusions that develop as a result of lymphatic blockage. The prognosis is uniformly poor (Morrison, 1984).

CYTOLOGICAL DIAGNOSIS

Differentiation of benign reactive mesothelium, mesothelioma, and adenocarcinoma can be extremely difficult. Moderate to high cellularity (5000 to 10,000 cells $\times$ 10^6/L.) is characteristic for cavity fluid from dogs affected with mesothelioma. Mesothelial cells predominate and have prominent anisokaryosis and hyperchromasia. Frequent aberrant mitosis may be seen. Clusters of mesothelial cells may resemble papillary adenocarcinomas. Cell borders are prominent. Huge microvilli can be seen in reactive and malignant mesothelial cells (Kwee, 1982). In humans the presence of large numbers of morulae, often with extensive cytoplasmic vacuolation within the morulae cells, is considered indicative of mesothelioma (Kwee, 1982). The nucleus is more frequently peripheral in cells from human mesotheliomas (Kwee, 1982). It was also suggested that malignant mesothelial cells had a more irregular and coarsely reticular chromatin pattern (Kwee, 1982). Prominent angular nucleoli may be present, and large secretory vacuoles may be seen. It is important to note that these cellular criteria describe alcohol-fixed Papanicolaou's stained mesothelial cells and not air-dried Romanowsky's stained cells.

Pericardial Effusions

CLINICAL DIAGNOSIS

Accumulation of fluid within the pericardial sac occurs in a small proportion of dogs with cardiac disease. Pericardial effusion is associated with congestive heart failure, uremia, bacterial and fungal infections, left atrial rupture, neoplasia, trauma, foreign bodies, and benign pericardial effusion (Berg, 1984). In 42 cases of pericardial effusion, 57% were due to neoplasia and of these 60% were hemangiosarcomas and 20% were chemodectomas (Berg, 1984). Some 19% of the 42 cases were benign idiopathic effusions and 14% were due to cardiac disease (Berg, 1984).

CYTOLOGICAL DIAGNOSIS

Pericardial effusions are classified, as for other cavity fluids, as transudative or exudative and according to the predominant cells present. Because of the contact with serosal surfaces and the continuous movement, there is marked mesothelial hyperplasia and exfoliation. The mesothelial cells exfoliate singly or in cell clusters with high N:C ratios, anisokaryosis, and cytoplasmic vacuolation mimicking several criteria of neoplasia. To further complicate interpretation, pericardial mesotheliomas have been diagnosed in three dogs that presented with recurring pericardial effusions (McDonough, 1992).

In a series of 21 dogs, pericardial fluid cytology was similar regardless of cause (Berg, 1984). The fluids were nonclotting and hemorrhagic (Berg, 1984). Reactive mesothelial cells, erythrophagocytosis, and heme pigments were commonly reported (Berg, 1984). In two cases, neoplastic cells were identified (Berg, 1984). Although neoplasia is a frequent cause of pericardial effusion, tumor cells are rarely identified in the fluid. In 19 dogs with idiopathic effusions the cell count and total protein were highly variable (Sisson, 1984). In 90% of these 19 dogs the cell count was less than 10,000 $\times 10^6$/L and included mesothelial cells and leukocytes in varying proportions (Sisson, 1984). In 50 pericardial fluids the protein concentration and total cell counts were highly variable, and cytological examination usually did not help differentiate neoplastic from benign effusions (Sisson, 1984). Of 18 dogs with pericardial effusion, 7 had neoplastic disease and 11 were nonneoplastic (Kerstetter, 1997). In 17 of 18 dogs the fluid was indicative of hemorrhage (Kerstetter, 1997). In one dog with lymphoma, malignant lymphocytes were identified in the pericardial fluid (Kerstetter, 1997). Reactive mesothelial cells are frequently confused with neoplastic cells.

References

Berg, R.J. and Wingfield, W. Pericardial effusion in the dog: a review of 42 cases. *J Am Anim Hosp Assoc* 20:721-729, 1984.

Birchard, S.J., Ware, W.A., Fossum, T.W., et al. Chylothorax associated with congestive cardiomyopathy in a cat. *J Am Vet Med Assoc* 189:1462-1465, 1986.

Birchard, S.J. and Bilkney, S.A. Chylothorax associated with dirofilariasis in a cat. *J Am Vet Med Assoc* 197:507-509, 1990.

Cowell, R.L., Tyler, R.D., and Meinkoth, J.H. Abdominal and thoracic fluid. In *Diagnostic Cytology of the Dog and Cat.* ed 2. R.L. Cowell and R.D. Tyler (eds). Mosby, St Louis, 1999.

Dow, S.W. and Jones, R.L. Anaerobic infections. Part 1. Pathogenesis and clinical significance. *Compend Cont Ed Pract* 9:711-718, 1987.

Dubielzig, R.R. Sclerosing mesothelioma in five dogs. *J Am Anim Hosp Assoc* 15:745-748, 1979.

Forrester, S.D., Troy, G.C., and Fossum, T.W. Pleural effusions: pathophysiology and diagnostic considerations. *Compend Cont Ed Pract* 10:121-135, 1988.

Forrester, S.D., Fossum, T.W., and Rogers, K.S. Diagnosis and treatment of chylothorax associated with lymphoblastic lymphosarcoma in four cats. *J Am Vet Med Assoc* 198:291-294, 1991.

Fossum, T.W. Feline chylothorax. *Compend Cont Ed Pract* 15:549-564, 1993.

Fossum, T.W. and Birchard, S.J. Chylothorax. In *Current Veterinary Therapy X, Small Animal Practice.* R.W. Kirk and J.D. Bonagura (eds). WB Saunders, Philadelphia, 1989.

Fossum, T.W., Birchard, S.J., and Jacobs, R.M. Chylothorax in 34 dogs. *J Am Vet Med Assoc* 188:1315-1318, 1986a.

Fossum, T.W., Forrester, S.D., Swenson, C.L., et al. Chylothorax in cats: 37 cases (1969-1989). *J Am Vet Med Assoc* 198:672-678, 1991.

Fossum, T.W., Hay, W.H., Boothe, H.W., et al. Chylous ascites in three dogs. *J Am Vet Med Assoc* 200:70-71, 1992.

Fossum, T.W., Jacobs, R.M., and Birchard, S.J. Evaluation of cholesterol and triglyceride concentrations in differentiating chylous and nonchylous pleural effusions in dogs and cats. *J Am Vet Med Assoc* 188:49-51, 1986b.

Hamm, H. Lipoprotein analysis in a chyloform pleural effusion: implications for pathogenesis and diagnosis. *Respiration* 58:294-300, 1991.

Harbison, M.L. and Godleski, J.J. Malignant mesothelioma in urban dogs. *Vet Pathol* 20:531-540, 1983.

Jonas, L.D. Feline pyothorax: a retrospective study of twenty cases. *J Am Anim Hosp Assoc* 19:865-871, 1983.

Kerstetter, K.K., Krahwinkel, D.J., Millis, D.L., et al. Pericardiectomy in dogs: 22 cases (1978-1994). *J Am Vet Med Assoc* 211:736-740, 1997.

Kwee, W.-S., Veldhuizen, R.W., Alons, C.A., et al. Quantitative and qualitative differences between benign and malignant mesothelial cells in pleural fluid. *Acta Cytologica* 26:401-406, 1982.

Marino, D.J. and Jaggy, A. Nocardiosis. *J Vet Intern Med* 7: 4-11, 1993.

McDonough, S.P., MacLachlan, N.J., and Tobias, A.H. Canine pericardial mesothelioma. *Vet Pathol* 29:256-260, 1992.

Meadows, R.L. and MacWilliams, P.S. Chylous effusions revisited. *Vet Clin Pathol* 23:54-62, 1994.

Meadows, R.L., MacWilliams, P.S., Dzata, G., et al. Chylothorax associated with cryptococcal mediastinal granuloma in a cat. *Vet Clin Pathol* 22:109-116, 1993.

Morrison, W.B. and Trigo, F.J. Clinical characterization of pleural mesothelioma in seven dogs. *Compend Cont Ed Pract* 6:342-348, 1984.

O'Brien, P.J. and Lumsden, J.H. The cytologic examination of body cavity fluids. *Semin Vet Med Surg (Small Anim)* 3:140-156, 1988.

Prasse, K.W. and Duncan, J.R. Laboratory diagnosis of pleural and peritoneal effusions. *Vet Clin North Am* 6:625-635, 1976.

Sisson, D., Thomas, W.P., Ruehl, W.W., et al. Diagnostic value of pericardial fluid analysis in the dog. *J Am Vet Med Assoc* 184:51-55, 1984.

Smith, D.A. and Hill, F.W.G. Metastatic malignant mesothelioma in a dog. *J Comp Pathol* 100:97-101, 1989.

Tyler, R.D. and Cowell, R.L. Evaluation of pleural and peritoneal effusions. *Vet Clin North Am Small Anim Pract* 19: 743-768, 1989.

Waddle, J.R. and Giger, U. Lipoprotein electrophoresis differentiation of chylous and nonchylous pleural effusions in dogs and cats and its correlation with pleural effusion triglyceride concentration. *Vet Clin Pathol* 19:80-85. 1990.

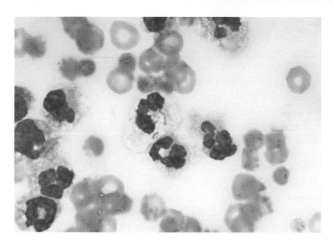

FIG. 9-1. Canine. Pleural fluid. Septic pleuritis. Three slightly degenerate neutrophils in the center of the field. Filamentous bacteria are present in the cytoplasm of one. Members of the *Actinomycetaceae* spp. often appear as long filamentous rods, typically phagocytized by neutrophils. (×400.)

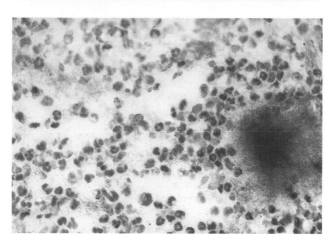

FIG. 9-2. Canine. Pleural fluid. Septic pleuritis. Background of neutrophils and macrophages with varying degrees of neutrophil nuclear degenerative change. There is a large colony of bacteria, consistent with *Actinomycetaceae* sp., which appear as a "sulfur" granule when fluid is aspirated. (×100.)

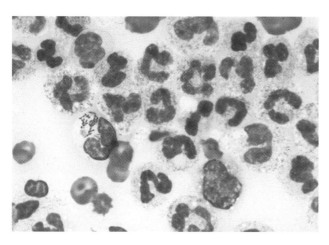

FIG. 9-3. Canine. Pleural fluid. Septic pleuritis. (Same case as Fig. 9-2.) Predominance of neutrophils with varying degrees of nuclear degeneration consistent with bacterial infection, especially if anaerobic species. With severe chromatolysis and swelling of nuclei neutrophils can resemble macrophages. (×400.)

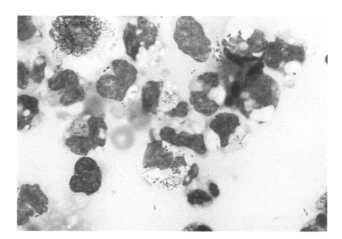

FIG. 9-4. Canine. Pleural fluid. Septic pleuritis. Mixed population of cells with phagocytized bacteria including filamentous and coccoid forms. Bacterial toxins contribute to the degree of neutrophil nuclear chromatolysis. (×500.)

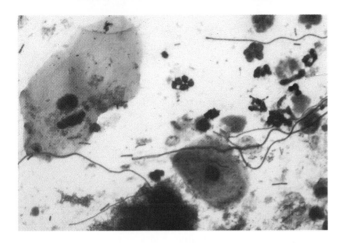

FIG. 9-5. Feline. Peritoneal fluid. Septic peritonitis associated with squamous cell carcinoma. Two intermediate to superficial squamous epithelial cells, neutrophils, and many pleomorphic bacteria. The location of these squamous epithelial cells is of greater significance than the nuclear morphology, in support of malignancy. Skin contamination must be ruled out. (×250.)

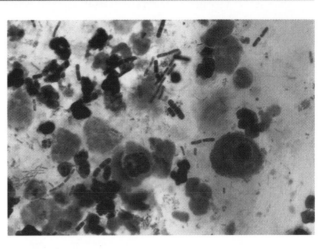

FIG. 9-6. Feline. Peritoneal fluid. Septic peritonitis associated with squamous cell carcinoma. (Same case as Fig. 9-5.) Cellular debris, degenerate neutrophils, pleomorphic bacteria, and a squamous epithelial cell with a very large hyperchromatic nucleus and nucleolus. Dysplasia and contamination must be considered when interpreting location and morphology of the squamous epithelial cells. (×400.)

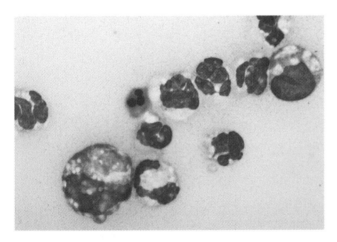

FIG. 9-7. Feline. Peritoneal fluid. Feline infectious peritonitis. Nucleated cell count was 5 × 10⁶/L, protein concentration was 51 g/L. A mixed population of neutrophils and macrophages with mild neutrophil nuclear degenerative changes. The pyknotic lobules in one neutrophil suggest aging versus bacterial lysis. (×400.)

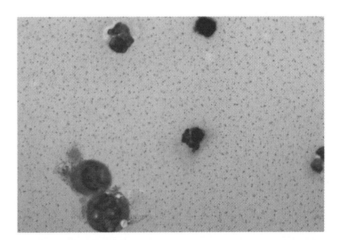

FIG. 9-8. Feline. Peritoneal fluid. Feline infectious peritonitis. Dense blue granular background suggests increased protein concentration. A low to moderate increase of various cell types is typical of FIP. (×400.)

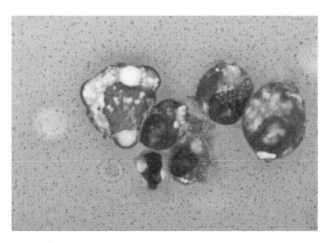

FIG. 9-9. Feline. Peritoneal fluid. Feline infectious peritonitis. (Same case as Fig. 9-8.) Dense background with fine granularity is consistent with increased protein concentration. Large, foamy macrophages, smaller mononuclear cells, and one neutrophil are visible. (×400.)

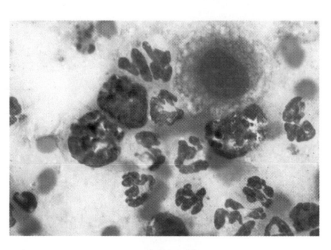

FIG. 9-10. Canine. Peritoneal fluid. Bile peritonitis. Neutrophils, macrophages containing green-black pigment, a mesothelial cell, erythrocytes, and a "dirty" background are consistent with bile peritonitis. Bile pigments can present as colors ranging from yellow to black and may be free or phagocytized. Free bile initiates a marked chemotactic response. (×400.)

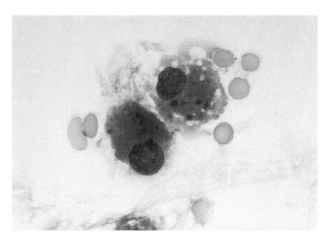

FIG. 9-11. Canine. Pleural fluid. Hemorrhagic effusion associated with carcinoma. Two nucleated cells contain hemosiderin-like pigment consistent with response to previous hemorrhage. (×400.)

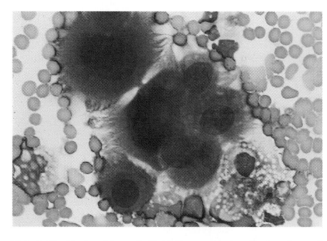

FIG. 9-12. Canine. Thoracic fluid. Hemorrhagic effusion. Several benign hyperplastic mesothelial cells illustrating anisocytosis, multinucleation, perinuclear fine pigmentation, and pink fibrillar appearance to cytoplasmic borders. (×250.)

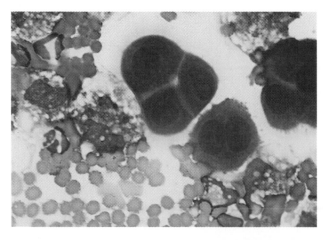

FIG. 9-13. Canine. Thoracic fluid. Hemorrhagic effusion. (Same case as Fig. 9-12.) Central hyperplastic mesothelial cells illustrating high N:C ratio, nuclear hyperchromasia, and binucleation. (×312.)

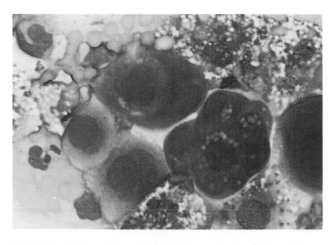

FIG. 9-14. Canine. Thoracic fluid. Hemorrhagic effusion. (Same case as Fig. 9-12.) Pleomorphic presentation of benign hyperplastic mesothelial cells. (×312.)

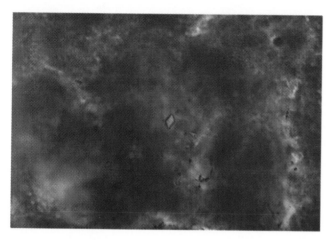

FIG. 9-15. Canine. Thoracic fluid. Hemorrhagic effusion. Dense background of cells with a small central hematoidin crystal. (×375.)

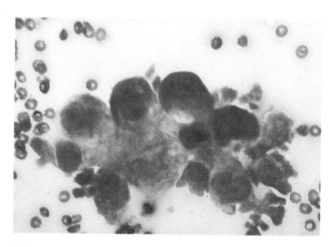

FIG. 9-16. Canine. Pleural fluid. Bronchogenic carcinoma. Polypoid arrangement of poorly differentiated epithelial cells, marked variation in cell and nuclear diameters, hyperchromatic nuclei, and multiple dark nucleoli. Papillary arrangement is consistent with exfoliating carcinoma. (×200.)

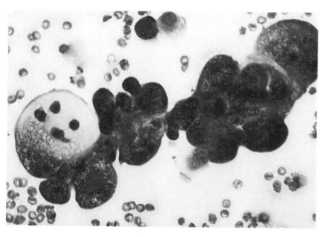

FIG. 9-17. Canine. Pleural fluid. Bronchogenic carcinoma. (Same case as Fig. 9-16.) Cluster of variable-sized epithelial cells, dense basophilic cytoplasm containing many small to large vacuoles, marked anisokaryosis, and prominent irregular nucleoli. The large vacuolated cell with aberrant mitosis suggests adenomatous origin. (×100.)

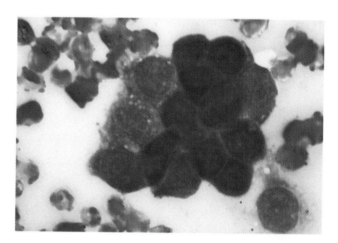

FIG. 9-18. Canine. Pleural fluid. Bronchogenic carcinoma. (Same case as Fig. 9-16.) A sheet of cells with prominent continuous cell borders, scant basophilic cytoplasm, and hyperchromatic nuclei with high N:C ratio is consistent with exfoliation of malignant epithelial cells. (×400.)

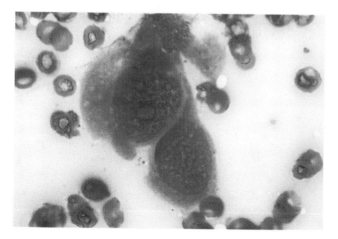

FIG. 9-19. Canine. Pleural fluid. Bronchogenic carcinoma. (Same case as Fig. 9-16.) Large epithelial cells with very large nuclei and high N:C ratio; multiple irregular nucleoli. Note size in comparison with red blood cells. (×400.)

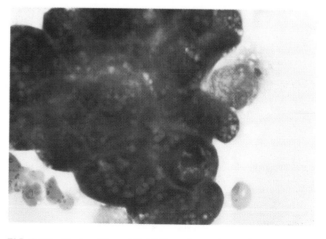

FIG. 9-20. Canine. Pleural fluid. Bronchogenic carcinoma. (Same case as Fig. 9-16.) Arrangement of cells, common borders, vacuolation, and high N:C ratio are consistent with malignant epithelial cells of papillary origin. (×400.)

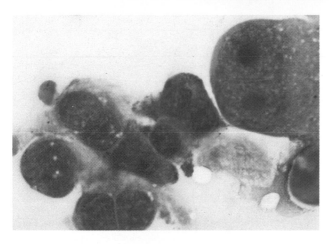

FIG. 9-21. Canine. Pleural fluid. Bronchogenic carcinoma. (Same case as Fig. 9-16.) Extreme anisokaryosis and high N:C ratio consistent with exfoliating malignant epithelial cells. (×400.)

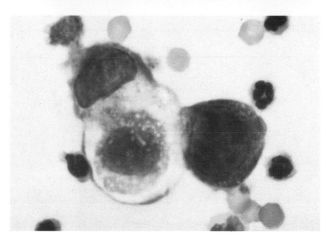

FIG. 9-22. Feline. Pleural fluid. Pulmonary carcinoma. Exfoliating malignant epithelial cells with marked anisokaryosis, hyperchromasia, and high N:C ratio. With the cellular criteria visible, malignancy can be diagnosed with assurance. (×500.)

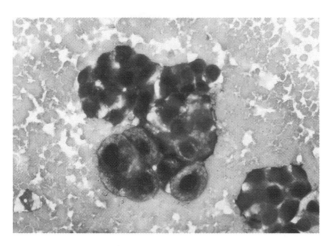

FIG. 9-23. Canine. Peritoneal fluid. Mammary carcinoma. Clusters of cells that vary in morphology, but all are consistent with epithelial origin. (×100.)

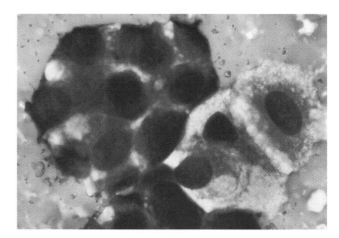

FIG. 9-24. Canine. Peritoneal fluid. Mammary carcinoma. (Same case as Fig. 9-23.) Large cells with round to oval nuclei, fine indistinct chromatin, indistinct large nucleoli, and some cytoplasmic vacuolation. Morphology of individual cells, including vacuolation and acinar arrangement, suggests exfoliation of adenocarcinoma. Because of potential misinterpretation of hyperplastic mesothelial cells strict criteria must be used to prevent a false-positive diagnosis of malignancy. (×400.)

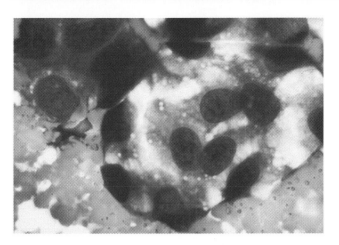

FIG. 9-25. Canine. Peritoneal fluid. Mammary carcinoma. (Same case as Fig. 9-23.) Acinar arrangement of epithelial cells. Clear to lightly staining cytoplasmic vacuolation suggests secretory capacity of primary cells. Imbibition of fluid can mimic the appearance of secretory vacuoles. (×400.)

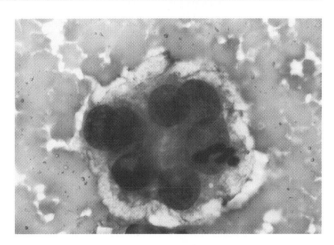

FIG. 9-26. Canine. Peritoneal fluid. Mammary carcinoma. (Same case as Fig. 9-23.) Acinar arrangement of epithelial cells suggests the glandular nature of the primary tumor, assuming hyperplastic mesothelial cells can be ruled out. (×400.)

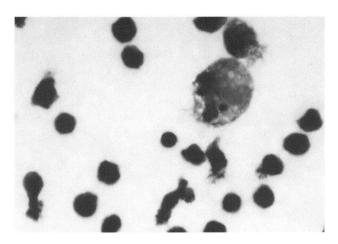

FIG. 9-27. Canine. Pleural fluid. Poor slide preparation and slow drying of the cells results in small, dark cells with loss of nuclear and cytoplasmic details. Better preservation of cells is required for interpretation. (×400.)

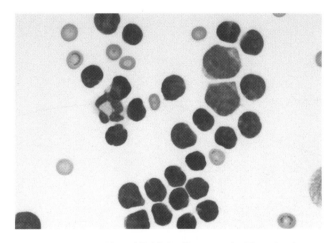

FIG. 9-28. Canine. Pleural fluid. Cardiomyopathy. The mixed population of small and large lymphocytes typical of cardiomyopathy contrasts with the homogeneous morphology observed with lymphoma. (×400.)

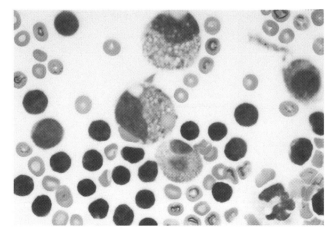

FIG. 9-29. Canine. Pleural fluid. Cardiomyopathy. Small lymphocytes; two macrophages, one exhibiting erythrocytophagy; an eosinophil, and neutrophil. If chylous effusion is present, vacuolation caused by lipids may be observed. (×400.)

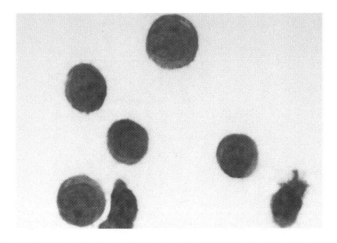

FIG. 9-30. Canine. Pleural fluid. Cardiomyopathy. Lymphocytes with uniform nuclear chromatin and some variation in cell size. Careful inspection is required to rule out lymphoma. (×500.)

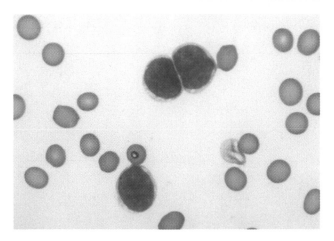

FIG. 9-31. Canine. Pleural fluid. Congestive heart failure. Large lymphocytes with uniform nuclear chromatin and one large nucleolus; not to be confused with lymphoma. (×500.)

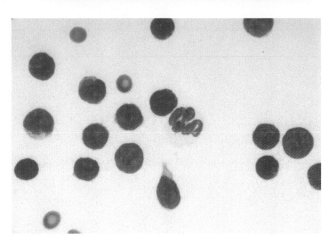

FIG. 9-32. Canine. Pleural fluid. Lymphocytic effusion of unknown cause. The predominant lymphocyte population was small with uniform nuclear chromatin and inconspicuous nucleoli. Based on morphology and an increase in triglycerides, chylothorax of undetermined origin was diagnosed. (×400.)

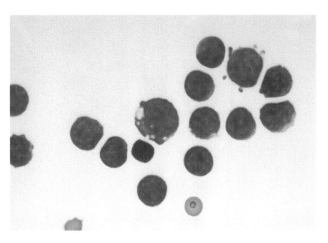

FIG. 9-33. Feline. Pleural fluid. Chylous effusion, lymphoma. Small and large lymphocytes with large, irregular nucleoli. The monomorphic large cells with high N:C ratio and multiple nucleoli suggest a diagnosis of malignancy. (×400.)

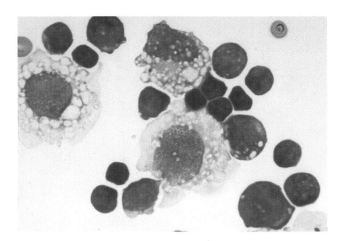

FIG. 9-34. Feline. Pleural fluid. Chylous effusion, lymphoma. (Same case as Fig. 9-33.) Small and large lymphocytes; three large, foamy macrophages. Macrophages and small lymphocytes can be observed in chylous effusions. The larger lymphocytes with high N:C ratio and irregular nucleoli should alert the cytologist to the possible diagnosis of lymphoma. (×400.)

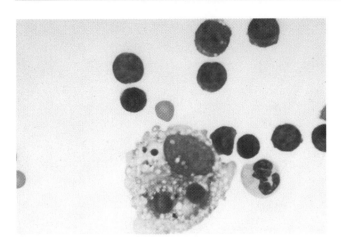

FIG. 9-35. Feline. Pleural fluid. Chylous effusion, lymphoma. (Same case as Fig. 9-33.) Small to medium lymphocytes. Cytophagy evident within the large macrophage. Although monomorphism is more characteristic for lymphoma, the cellular response to effusion and possible necrosis must be distinguished from the primary disease. (×400.)

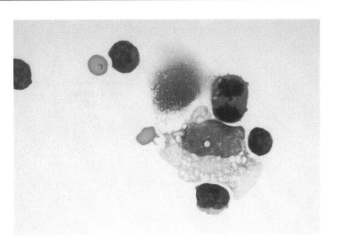

FIG. 9-36. Feline. Pleural fluid. Chylous effusion, lymphoma. (Same case as Fig. 9-33.) Small lymphocyte with mitosis, large macrophage, and bare nucleus. Although mitotic nuclei may be observed within benign and malignant lymphocyte populations, they are more common in lymphoma. Tumor cells tend to be more fragile, resulting in increased prevalence of nuclear debris. (×400.)

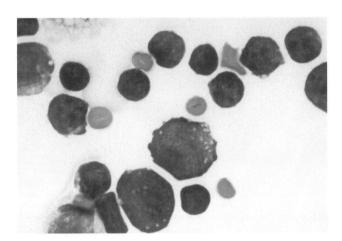

FIG. 9-37. Feline. Pleural fluid. Chylous effusion, lymphoma. (Same case as Fig. 9-33.) Two populations of lymphocytes; large lymphocytes with high N:C ratio, prominent nucleoli, and basophilic cytoplasm and smaller lymphocytes with retiform chromatin. In this case, the former cells provide greater indication of the primary diagnosis. (×500.)

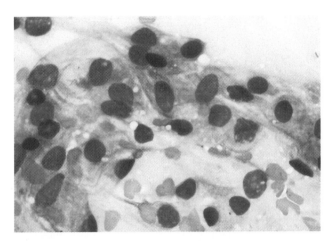

FIG. 9-38. Canine. Imprint. Liver surface. Loosely cohesive large cells consistent with benign nonreactive mesothelium as frequently observed within imprints or FNAs of internal organs. (×250.)

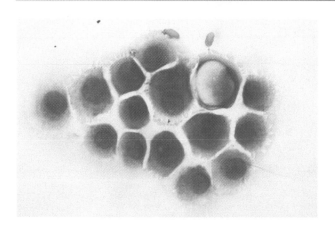

FIG. 9-39. Canine. Pleural fluid. Congestive heart failure. Close aggregation of benign mesothelial cells. The large cytoplasmic vacuole, resembling a signet ring cell associated with adenocarcinomas, is frequently observed in mesothelial cells, possibly caused by imbibition of fluid. (×200.)

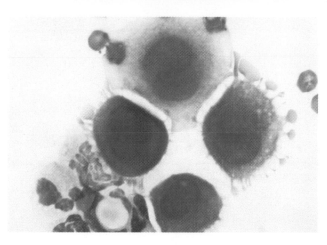

FIG. 9-40. Canine. Pleural fluid. Congestive heart failure. (Same case as Fig. 9-39.) Mesothelial cell hyperplasia, as indicated by hyperchromasia and binucleation, is frequently observed with chronic effusions in dogs. The cytoplasmic pseudopodia are artifacts associated with air drying. (×400.)

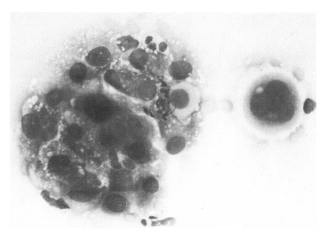

FIG. 9-41. Canine. Pericardial fluid. Benign idiopathic pericardial effusion. Benign hyperplasia of mesothelial cells illustrating cluster formation, which may be mistaken for exfoliating adenocarcinoma. (×200.)

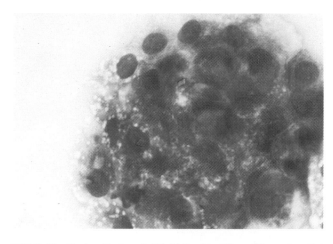

FIG. 9-42. Canine. Pericardial fluid. Benign idiopathic pericardial effusion. (Same case as Fig. 9-41.) A large cluster of benign mesothelial cells, with cytoplasmic vacuolation and hematoidin pigment. (×250.)

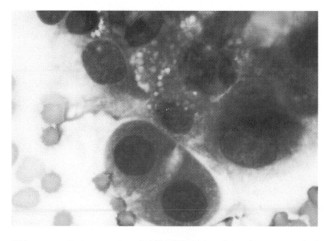

FIG. 9-43. Canine. Pericardial fluid. Benign idiopathic pericardial effusion. (Same case as Fig. 9-41.) Benign hyperplasia of mesothelial cells. The intracytoplasmic pigment, likely hemosiderin, is observed with chronic hemorrhagic effusions. (×400.)

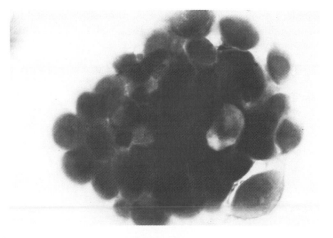

FIG. 9-44. Canine. Pleural fluid. Benign hemorrhagic effusion. Lung torsion with hemorrhage. Closely aggregated round cells with large nuclei, hyperchromasia, high N:C ratio, and multinucleation mimicking exfoliating neoplastic epithelial cells. (×200.)

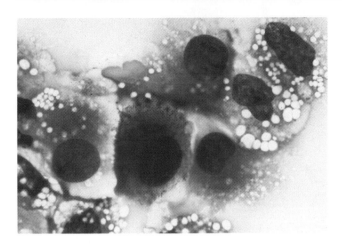

FIG. 9-45. Canine. Pleural fluid. Benign hemorrhagic effusion. Lung torsion with hemorrhage. (Same case as Fig. 9-44.) Hyperplastic benign mesothelial cells and macrophages. (×400.)

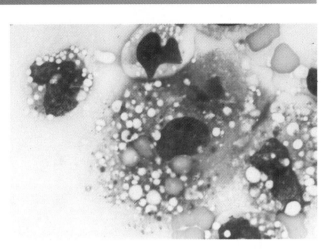

FIG. 9-46. Canine. Pleural fluid. Benign hemorrhagic effusion. Lung torsion with hemorrhage. (Same case as Fig. 9-44.) Large vacuolated macrophage, with erythrocytophagy and fine granulation resulting from hemosiderin accumulation or cell debris. (×400.)

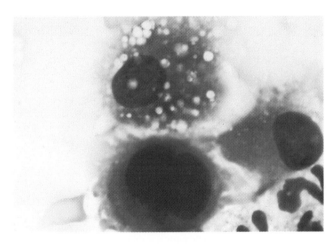

FIG. 9-47. Canine. Pleural fluid. Benign hemorrhagic effusion. Lung torsion with hemorrhage. (Same case as Fig. 9-44.) Binucleated mesothelial cell with macrophages and neutrophil. (×400.)

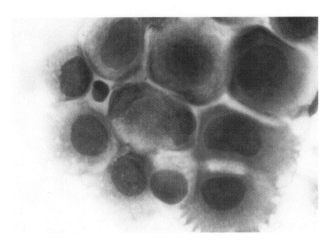

FIG. 9-48. Canine. Peritoneal fluid. Benign nonseptic effusion. Loosely cohesive aggregation of hyperplastic mesothelial cells. Many morphological criteria are present that in most other cell types would be consistent with malignancy. (×400.)

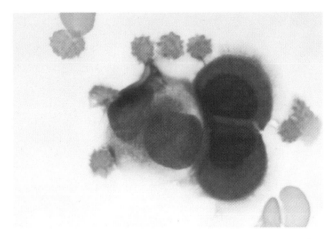

FIG. 9-49. Canine. Peritoneal fluid. Benign nonseptic effusion. (Same case as Fig. 9-48.) Benign hyperplastic mesothelial cells. Note nuclear hyperchromasia and common border between the cells. (×500.)

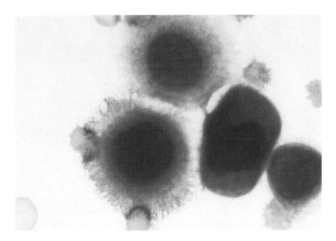

FIG. 9-50. Canine. Peritoneal fluid. Benign nonseptic effusion. (Same case as Fig. 9-48.) Benign hyperplastic mesothelial cells. The bright pink halo surrounding two of the mesothelial cells is an artifact of preparation. (×500.)

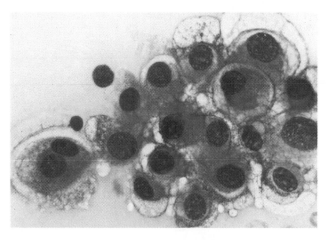

FIG. 9-51. Canine. Peritoneal fluid. Mesothelioma. Loosely cohesive mesothelial cells with moderate N:C ratio. Benign reactive hyperplasia and mesothelioma can be extremely difficult to differentiate on the basis of cytomorphology. (×250.) (Courtesy Duane F. Brobst, 1988.)

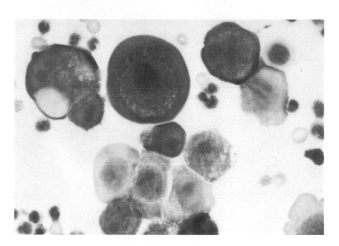

FIG. 9-52. Canine. Peritoneal fluid. Mesothelioma. High cellularity is common with mesothelioma. Mesothelial cells have marked anisokaryosis, hyperchromasia, and high N:C ratio. (×250.)

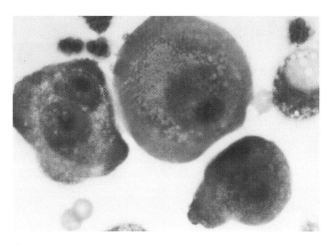

FIG. 9-53. Canine. Peritoneal fluid. Mesothelioma. (Same case as Fig. 9-52.) Large mesothelial cells with prominent nucleoli and cytoplasmic vacuolation. (×400.)

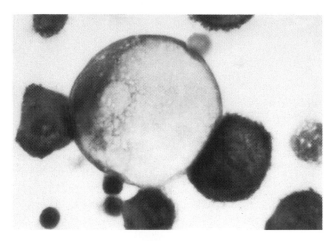

FIG. 9-54. Canine. Peritoneal fluid. Mesothelioma. (Same case as Fig. 9-52.) Mesothelial cells with hyperchromasia, high N:C ratio, and prominent nucleoli. One cell has a large cytoplasmic vacuole, creating the signet ring appearance associated with secretory epithelial cells. (×400.)

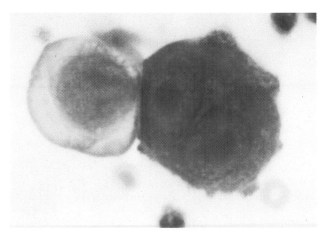

FIG. 9-55. Canine. Peritoneal fluid. Mesothelioma. (Same case as Fig. 9-52.) Large mesothelial cells with marked variation in appearance. Binucleated cell has large, irregular nucleoli and hyperchromasia. (×500.)

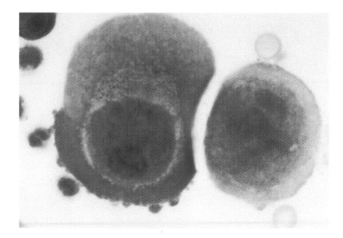

FIG. 9-56. Canine. Peritoneal fluid. Mesothelioma. (Same case as Fig. 9-52.) Bizarre appearance of mesothelial cells with unusual nuclear morphology and mitotic figure. Perinuclear vacuolation suggests secretory cell function. The accumulating abnormalities assist differentiation of benign hyperplasia and malignancy. (×400.)

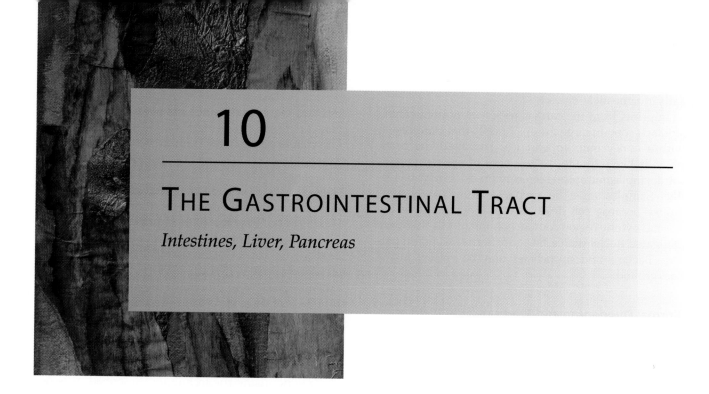

10

THE GASTROINTESTINAL TRACT

Intestines, Liver, Pancreas

Cytological examination is used less frequently for examination of the gastrointestinal tract than for organ systems that are more accessible. Both primary and secondary diseases of the digestive system can be diagnosed using suitable methods as outlined below. Rectal scrapings are used to diagnose localized lesions of the rectum or diseases of the lower colon. In conditions that diffusely affect the gastrointestinal tract, a rectal scraping may reflect the disease process and obviate the necessity for an intestinal surgical biopsy. Diagnosis of histoplasmosis, prototothecosis, *Balantidium coli* infection, eosinophilic colitis, and lymphosarcoma can be made using rectal scrapings. Aspiration biopsy of the liver is frequently diagnostic.

■ GASTROINTESTINAL TRACT

TECHNIQUES

The primary limitation to cytological investigation of diseases involving the gastrointestinal tract is the access to representative cells. Aspiration biopsies may be performed directly through the abdominal wall. Large intraabdominal lesion biopsies can be guided by palpation, whereas small lesions are more likely successful if biopsies are guided using imaging techniques. Imprints of surgical biopsy material or rectal scrapings are used to investigate systemic diseases affecting the gastrointestinal tract.

Rectal mucosal scrapings are performed using an instrument such as a small chemistry spatula. The rectum should be free of feces. The spatula is inserted into

the rectum using digital guidance. Scrapings must be done firmly to remove the surface epithelium and penetrate the lamina propria (Rakich, 1999). Lubricant should not be used because its staining properties can mask cytological details (Rakich, 1999). There is increased risk of perforation in conditions in which the colon is thin and friable (Rakich, 1999). The material scraped off the mucosal surface is spread onto a glass slide and stained.

Normal Esophagus (Figs. 10-1 to 10-5)

Scrapings of canine mid-region esophagus contain angular cells with distinct cytoplasmic boundaries, round nuclei, and a low N:C ratio. Squamous differentiation is apparent within the cytoplasm. Indistinct fine cytoplasmic vacuolation and occasional basophilic cytoplasmic pigment may be visible. Impression smears may contain superficial cellular debris and bacteria compatible with partially digested food.

Normal Stomach (Figs. 10-6 to 10-11)

Cytology is not used frequently for examining lesions of the stomach in dogs and cats. Stomach washes are performed under general anesthesia. Interest has increased with greater access to endoscopes for visual and brush biopsy examination. The controversy regarding the clinical significance of *Helicobacter* organisms has led to increased interest in examinations for the presence of these organisms. Occasionally stomach washings are performed, but the interpretive experience of the authors is limited. Impression smears of surgical biopsy samples can complement the histological diagnosis and provide early diagnostical clues.

Imprints from the cardiac region of normal canine stomach contain large groups of cells that can present with a honeycomb appearance. The overlying basophilia is likely due to the presence of normal mucus. Intracytoplasmic apical secretory products may be visible. Samples must be prepared immediately after biopsy because cell death is rapid. Scrapings of the normal pyloric region contain columnar cells that have elongated nuclei with a fine cribriform chromatin pattern. Bacteria and spirochetes may be present in the background.

Normal Duodenum and Jejunum (Figs. 10-12 to 10-14)

Impression smears made from fresh normal canine duodenal biopsies contained tissue fragments, lymphoid cells, a few neutrophils, and eosinophils (Tobey, 1984). Bacteria were not observed (Tobey, 1984). Imprints from the jejunum contain mucosal cells arranged in a typical honeycomb relationship. The mucosal epithelial cells are cuboidal with visible cell borders, moderate N:C ratio, and cytoplasmic basophilia. Nuclei are 1½ erythrocytes in diameter. Small, indistinct, multiple nucleoli are apparent. Coccobacilli are present in the background.

Normal Colon (Figs. 10-15 to 10-18)

Imprints and rectal scrapings of normal colon contain similar cells. The mucosal epithelial cells have basilar located nuclei and moderate N:C ratio. Some cells demonstrate apical mucus production and cytoplasmic vacuolation.

Normal Rectal Scrapings

The normal rectal scraping consists of columnar epithelial cells, acellular debris, mucus, and a mixed population of bacteria (Rakich, 1999). Squamous cells are present with inadvertent scraping of the rectum (Rakich, 1999). Low numbers of lymphocytes, plasma cells, and neutrophils may be present (Rakich, 1999). If a lymphoid follicle is accidentally scraped, a heterogeneous population of lymphocytes may be present (Rakich, 1999).

INFLAMMATORY CONDITIONS OF THE GASTROINTESTINAL TRACT (Figs. 10-19 and 10-20)

CLINICAL AND CYTOLOGICAL DIAGNOSES

Any inflammatory disease that affects the intestine can theoretically be diagnosed from brush biopsies or from impression smears of the biopsy sample. *Histoplasma*

and *Prototheca* organisms are easily identified when present. A predominance of lymphocytes and plasma cells and increased eosinophils is expected with lymphocytic-plasmacytic enteritis in dogs (Jacobs, 1990).

Rectal scrapings have been used to diagnose colitis caused by infectious agents, including *Cryptococcus neoformans, Prototheca, Histoplasma,* and *Balantidium. Balantidium* is a large, ciliated protozoa that can infect dogs after ingestion of pig feces (Rakich, 1999). *Balantidium* trophozoites are 40 to 80 μ by 25 to 45 μ. They have a large, oval nucleus and a unique spiral arrangement for the rows of cilia (Rakich, 1999). Large cysts (60 μ) may be seen (Rakich, 1999).

Neutrophils were present in the mucosal scrapings from 88% of dogs with colitis and 93% of the control population (Houston, 1988). Irritation from the enema administered before the scraping and variation in mucosal scraping techniques were suggested as possible explanations for the neutrophils (Houston, 1988). Rectal scraping, using the techniques described, was not concluded to be useful for assisting diagnosis of clinical colitis (Houston, 1988).

NEOPLASTIC DISEASE

Gastrointestinal tumors account for 2% of all neoplasms in the dog and cat (Couto, 1992). Two thirds of these are malignant (Couto, 1992). A male predisposition to adenocarcinomas is noted in the dog (Birchard, 1986; Patnaik, 1977).

Gastric Neoplasia

CLINICAL AND CYTOLOGICAL DIAGNOSES

In the dog, gastric tumors accounted for 17% of 350 canine gastrointestinal neoplasms (Couto, 1992). Approximately 60% of these were gastric carcinomas (Birchard, 1986; Couto, 1992). Tumors limited to the gastric wall without serosal invasion have the best prognosis. Prolonged survival times are possible, although local lymph node metastases are common in the dog (Couto, 1992). Surgical excision is the best approach to therapy (Couto, 1992).

Gastric neoplasia appears to be rare in the cat. Of 40 reported feline gastrointestinal neoplasms, none were gastric in origin (Couto, 1992).

Cytological reports of gastric neoplasia are rare. The usual criteria of malignancy should be applied.

Intestinal Neoplasms—Nonlymphoid (Figs. 10-21 to 10-36)

CLINICAL DIAGNOSIS

Several surveys of gastrointestinal neoplasia in the dog and cat are reported. (Birchard, 1986; Couto, 1992; Patnaik, 1977). Of 64 neoplasms of the canine small and large intestine reported in one study, 34 were adenocarcinomas, 19 were leiomyosarcomas, 5 were lymphosarcomas, 4 were carcinoids, and 2 were benign stromal masses (Patnaik, 1977). The rectum was the most common site for adenocarcinomas, followed by the colon and duodenum (Patnaik, 1977). In a study including 32 dogs and 14 cats with nonlymphoid intestinal neoplasms, 53% were adenocarcinomas, 19% were leiomyosarcomas, 13% were fibrosarcomas, 9% were leiomyomas, 3% were undifferentiated sarcomas, and 3% were benign polyps (Birchard, 1986). In the dog the frequency of adenocarcinoma in the colon equaled that of the duodenum, jejunum, and ileum combined (Birchard, 1986). In the cat, carcinomas were equally represented in the jejunum, ileum, and colon (Birchard, 1986).

The prognosis is poor for all malignant tumors of the intestinal tract (Couto, 1992).

CYTOLOGICAL DIAGNOSIS

Cytological descriptions for carcinomas of the gastrointestinal tract are limited. Based on minimal experience the usual cytological criteria of malignancy apply. Cells are frequently very anaplastic and have large, bizarre nucleoli, hyperchromasia, and a very high N:C ratio. Anisokaryosis may be prominent. Occasionally the cytoplasm contains a large secretory vacuole, likely representing mucus production.

Neuroendocrine Tumors (Figs. 10-37 to 10-44)

CLINICAL DIAGNOSIS

Neuroendocrine tumors, variably called carcinoid tumors, argentaffin tumors, and amine precursor uptake and decarboxylation (APUD) tumors, arise from specialized endocrine or paracrine cells that can be found in various organs in the body (Barker, 1993). These tumors, although rare, most commonly present in the intestine, liver, adrenal gland, pancreas, and heart of the dog. They are uncommon in the cat. These tumors are often locally invasive and may metastasize. The prognosis is poor.

CYTOLOGICAL DIAGNOSIS

Neuroendocrine tumors have several characteristic cytological features; however, differentiation between the various sites of origin is not possible. Immunocytochemical features can be used histologically to confirm the presence of argyrophilic granules. Smears from neuroendocrine tumors are usually highly cellular. Smear preparation must be done with great care because in most preparations bare nuclei vastly outnumber intact cells (Blue, 1999). Intact cells have round central nuclei and dense nuclear chromatin (Blue, 1999). The cells have a fairly even monotonous appearance and often appear enmeshed in a blue to pink background material. A mosaic pattern has been described in imprints (Blue, 1999). Cytoplasmic

vacuolation may be prominent, and N:C ratio is usually low.

Gastrointestinal Lymphoma

The clinical/cytological description of gastrointestinal lymphoid neoplasia is in Chapter 5.

■ LIVER

In the dog and cat, biochemical tests are used for the initial investigation of suspected liver disease. Cytological examination is used for subsequent differentiation of selected types of liver disease. Blind FNA biopsies are often adequate for detecting diffuse lesions. Imaging procedures are required for directing reliable fine-needle biopsies of focal lesions. Impression smears of core or surgical biopsy imprints provide independent assessment or enhance histological interpretation of liver lesions. FNA biopsies are used for initial investigation of a few specific liver disorders, before surgical biopsy, because of the low risk, low cost, and ease with which FNA biopsies can be obtained.

TECHNIQUES

FNA biopsy of dog or cat liver is made with the animal either standing or in right lateral recumbency. For a suspect diffuse lesion the left twelfth or thirteenth intercostal space is the site of entry. For a focal lesion, the intercostal space is selected from imaging information. The biopsy site is prepared as for a surgical approach. The biopsy needle is directed craniomedially into the liver. Suction is applied using the attached syringe. The needle tip is advanced and withdrawn several times while the needle tip remains within the organ. When withdrawn, a change in needle tip direction may be made to increase sampling area. The changes in direction should be limited to minimize tissue laceration. In advanced liver disease, clotting abnormalities may lead to hemorrhage. Coagulation profiles and platelet counts should be determined before liver biopsy, especially if a core biopsy technique is used. Complications from liver fine-needle biopsy are rare.

NORMAL LIVER (Figs. 10-45 to 10-53)

An aspiration biopsy of normal liver should produce a moderately cellular slide. The majority of cells are hepatocytes, single or in clumps, with distinct cell margins. In the dog, hepatocytes are 4 to 5 times the size of a red blood cell. Nuclei are round with one prominent nucleolus. Hepatocyte cytoplasm is lightly basophilic and has a fine pink to blue granularity representing endoplasmic reticulum. A few hepatocytes obtained from normal liver may be binucleate or have macronucleoli or cytoplasmic vacuolation. Small amounts of blue-green intrahepatic or intracanalicular bile pigment may be visible. Small clusters of biliary epithelial cells and occasionally endothelial cells or differentiating hematopoietic cells may be present. Biliary epithelial cells are usually smaller than hepatocytes and are round and regular in appearance with prominent cell margins.

NONNEOPLASTIC DISEASE

Nonneoplastic changes that can be diagnosed using cytology include glucocorticoid-induced hepatopathy, feline hepatic lipidosis, feline cholangitis or cholangiohepatitis, nonspecific inflammatory lesions of the liver, and disseminated infectious agents (e.g., histoplasmosis and infectious canine hepatitis).

Feline Hepatic Lipidosis (Figs. 10-54 to 10-58)

CLINICAL DIAGNOSIS
In feline hepatic lipidosis, triglycerides accumulate within hepatocytes. This syndrome affects obese cats of any age. The average age was 4.6 years in a study including 45 cats (Hubbard, 1992). Most cats presented with depression, anorexia, and icterus (Center, 1993a). Serum alkaline phosphatase activity and bilirubin concentration were consistently increased (Hubbard, 1992). Hepatic lipidosis is associated with a decrease in endoplasmic reticulum, glycogen, Golgi complexes, and peroxisomes (Center, 1993b). Cytoskeletal injury has been suggested as the cause of the cholestasis (Center, 1993b). Lipidosis is also reported in cats with α-mannosidosis and sphingomyelin lipidosis (Baker, 1987; Jezyk, 1986).

CYTOLOGICAL DIAGNOSIS
Because hepatic lipidosis can be confirmed readily using FNA biopsy, anesthesia and surgical biopsy are not required (Hubbard, 1992). Hepatocytes contain small, clear vacuoles representing lipid accumulation. Vacuoles are numerous throughout the cytoplasm. Frequently, hepatocytes contain fine intracytoplasmic granular clumps of blue-green pigment representing bile accumulation. In severely icteric cats, bile may fill the intracanalicular spaces. Multiple large vacuoles have been designated macrovesicular fat, whereas multiple small vacuoles have been designated microvesicular (Meyer, 1999). Occasionally, large, discrete vacuoles may displace the nucleus peripherally.

The cytological diagnosis was correct in 13 cats with histologically confirmed feline hepatic lipidosis (Kristensen, 1984).

Feline Hepatic Cholangitis or Cholangiohepatitis

CLINICAL DIAGNOSIS
In cats, cholangiohepatitis is a well-documented syndrome characterized by inflammatory changes originating in the periportal region and extending into the hepatic lobules. The cholangiohepatitis may be suppurative (cholangiohepatitis) or lymphocytic (lymphocytic portal hepatitis) (Gagne, 1996; Prasse, 1982; Shaker, 1991).

CYTOLOGICAL DIAGNOSIS
With suppurative cholangitis, aspirates contain hepatocytes, many neutrophils, and possibly bacteria. Differentiation of acute and chronic suppurative hepatitis is not possible using FNA biopsies. With lymphocytic cholangitis there are moderate numbers of lymphocytes and plasma cells interspersed with hepatocytes (Prasse, 1982). Histology may be required to differentiate lymphocytic cholangitis from well-differentiated lymphoma (Meyer, 1999). Intrahepatic and intracanalicular cholestasis may be prominent with both lesions.

Glucocorticoid Hepatopathy (Figs. 10-59 to 10-60)

CLINICAL DIAGNOSIS
In dogs, an increase in glucocorticoids from endogenous lesions, or exogenous administration, will lead to glycogen accumulation and increased liver related serum enzyme activity.

CYTOLOGICAL DIAGNOSIS
The glycogen deposits appear as clear cytoplasmic vacuoles within hepatocytes. It is reported that glycogen accumulation creates a "feathery" appearance to the cytoplasm, with vacuoles "laced with wisps of blue cytoplasm" (Meyer, 1999). This indistinct vacuolar change contrasts with the "crisper" vacuolar outline observed with hepatic lipidosis (Meyer, 1999).

Nonspecific Inflammatory Liver Disease

CLINICAL AND CYTOLOGICAL DIAGNOSES
Blind FNA biopsies will allow identification of the predominant cells associated with hepatic inflammatory processes. Histological examination is required to determine the architectural location and extent of the inflammatory process necessary for differentiation and prognosis of many lesions. Use of advanced imaging techniques will improve the diagnostic utility of FNA biopsy for focal liver lesions. In 36 liver specimens, correlation between histopathology and FNA was low at 20% (Kristensen, 1984). Histology and tissue core biopsy correlation was 75% (Kristensen, 1984). In each of the five cases classified from cytological examination as cholestatic, there was histological confirmation (Kristensen, 1984).

Infectious Canine Hepatitis

CLINICAL AND CYTOLOGICAL DIAGNOSES

Canine adenovirus type 1 is the etiological agent of infectious canine hepatitis. Clinically, signs can vary from an inapparent infection to peracute overwhelming viremia (Kelly, 1993). This virus has a tropism for endothelium, hepatic parenchyma, and mesothelium (Kelly, 1993). Eosinophilic intranuclear inclusions are readily visible with H&E staining and considered to be pathognomonic for canine infectious hepatitis. Staining characteristics may be less distinct and will vary with Romanowsky's stains.

Extramedullary Hematopoiesis (Figs. 10-61 and 10-62)

CLINICAL AND CYTOLOGICAL DIAGNOSES

The occasional hematopoietic precursor cell may be observed in normal liver. When there is bone marrow stress, these precursor cells may increase dramatically and include blast stages of the granulocytic, erythrocytic, and megakaryocytic series. The later stages of each cell line predominate, as in bone marrow. Rubricytes are often prominent in cases of chronic anemia.

Aspiration biopsies of the liver are useful in identifying diseases involving blood because of the highly vascular nature. Thus leukemic animals frequently present with large numbers of blastic cells in liver aspirates.

Copper Toxicity in Bedlington and West Highland White Terriers (Figs. 10-63 and 10-64)

CLINICAL AND CYTOLOGICAL DIAGNOSES

Accumulation of copper in the liver of Bedlington terriers and West Highland white terriers leads to chronic active hepatitis and progressive liver failure (Thornnburg, 1990; Twedt, 1979). FNA of affected liver reveals low numbers of mixed inflammatory cells intermixed with hepatocytes (Scott, 1991). Hepatocytes contain pale green refractile granules that are rubeanic acid stain–positive and are consistent with copper (Scott, 1991).

NEOPLASTIC LESIONS OF THE LIVER (Figs. 10-65 and 10-66)

Nodular Hyperplasia, Hepatic Adenoma, or Adenocarcinoma

CLINICAL DIAGNOSIS

In the dog and cat, hepatocellular carcinomas are rare (Kelly, 1993; Patnaik, 1981a). Neoplasms of the liver and biliary tract account for 0.6% to 1.3% of all neoplasms in the dog, and 1.5% to 2.0% in the cat (Patnaik, 1980; Patnaik, 1992). In the dog, 50% of hepatic neoplasms are hepatocellular in origin with predisposition for the left hepatic lobe (Kelly, 1993; Patnaik,

1981a). Metastasis is reported in 61% of dogs with hepatocellular carcinoma (Patnaik, 1980). In cats, hepatocellular carcinomas account for 19% of all hepatic neoplasms (Patnaik, 1992).

CYTOLOGICAL DIAGNOSIS

Differentiation of a hepatoma from a well-differentiated carcinoma can be difficult histologically and is often impossible cytologically. Histological evidence of venous invasion is an important criterion unavailable to the cytologist. Hepatocytes from benign hyperplastic or regenerative liver lesions often have considerable inherent variability, with large, binucleate cells containing a large, prominent nucleolus. Diagnosis of hepatocellular carcinoma should be reserved for lesions from an obvious liver mass that has highly anaplastic cytological changes. Malignant hepatocytes frequently have a high N:C ratio and one to three prominent nucleoli and may have bizarre multinucleate forms. In 11 cases diagnosed cytologically as neoplasia in dogs and cats, 10 were confirmed histologically (Kristensen, 1984).

Cholangiocellular Adenoma or Carcinoma (Figs. 10-67 to 10-69)

CLINICAL DIAGNOSIS

In cats, approximately 53% of hepatic neoplasms are of intrahepatic bile duct origin and 11% involve the extrahepatic bile duct (Patnaik, 1992). In dogs this percentage is lower at approximately 20% (Patnaik, 1981b). A metastatic rate of 88% is reported in affected dogs (Patnaik, 1980).

CYTOLOGICAL DIAGNOSIS

In dogs and cats the diffuse nature of bile duct carcinomas increases the potential for cytological detection (Kelly, 1993). The cells are cuboidal and have moderate anisokaryosis, high N:C ratio, and usually one large nucleolus (Kelly, 1993). Acinar and trabecular/papillary formations are common.

Metastatic Neoplasms of the Liver (Figs. 10-70 to 10-73)

CLINICAL AND CYTOLOGICAL DIAGNOSES

Metastatic neoplasms can be detected within liver aspiration biopsies, but differentiation of tumor origin may be difficult depending on the distinctiveness of the cell type and stage of differentiation, for example, mast cell tumor and lymphosarcoma.

■ PANCREAS

Cytological examination of the pancreas is rarely performed. However, with aspiration biopsy of an abdominal mass a diagnosis of pancreatic neoplasia must be considered. As well, pancreatic origin must be considered when septic or nonseptic effusions are encountered in abdominocentesis.

NORMAL PANCREAS (Figs. 10-74 to 10-76)

Cytological preparations of pancreatic tissue frequently contain large numbers of "lytic" cells or ruptured cellular material. The extreme fragility of the cells combined with the cellular proteolytic activity leads to rapid cell degradation after death. Imprints obtained from healthy dogs within 30 seconds of euthanasia displayed significant cellular deterioration. Loss of cytoplasmic and nuclear detail was prominent. An acinar cellular arrangement was occasionally visible. Intact cells had indistinct cellular borders and basophilic finely granular cytoplasm, reflecting the functional activity of the cells. Cytoplasmic vacuolation was variable. Several cohesive cell clusters contained prominent cytoplasmic vacuolation, which may represent islet cells. Nuclei were small with indistinct nucleoli.

NONNEOPLASTIC DISEASE

CLINICAL AND CYTOLOGICAL DIAGNOSES

Nonneoplastic conditions of the pancreas are rarely diagnosed cytologically. A nonseptic peritonitis, diagnosed with abdominocentesis, may be associated with acute pancreatitis.

NEOPLASTIC DISEASE

Pancreatic Carcinoma (Figs. 10-77 to 10-80)

CLINICAL DIAGNOSIS

Neoplasia of the pancreas is not uncommon in the dog and is infrequently seen in the cat (Jubb, 1993). These tumors have an aggressive behavior and are inevitably fatal.

CYTOLOGICAL DIAGNOSIS

Samples from pancreatic carcinomas frequently contain cellular debris and inflammatory cells as a result of tumor necrosis and often intestinal contamination. Sepsis is common. Intact neoplastic cells demonstrate the usual features of malignancy with high N:C ratio, anisokaryosis, and hyperchromasia. Cytoplasmic details are often indistinct, although a prominent blue granularity is common. Frequently these tumors display a dirty gray-blue background (material), representing proteolytic cellular degradation.

Islet Cell Neoplasms (Figs. 10-43 and 10-44)

CLINICAL DIAGNOSIS

Tumors of the islet cells are an uncommon diagnosis in dogs and rarely reported in cats (Jubb, 1993). Islet cells and other neuroendocrine cells within the pancreas are part of the APUD system in the body. These tumors may produce several different polypeptide hormones and as such clinical signs can vary. However, the most frequently diagnosed of these tumors is insulinoma. This tumor is associated with excess insulin production and clinical signs relate to hypoglycemia. These tumors can be benign or malignant (Jubb, 1993).

CYTOLOGICAL DIAGNOSIS

Although these tumors are rarely diagnosed cytologically within the pancreas, metastatic disease, frequently in the liver, is occasionally seen. These tumors have a typical neuroendocrine appearance, as described previously in this chapter.

References

Baker, H.J., Wood, P.A., and Wenger, D.A., et al. Sphingomyelin lipidosis in a cat. 1. Clinicopathological and biochemical studies. *Vet Pathol* 24:386-391,1987.

Barker, I. K. and Van Dreumel, A. A. The alimentary system. In *Pathology of Domestic Animals*. ed 4. K.V.F. Jubb, P.C. Kennedy, and N. Palmer (eds). Academic Press, San Diego, 1993.

Birchard, S.J., Guillermo Couto, C., and Johnson, S. Nonlymphoid intestinal neoplasia in 32 dogs and 14 cats. *J Am Anim Hosp Assoc* 22:533-537, 1986.

Blue, J.T., French, T.W., and Meyer, D.J. The liver. In *Diagnostic Cytology and Hematology of the Dog and Cat*. ed 2. R.L. Cowell, R.D. Tyler, and J.H. Meinkoth (eds). Mosby, St Louis, 1999.

Center, S.A., Crawford, M.A., Guida, L., et al. A retrospective study of 77 cats with severe hepatic lipidosis: 1975-1990. *J Vet Intern Med* 7:349-359, 1993a.

Center, S.A., Guida, L., Zanelli, M.J., et al. Ultrastructural hepatocellular features associated with severe hepatic lipidosis in cats. *Am J Vet Res* 54:724-731, 1993b.

Couto, G.C. Gastrointestinal neoplasia in dogs and cats. In *Current Veterinary Therapy XI, Small Animal Practice*. R.W. Kirk and J.D. Bonagura (eds). WB Saunders, Philadelphia, 1992.

Gagne, J.M., Weiss, D.J., and Armstrong, P.J. Histopathologic evaluation of feline inflammatory liver disease. *Vet Pathol* 33:521-526, 1996.

Houston, D.M. *An integrated study of colonic disease in the dog*. Master's thesis, University of Guelph, Guelph, Ontario, 1988.

Hubbard, B.S. and Vulgamott, J.C. Feline hepatic lipidosis. *Compend Cont Ed Pract* 14:459-465, 1992.

Jacobs, G., Collins-Kelly, L., Lappin, M., et al. Lymphocytic-plasmacytic enteritis in 24 dogs. *J Vet Intern Med* 4:45-53, 1990.

Jezyk, W.F., Haskins, M.E., and Newman, L.R. Alpha-mannosidosis in a Persian cat. *J Am Vet Med Assoc* 189:1483-1485, 1986.

Jubb, K.V.F. The pancreas. In *Pathology of Domestic Animals*. ed 4. K.V.F. Jubb, P.C. Kennedy, and N. Palmer (eds). Academic Press, San Diego, 1993.

Kelly, W.R. The liver and biliary system. In *Pathology of Domestic Animals.* ed 4. K.V.F. Jubb, P.C. Kennedy, and N. Palmer (eds). Academic Press, San Diego, 1993.

Kristensen, A.T., Weiss, D.J., and Klausner, J.S. Evaluation of hepatic cytology as a diagnostic tool in canine and feline hepatic disease. *Vet Clin Pathol* 18:12, 1984 (abstract).

Meyer, D.J. and French, T.W. The liver. In *Diagnostic Cytology of the Dog and Cat.* ed 2. R.L. Cowell, R.D. Tyler, and J.H. Meinkoth (eds). Mosby, St Louis, 1999.

Patnaik, A.K. Morphological and immunocytochemical study of hepatic neoplasms in cats. *Vet Pathol* 29:405-414, 1992.

Patnaik, A.K., Hurvitz, A.I., and Johnson, G.F. Canine gastrointestinal neoplasms *Vet Pathol* 14:547-555, 1977.

Patnaik, A.K., Hurvitz, A.I., and Lieberman, P.H. Canine hepatic neoplasms: a clinicopathologic study. *Vet Pathol* 17:553-564, 1980.

Patnaik, A.K., Hurvitz, A.I., Lieberman, P.H., et al. Canine hepatocellular carcinoma. *Vet Pathol* 18:427-438, 1981a.

Patnaik, A.K., Hurvitz, A.I., Lieberman, P.H., et al. Canine bile duct carcinoma. *Vet Pathol* 18:439-444, 1981b.

Prasse, K.W., Mahaffey, E.A., DeNovo, R., et. al. Chronic lymphocytic cholangitis in three cats. *Vet Pathol* 19:99-108, 1982.

Rakich, P.M. and Latimer, K.S. Rectal mucosal scrapings. In *Diagnostic Cytology and Hematology of the Dog and Cat.* ed 2. R.L. Cowell, R.D. Tyler, and J.H. Meinkoth (eds). Mosby, St Louis, 1999.

Scott, M.A. *Case 12.* ASCVP Slide Review Session, Orlando, Florida, 1991.

Shaker, E.H., Zawie, D.A., Garvey, M.S., et. al. Suppurative cholangiohepatitis in a cat. *J Am Anim Hosp Assoc* 27: 148-150, 1991.

Thornnburg, L.P., Shaw, D., Raisbeck, M., et. al. Hereditary copper toxicosis in West Highland white terriers. *Vet Pathol* 23:148-154, 1990.

Tobey, J.C., Willard, M.D., and Krehbiel, J.D. Comparison of cytologic and histopathologic evaluations of duodenal biopsies. *Vet Clin Pathol* 18:13, 1984 (abstract).

Twedt, D.C., Sternlieb, I., and Gilbertson, S.R. Clinical, morphological, and chemical studies on copper toxicosis of Bedlington terriers. *J Am Vet Med Assoc* 175:269-275, 1979.

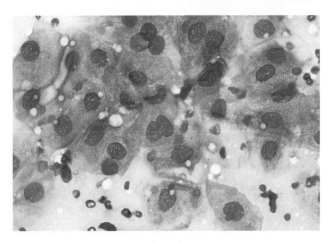

FIG. 10-1. Canine. Imprint. Normal mid-region esophagus. Large cells with angular, distinctive borders, round nuclei, and low N:C ratio consistent with squamous differentiation. (×100.)

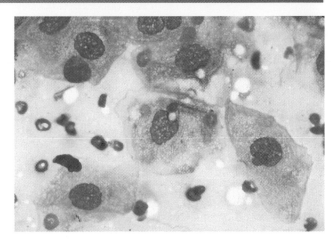

FIG. 10-2. Canine. Imprint. Normal mid-region esophagus. (Same case as Fig. 10-1.) Slightly higher magnification illustrating indistinct, fine cytoplasmic vacuolation and nuclear chromatin pattern. (×250.)

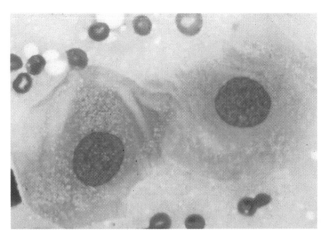

FIG. 10-3. Canine. Imprint. Normal mid-region esophagus. (Same case as Fig. 10-1.) Two epithelial cells demonstrating low N:C ratio and fine cytoplasmic vacuolation. Nuclear diameter approximates 2 to 3 erythrocytes. Nucleoli are small and indistinct. (×400.)

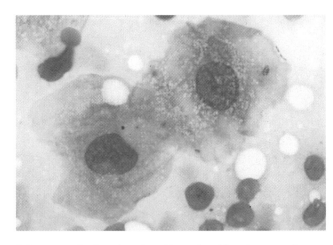

FIG. 10-4. Canine. Imprint. Normal mid-region esophagus. (Same case as Fig. 10-1.) Basophilic cytoplasmic pigment is consistent with melanin precursors. (×400.)

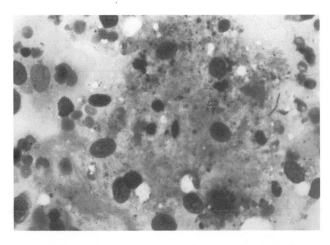

FIG. 10-5. Canine. Imprint. Normal mid-region esophagus. (Same case as Fig. 10-1.) Cellular debris and bacteria is consistent with lumen contents including partially digested food. (×200.)

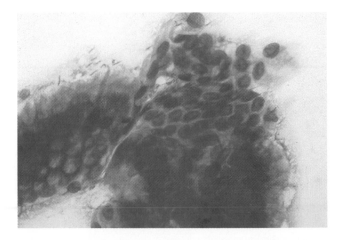

FIG. 10-6. Canine. Imprint. Cardiac region of normal stomach. Honeycomb appearance of mucosal epithelial cells with suggestion of apical secretory products and overlying bacteria. A vertical and horizontal view of glandular cells is presented. (×100.)

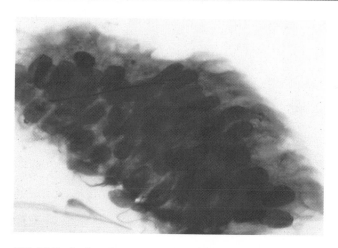

FIG. 10-7. Canine. Scraping. Cardiac region of normal stomach. (Same case as Fig. 10-6.) Superficial basophilic mucus could be confused with cilia. (×250.)

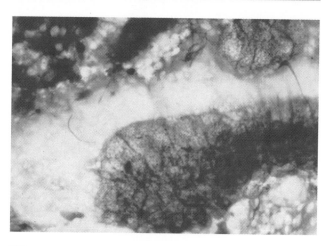

FIG. 10-8. Canine. Imprint. Normal stomach. Fine, indistinct apical vacuolation is consistent with secretory activity of epithelial cells. (×200.)

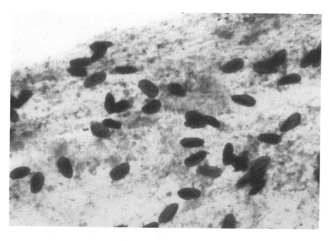

FIG. 10-9. Canine. Imprint. Normal stomach, pyloric region. The background debris contains degenerating cells with oval-shaped nuclei. Although the slides were prepared within 5 minutes of death, rapid cell degeneration may be expected where proteolytic enzymes are produced locally. (×200.)

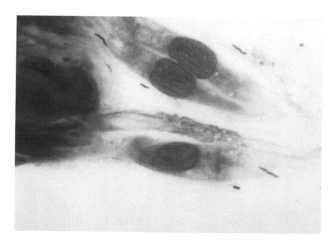

FIG. 10-10. Canine. Scraping. Normal pylorus. Intact columnar cells with elongated nuclei and fine cribriform chromatin pattern. A few bacteria, some spiriliform, are visible in the background. (×400.)

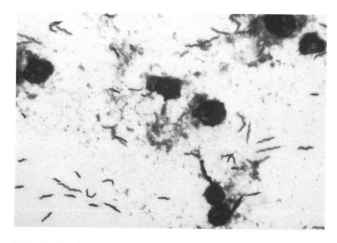

FIG. 10-11. Canine. Imprint. Normal pylorus. A few degenerate cells with a background of prominent spiriliform bacteria consistent with *Helicobacter* sp. (×200.)

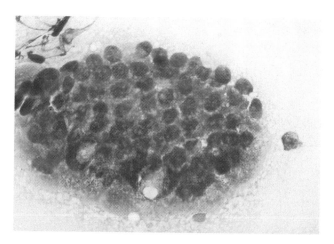

FIG. 10-12. Canine. Scraping. Normal jejunum. Basilar honeycomb arrangement of mucosal cells. (×100.)

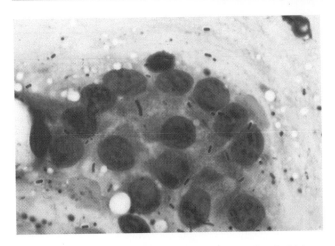

FIG. 10-13. Canine. Imprint. Normal jejunum. Small, cuboidal epithelial cells with visible cell borders, moderate N:C ratio, homogeneous basophilic cytoplasm, and small, multiple indistinct nucleoli. (×400.)

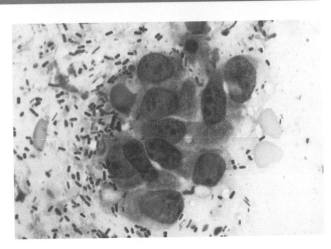

FIG. 10-14. Canine. Imprint. Normal jejunum. (Same case as Fig. 10-13.) Cuboidal epithelial cells with nuclear diameters about 1½ to 2 erythrocytes. There are many coccobacilli in the background. (×400.)

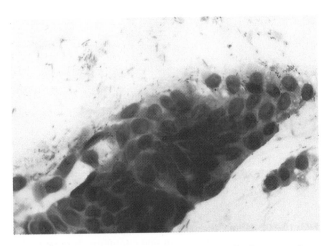

FIG. 10-15. Canine. Imprint. Normal colon. Colonic mucosal epithelial cells. (×200.)

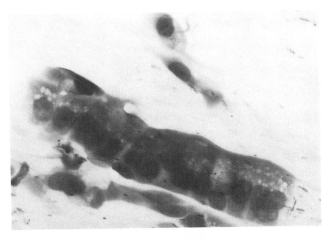

FIG. 10-16. Canine. Imprint. Normal colon. (Same case as Fig. 10-15.) Lateral view of mucosal epithelial cells illustrating basilar nuclei and apical mucus production. (×250.)

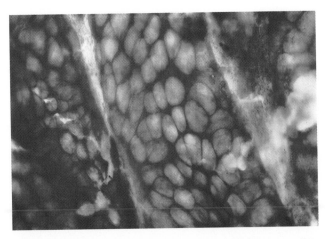

FIG. 10-17. Canine. Imprint. Normal colon. (Same case as Fig. 10-15.) Honeycomb appearance created by mucus-producing cells. (×100.)

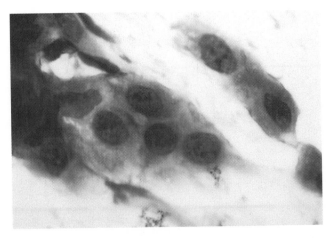

FIG. 10-18. Canine. Imprint. Normal colon. (Same case as Fig. 10-15.) Round to cuboidal epithelial cells without the typical columnar secretory epithelial cell appearance. (×400.)

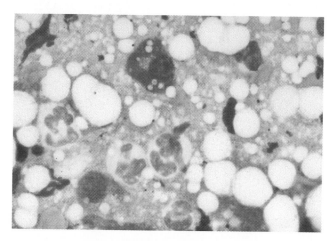

FIG. 10-19. Feline. Fine needle. Mass at ileocecal junction. Steatitis. Large, clear vacuoles; dense, irregular, dirty background; and neutrophils are consistent with steatitis. Loss of cellular detail and indistinct staining may be associated with necrosis or autolysis. (×400.)

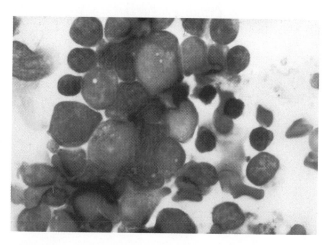

FIG. 10-20. Canine. Imprint. Mesenteric lymph node. Chronic enteritis. Heterogenous population of lymphocytes with increased large "blastic" lymphocytes, suggesting response to antigenic stimulation. (×400.)

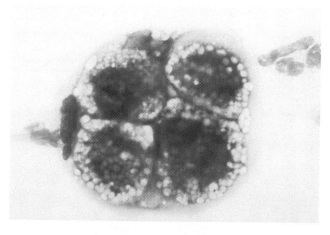

FIG. 10-21. Canine. Peritoneal fluid. Duodenal adenocarcinoma. A cluster of epithelial cells with marked anisokaryosis, increased N:C ratio, and cytoplasmic vacuolation consistent with exfoliating secretory epithelial cells. (×100.)

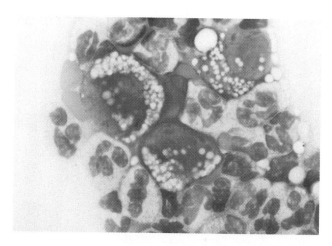

FIG. 10-22. Canine. Abdominal fluid. Duodenal adenocarcinoma. (Same case as Fig. 10-21.) The large vacuolated cells are consistent with secretory epithelial cells. These cells have a high N:C ratio and numerous intracytoplasmic vacuoles. There are numerous neutrophils and a few macrophages. Observation of these large cells, single and in clusters, is consistent with a cytological diagnosis of carcinoma. (×400.)

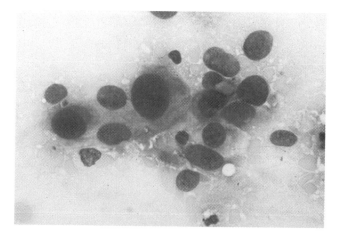

FIG. 10-23. Canine. Imprint. Colonic adenocarcinoma. Epithelial cells with marked anisocytosis, anisokaryosis, and a moderate amount of basophilic cytoplasm. (×100.)

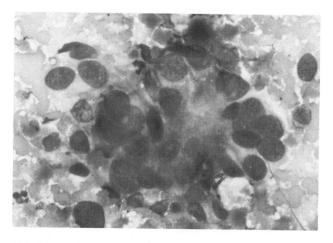

FIG. 10-24. Canine. Imprint. Colonic adenocarcinoma. (Same case as Fig. 10-23.) Cluster of epithelial cells, suggesting acinar origin. The cells have indistinct cytoplasmic borders and marked anisokaryosis. (×200.)

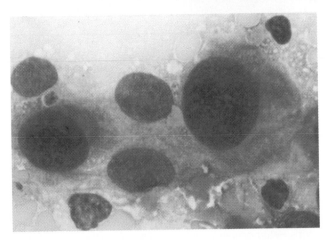

FIG. 10-25. Canine. Imprint. Colonic adenocarcinoma. (Same case as Fig. 10-23.) Epithelial cells with a moderate amount of basophilic cytoplasm, indistinct borders, marked hyperchromasia, anisocytosis and anisokaryosis, and multiple nucleoli. (×400.)

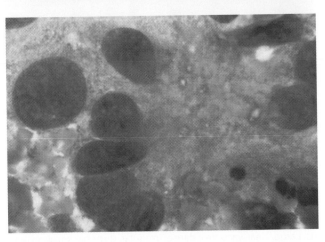

FIG. 10-26. Canine. Imprint. Colonic adenocarcinoma. (Same case as Fig. 10-23.) Similar epithelial cells containing basophilic vacuolation, suggesting secretory activity. (×400.)

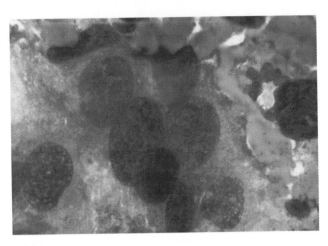

FIG.10-27. Canine. Imprint. Colonic adenocarcinoma. (Same case as Fig. 10-23.) Large epithelial cells with indistinct cytoplasmic borders, marked anisokaryosis, and multiple, prominent nucleoli. (×400.)

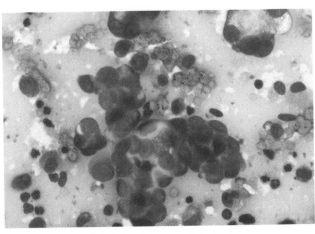

FIG. 10-28. Canine. Imprint. Intestinal carcinoma. Exfoliating epithelial cells, suggesting acinar origin. The anisokaryosis, hyperchromasia, and disorganization of adjoining cells are consistent with malignancy. (×100.)

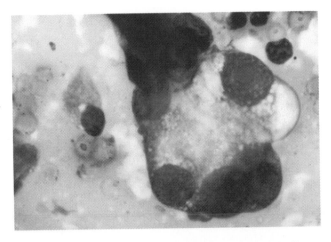

FIG. 10-29. Canine. Imprint. Intestinal adenocarcinoma. (Same case as Fig. 10-28.) A cluster of epithelial cells with cytoplasmic clear areas, suggesting secretory product. There is anisokaryosis with prominent nucleoli. (×400.)

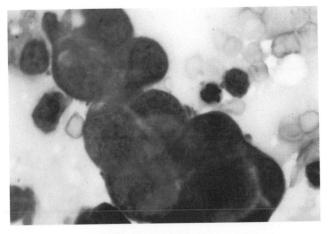

FIG. 10-30. Canine. Imprint. Intestinal carcinoma. (Same case as Fig. 10-29.) A "frond" of epithelial cells illustrating adjoining cell borders, high N:C ratio, hyperchromasia, and anisokaryosis. (×400.)

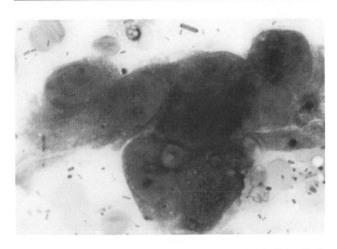

FIG. 10-31. Canine. Imprint. Rectal carcinoma. Epithelial cells illustrating several criteria of malignancy, including increased N:C ratio, hyperchromasia, and prominent, variable-sized nucleoli. Mixed bacteria are present in the background. (×400.)

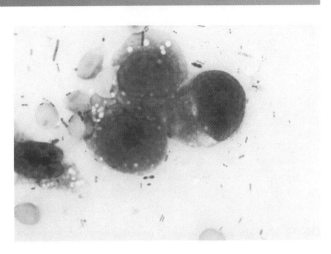

FIG. 10-32. Canine. Imprint. Rectal carcinoma. (Same case as Fig. 10-31.) Three epithelial cells with high N:C ratio and prominent nucleoli. Slight cytoplasmic vacuolation is observed. (×400.)

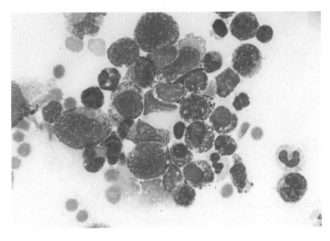

FIG. 10-33. Canine. Abdominal fluid. Colonic mass. Eosinophilic sarcoma. Round cells are primarily promyelocytic to mature eosinophils. Granulocytic sarcoma is a solid tumor mass of the myeloid series. (×250.)

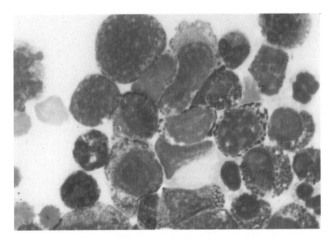

FIG 10-34. Canine. Abdominal fluid. Colonic mass. Eosinophilic sarcoma. (Same case as Fig. 10-33.) Precursor cells and differentiation of eosinophilic series are indicated by the eosinophilic granulation and progression of nuclear lobulation. (×400.)

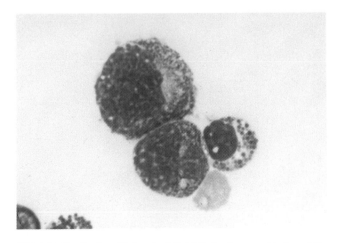

FIG. 10-35. Canine. Abdominal fluid. Colonic mass. Eosinophilic sarcoma. (Same case as Fig. 10-33.) Eosinophil precursors, typical of most cells in the mass. (×500.)

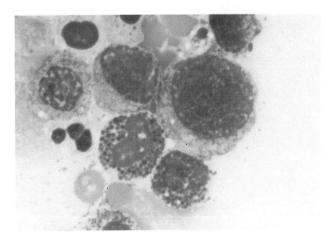

FIG. 10-36. Canine. Abdominal fluid. Colonic mass. Eosinophilic sarcoma. (Same case as Fig. 10-33.) Granulation and lobulation of developing eosinophils are prominent. (×500.)

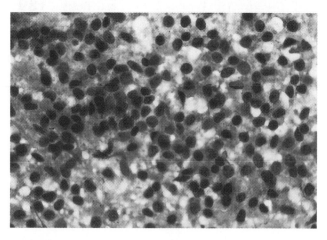

FIG. 10-37. Canine. Imprint. Heart base. Neuroendocrine tumor. Loosely aggregated round to spindle cells with pale cytoplasm and indistinct borders. (×160.)

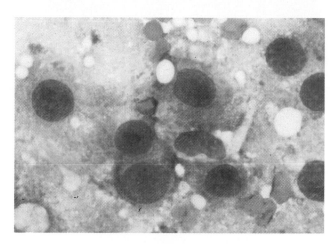

FIG. 10-38. Canine. Imprint. Carotid body tumor. Cells have round nuclei with indistinct round nucleoli and prominent chromocenters and finely granular basophilic cytoplasm. (×400.)

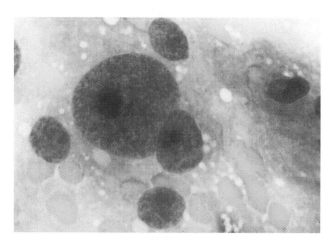

FIG. 10-39. Canine. Imprint. Carotid body tumor. Prominent anisokaryosis. Large, round nuclei with fine chromatin pattern, prominent nucleoli, and pale, indistinct cytoplasm. (×500.)

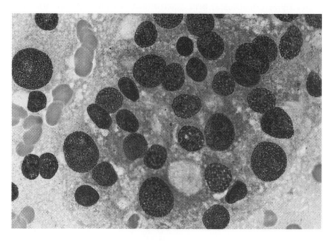

FIG. 10-40. Canine. Fine needle. Cranial abdominal mass. Neuroendocrine tumor. The cells present have lightly basophilic, mildly vacuolated cytoplasm and poor delineation of cytoplasmic borders. The nuclei are hyperchromatic and have a prominent fine to coarse chromatin pattern and marked anisokaryosis. The histological diagnosis was insulinoma. (×400.)

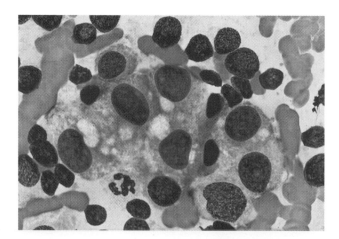

FIG. 10-41. Canine. Fine needle. Cranial abdominal mass. Neuroendocrine tumor. (Same case as Fig 10-40.) Acinar arrangement of cells and degree of anisokaryosis support interpretation of malignant transformation of secretory epithelial cells compatible with neuroendocrine tumor. (×400.)

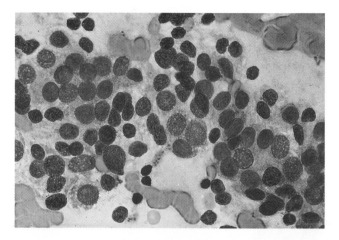

FIG. 10-42. Canine. Imprint. Abdominal mass. Neuroendocrine tumor. Loosely cohesive cells with round nuclei, mild anisokaryosis, and lightly basophilic cytoplasm. This cellular arrangement is common to neuroendocrine tumors. (×200.)

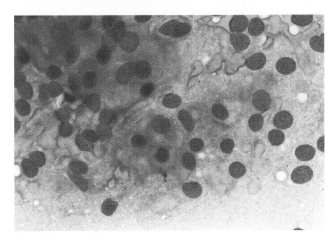

FIG. 10-43. Canine. Imprint. Pancreas. Islet cell tumor. Dispersed cells with delicate cytoplasm and round nuclei with mild anisokaryosis. There is a suggestion of a follicular pattern. (×200.)

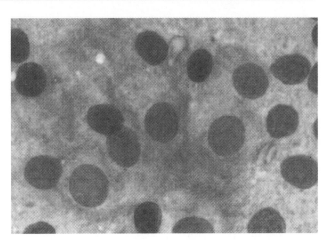

FIG. 10-44. Canine. Imprint. Pancreas. Islet cell tumor. (Same case as Fig. 10-43.) Increased magnification of cells demonstrating low N:C ratio and mild nuclear variability. (×400.)

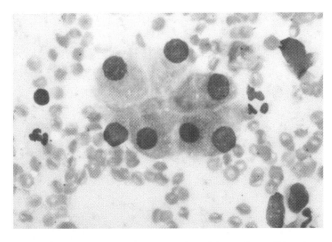

FIG. 10-45. Canine. Fine needle. Normal liver. The cell borders, moderate density, abundant basophilic cytoplasm, and dark, round nuclei are typical of normal hepatocytes. Note size relative to erythrocytes. (×250.)

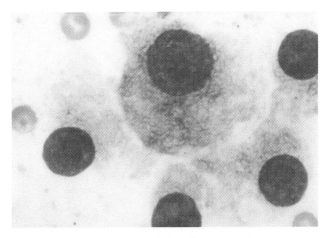

FIG. 10-46. Canine. Fine needle. Normal liver. Hepatocytes are round and have basophilic cytoplasm, nuclei with smooth to coarse chromatin patterns, and large nucleoli. The basophilic granularity within the cytoplasm is associated with the content and activity of the endoplasmic reticulum. (×500.)

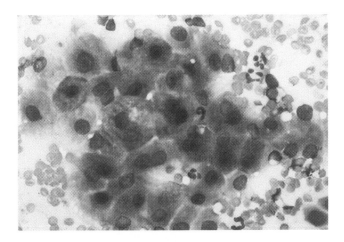

FIG. 10-47. Canine. Fine needle. Normal liver. Large round cells with abundant basophilic cytoplasm, round central to eccentric nuclei, and indistinct to prominent large nucleoli are consistent with normal hepatocellular morphology. Note the few neutrophils present. (×100.)

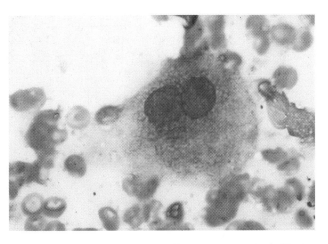

FIG. 10-48. Canine. Fine needle Normal liver. Binucleated hepatocyte illustrating light-staining areas and basophilic granularity within the cytoplasm, presumably RNA. (×400.)

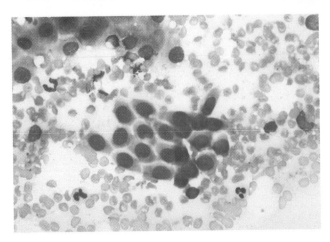

FIG. 10-49. Canine. Imprint. Normal liver. Small sheet of large, loosely adherent round to elongated epithelial cells with large oval nuclei. These cells appear to be of ductal origin. (×100.)

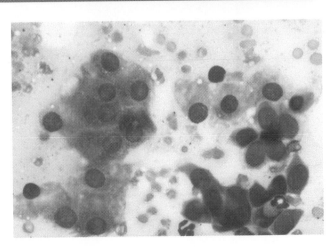

FIG. 10-50. Canine. Imprint. Normal liver. Hepatocytes, single and in sheets, contrast with the elongated cells, which are morphologically similar to the lining cells illustrated in Fig. 10-49. (×160.)

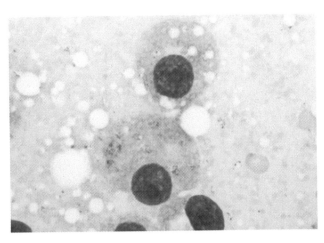

FIG. 10-51. Canine. Fine needle. Normal liver. Occasional intracytoplasmic granules of bile pigment can be seen in most normal livers. (×500.)

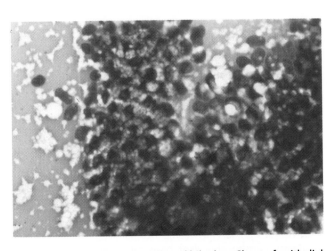

FIG. 10-52. Canine. Imprint. Normal bile duct. Sheet of epithelial cells, likely ductular in origin, with intracellular and extracellular vacuolation contributing to honeycomb appearance. (×160.)

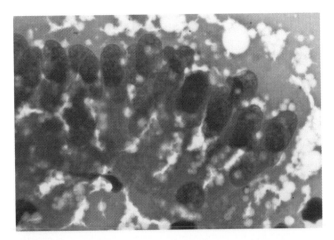

FIG. 10-53. Canine. Imprint. Normal bile duct. Columnar cells with indistinct borders, basophilic amorphous cytoplasm, basilar elongated nuclei, and indistinct nucleoli. (×400.)

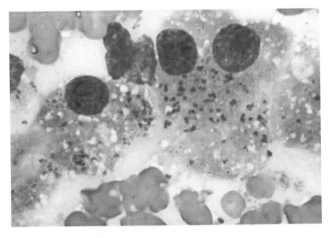

FIG. 10-54. Feline. Fine needle. Fatty liver. Swollen hepatocytes contain small clear vacuoles representing lipid accumulation and fine intracytoplasmic granular clumps of bile pigment. (×500.)

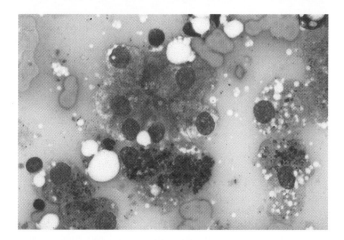

FIG. 10-55. Feline. Fine needle. Fatty liver. Focal areas of hepatocytes containing blue-green intracellular bile pigment can be prominent in fatty liver. (×250.)

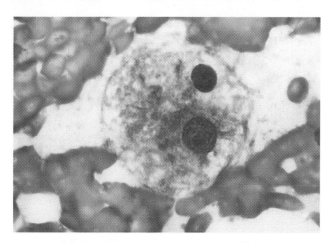

FIG. 10-56. Feline. Imprint. Fatty liver. A large hepatocyte, possibly binucleated, with multiple small clear areas consistent with lipid accumulation. (×100.)

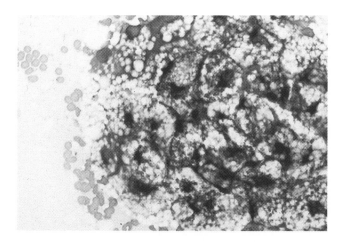

FIG. 10-57. Feline. Fine needle. Fatty liver. Hepatocytes with extensive cytoplasmic vacuolation consistent with fatty infiltration. (×100.)

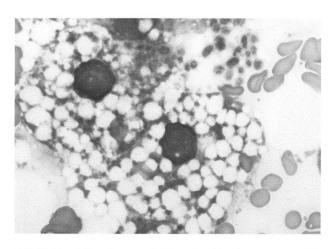

FIG. 10-58. Feline. Fine needle. Fatty liver. Two hepatocytes with large cytoplasmic vacuoles. Hepatocyte lipid accumulation in this cat was extensive. (×400.)

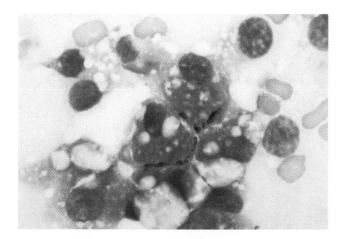

FIG. 10-59. Canine. Imprint. Glucocorticoid hepatopathy. Dark green-black pigment between hepatocytes is consistent with canalicular cholestasis. Canalicular bile may be observed within normal liver but is increased with cholestasis. (×400.)

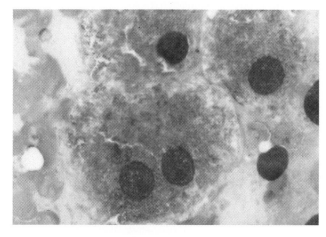

FIG. 10-60. Canine. Fine needle. A binucleated hepatocyte with indistinct intracytoplasmic blue-green pigment contrasts with the distinct blue-green granules visible in Fig. 10-59 and is consistent with early bile accumulation. (×400.)

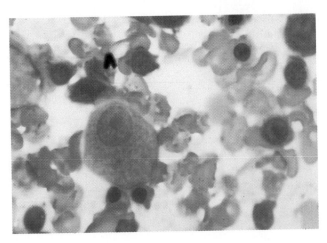

FIG. 10-61. Canine. Imprint. Liver. Extramedullary hematopoiesis (EMH). A normal hepatocyte is surrounded by erythroid and myeloid precursors. This is a common observation in the liver of young animals and less commonly in older animals with bone marrow stress. (×400.)

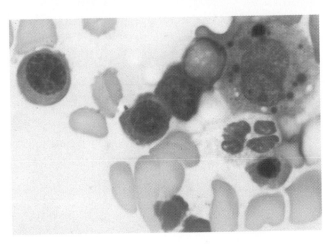

FIG. 10-62. Canine. Imprint. Liver. Extramedullary hematopoiesis. Erythroid precursors surround a large macrophage/Kupffer's cell. Intracytoplasmic cell remnants and hemosiderin suggest consumption or destruction of the erythrocyte series. Liver aspiration biopsy can assist investigation of hematopoietic disorders. (×500.)

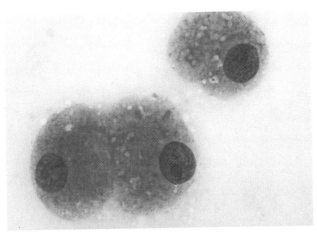

FIG. 10-63. Canine. Imprint. Liver. Copper-associated hepatitis. Hepatocytes contain many blue-green refractile cytoplasmic granules. These granules stained positive with rubeanic acid and represent copper accumulation. (×400.) (Courtesy M.A. Scott, 1991.)

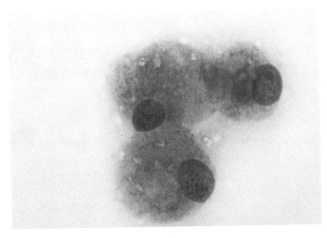

FIG. 10-64. Canine. Imprint. Liver. Copper-associated hepatitis. (Same case as Fig. 10-63.) Hepatocytes contain many refractile blue-green granules and some large diffuse aggregates of blue-green pigment. (×400.) (Courtesy M.A. Scott, 1991.)

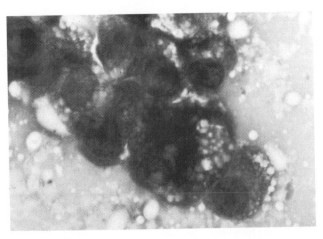

FIG. 10-65. Feline. Imprint. Hepatic carcinoma. A cluster of hepatocytes with cytoplasmic vacuolation, marked anisokaryosis, and prominent nucleoli. (×500.)

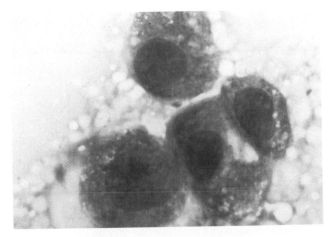

FIG. 10-66. Feline. Imprint. Hepatic carcinoma. Hepatocytes with prominent anisokaryosis and hyperchromasia. The N:C ratio is markedly increased in two hepatocytes as assessed by comparison with more normal-appearing cells. (×500.)

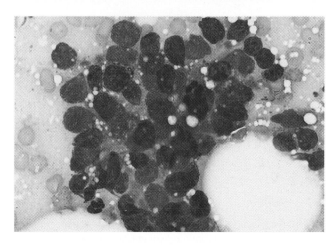

FIG. 10-67. Canine. Imprint. Cholangiocarcinoma. A dense cluster of epithelial cells with high N:C ratio, mild anisokaryosis, and occasional cytoplasmic vacuolation. (×100.)

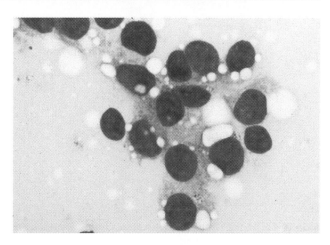

FIG. 10-68. Canine. Fine needle. Cholangiocarcinoma. A sheet of cuboidal, loosely aggregated epithelial cells. Nuclei have one or two small nucleoli. Cytoplasm is gray-blue with an indistinct outline and occasional vacuolation. (×400.)

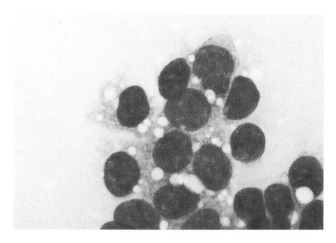

FIG. 10-69. Canine. Fine needle. Cholangiocarcinoma. (Same case as Fig. 10-68.) Similar cells, suggesting acinar arrangement. A pure population of these cells would alert the cytologist to an epithelial neoplasm, although its status as benign or malignant would be difficult to determine. (×500.)

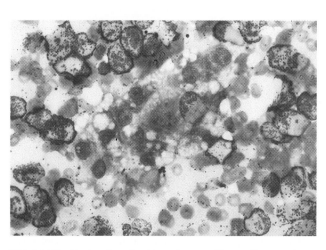

FIG. 10-70. Canine. Imprint. Hepatic mass. Mast cell tumor. Low-power view of faintly staining hepatocytes surrounded by many granulated mast cells. Normal liver tissue contains a few mast cells, but the concentration observed confirms metastasis or de novo mast cell tumor formation. (×200.)

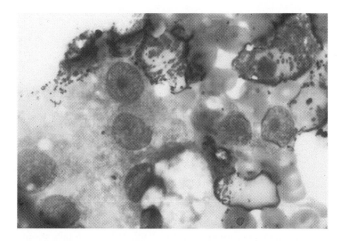

FIG. 10-71. Canine. Imprint. Hepatic mass. Mast cell tumor. Hepatocytes surrounded by several mast cells. Additional staining time may be required when cellularity is increased. (×400.)

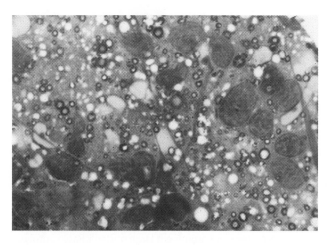

FIG. 10-72. Feline. Imprint. Liver. Large granular lymphoma. Blue-gray background is overlaid with dispersed granules from ruptured cells. (×400.)

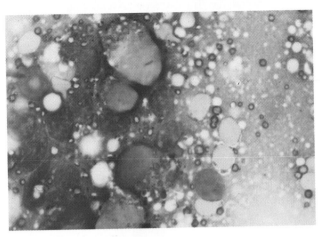

FIG. 10-73. Feline. Imprint. Liver. Large granular lymphoma. There are several large, round cells with understained nuclei and prominent intracytoplasmic magenta granules consistent with large granular lymphocytes. (×500.)

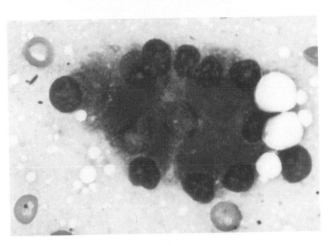

FIG. 10-74. Canine. Imprint. Normal pancreas. Acinar arrangement of pancreatic cells with indistinct borders, basophilic finely granular cytoplasm, small nuclei, and indistinct nucleoli. (×400.)

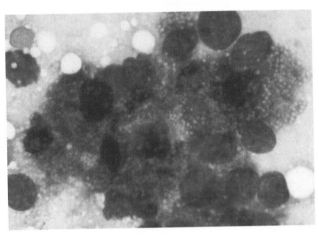

FIG. 10-75. Canine. Imprint. Normal pancreas. Cluster of cells with granular cytoplasm indicative of functional activity. Cytological detail of pancreatic cells is often poor, presumably because of the influence of proteolytic enzymes. (×400.)

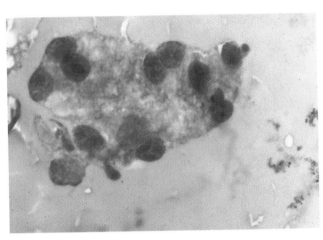

FIG. 10-76. Canine. Imprint. Normal pancreas. Impression smear made immediately after euthanasia. Cluster of cells with indistinct borders and foamy cytoplasm, presumably of islet cell origin. (×400.)

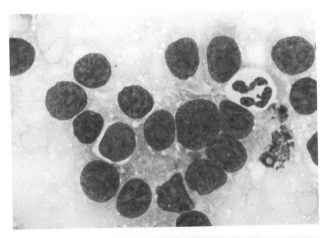

FIG. 10-77. Canine. Imprint, postmortem. Pancreas. Pancreatic carcinoma. Acinar arrangement of large nuclei; with a coarse chromatin pattern and prominent large nucleoli. Rapid autolysis resulting from release of proteolytic enzymes can alter chromatin pattern, prominence of nucleoli, and cytoplasmic details. (×400.)

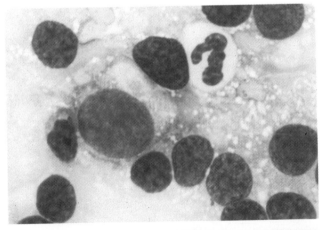

FIG. 10-78. Canine. Imprint, postmortem. Pancreas. Pancreatic carcinoma. (Same case as Fig. 10-77.) Marked anisokaryosis, variation in nuclear chromatin and nucleoli. Nuclear details should only be evaluated in intact cells. (×500.)

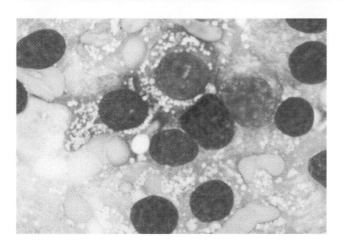

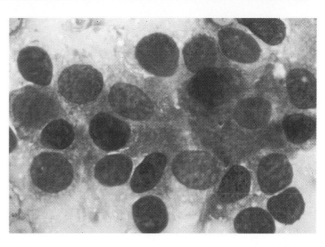

FIG. 10-79. Canine. Imprint, postmortem. Pancreas. Pancreatic carcinoma. (Same case as Fig. 10-77.) Nuclear details are similar in intact cells; cytoplasmic vacuolation is consistent with secretory cells. (×500.)

FIG. 10-80. Canine. Imprint, postmortem. Pancreatic carcinoma. (Same case as Fig. 10-77.) Cluster of cells suggests acinar formation. Blue-gray cytoplasmic granulation is prominent. (×400.)

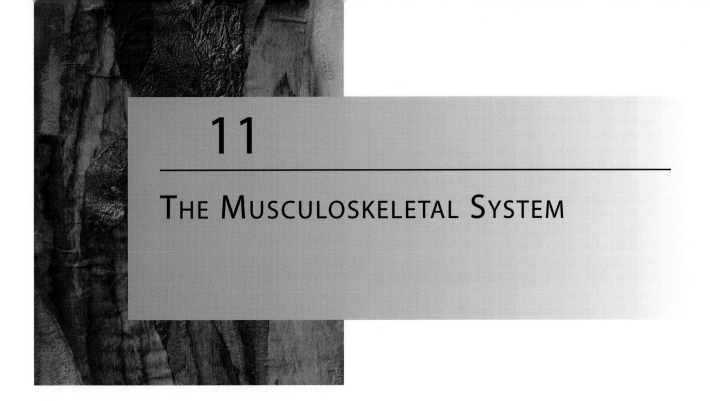

11

THE MUSCULOSKELETAL SYSTEM

Cytological examination of the musculoskeletal system is generally restricted to evaluation of muscle, bone, and synovial fluid. Synovial fluid cytological evaluation is presented in Chapter 12. Because of the prevalence of tumors of the skeleton, cytologists spend a great deal of time considering the appearance of benign and malignant progenitor cells of bone and cartilage. Muscular samples, although readily accessible, are seldom examined.

Several stromal tumors that can affect the muscular and bony tissues are considered in Chapter 4, including hemangiosarcoma and fibrosarcoma.

TECHNIQUE

Both inflammatory and neoplastic diseases of the bone can be readily diagnosed with aspiration techniques. Fine-needle aspirations are performed as previously described in Chapter 2. Because of the nature of bony lesions, needle penetration into the tissue is often perceived as a problem. Our experience suggests that most bony tumors can be adequately sampled with a 22-gauge needle using repeated aspirations. In very firm lesions, taking three to four aspirates from different sites is suggested to obtain adequate cellular material for diagnosis. Occasionally, bone lysis and necrosis caused by tumor or osteomyelitis is so advanced that the needle readily slips into the lesion. This prime biopsy site may be identified as a radiolucent area in radiographs where acquisition of diagnostic material is most probable (Stirtzinger, 1988). Aspirate samples from the lesion periphery may yield only reactive osteoblasts (Stirtzinger, 1988).

Cytological examination of biopsy material can be useful during a surgical procedure. It is often prefer-

able to use a scraping technique rather than imprints to enhance exfoliation because of the intercellular adhesion between stromal cells.

NORMAL TISSUE (Figs. 11-1 to 11-4)

Normal bony tissue is rarely examined. Cytologists must become familiar with the morphological appearance of osteoblasts, chondroblasts, osteoclasts, and fibroblasts within proliferative bone involving benign and malignant lesions. Examination of stromal tissue is one of the more difficult tasks for the cytopathologist because of the extreme proplastic changes observed in reactive stromal cells, often closely mimicking malignancy. As well, because soft tissue and bone tumors arise from embryonic mesoderm differing only in their final cell products and function, anaplastic cells may not be readily differentiated on morphology (Stirtzinger, 1988).

In normal tissue and reactive bone, fine-needle aspirates have very low cellularity. Scrapings may be required to harvest adequate cells for diagnosis. Many slides will contain only 5 to 10 stromal cells. These cells may be a combination of osteoblasts, chondroblasts, reactive fibroblasts, and, rarely, osteoclasts. Unidentifiable stromal cells may also be part of the picture. The presence of intercellular matrix is variable but aids in identifying the tissue of origin.

As a rule, benign stromal cells do not usually exceed the diameter of two to three homologous erythrocytes (Stirtzinger, 1988). Osteoblasts typically have abundant cytoplasm with oval eccentric nuclei and a prominent Golgi zone. Nucleoli are small and indistinct. Fine pink granulation may be present in the cytoplasm, as in all stromal cells. As is typical of all stromal populations, cell outlines are usually indistinct with cytoplasmic margins fading into the background. No organized cell clusters with distinct cell borders, typical of epithelium, are seen.

Chondroblasts have a similar appearance to osteoblasts but with a rounder nucleus and even distribution of cytoplasm. Nucleoli are rare and if present are small, single, and regular. Cytoplasm is faintly basophilic and may contain variable numbers of metachromatic granules and occasional vacuolation. Large cytoplasmic metachromatic granules are characteristic of chondroblasts but are not always present. Association with bright pink extracellular matrix is characteristic if present.

Osteoclasts are large, multinucleate cells easily identified cytologically. These cells originate from the mononuclear cell line (Mahaffey, 1999). Osteoclasts are very large with irregular cytoplasmic margins, 6 to 10 nuclei, and abundant cytoplasm (Mahaffey, 1999).

NORMAL MUSCLE

Aspiration of normal skeletal muscle is an uncommon clinical request. However, muscle fibers occasionally appear as contaminants when aspirating other tissues. Normal muscle has a characteristic appearance. With Wright's stain, muscle fibers are turquoise blue to green. Fibers are elongate with small, regular, cigar-shaped nuclei lining the periphery of the fiber.

NONNEOPLASTIC DISEASE (Figs. 11-5 to 11-9)

Osteomyleitis/Fracture

CLINICAL AND CYTOLOGICAL DIAGNOSES
Inflammatory lesions of bone are occasionally examined using cytological techniques. Many infectious agents are associated with osteomyelitis, including *Actinomyces, Staphylococcus,* and *Streptococcus* spp. (Mahaffey, 1999). The deep mycosis, such as with *Blastomyces, Histoplasma,* and *Coccidioides,* may be observed within aspirate slides. The cellular response to inflammation is similar to other tissues with a mixture of neutrophils, macrophages, and reactive stroma. If there is new bone formation, osteoblasts, chondroblasts, and osteoclasts may be part of the cytological picture. Reactive osteoblasts differ from malignant cells in that they lack nuclear features of malignancy and are uniform in size (Mahaffey, 1999). The cells have abundant cytoplasm and fine nuclear chromatin patterns. More differentiated benign cells may have a single prominent regular nucleolus (Stirtzinger, 1988).

Coccidioides samples typically contain many macrophages and multinucleated cells intermixed with the occasional organism (Mahaffey, 1999). Osteoclasts may be present.

Aspirates taken from a maturing fracture callus are low in cellularity. Osteoblasts predominate, but occasional reactive fibroblasts may be seen. Again, the low N:C ratio and regular size of the nuclei help differentiate the proplastic (hyperplastic) response of healing from malignancy.

NEOPLASTIC DISEASE (Figs. 11-10 to 11-16)

Osteosarcoma

CLINICAL DIAGNOSIS
Primary bone tumors account for 3% to 4% of all canine malignancies (LaRue, 1986). Osteosarcomas account for 80% of bone tumors in the dog and 50% in the cat (Palmer, 1993; Probst, 1982). Osteosarcomas develop mainly in the medullary shaft of long bones, especially the radius. They have a high propensity for metastasis and therefore a guarded prognosis (Straw, 1995). It is assumed that all dogs have undetectable metastasis at the time of diagnosis (Straw, 1995). The incidence for osteosarcoma is highest in large and giant breeds of dogs, in which the average age at presentation is 7 years (Straw, 1995). Dogs often present with a slowly progressive lameness. Without treatment, median survival time is 1 to 2 months (Straw, 1995). With amputation alone the median survival is 162 days with death caused by lung metastasis and resulting euthanasia (Straw, 1995).

In a series of cats with 395 neoplasms, 5% of tumors originated in bone (Bitetto, 1987). Osteosarcoma accounted for 15 of 24 primary bone tumors in cats (Liu, 1974), and 9 of 15 originated in the long bones and 3 in the skull (Liu, 1974). Of 12 appendicular osteosarcomas in the cat that were treated with amputation, most cats lived longer than 4 years postsurgically (Bitetto, 1987; Liu, 1974). The prognosis in the cat appears to be slightly better than in dogs (Bitetto, 1987; Liu, 1974).

CYTOLOGICAL DIAGNOSIS
Cell harvest from chondrosarcoma and osteosarcoma varies depending on area sampled and accessibility of radiolucent areas. Sedation is not usually required unless the area is particularly painful. A dense outer shell of bone may limit access to sample areas, and sedation may be required to allow probing for an appropriate site.

With a good cell harvest a diagnosis of osteosarcoma can be made in most cases. Cellular appearances vary from the well-differentiated sarcoma with cells exhibiting only mild criteria of malignancy to the opposite end of the spectrum, in which cells demonstrate extreme abnormalities associated with malignancy. Osteoblasts, the malignant cell type, can have marked variation in cell and nuclear size. The N:C ratio is high, hyperchromasia is prominent, and anisokaryosis can be marked. Nucleoli are often large and irregular and may be multiple. Highly basophilic cytoplasm is usually asymmetrically arranged and may be flame shaped (Stirtzinger, 1988). Nonspecific cytoplasmic granulation may be prominent or absent. In well-differentiated osteosarcomas, cell definition may be more pronounced and cells appear to aggregate or cluster; however, if carefully examined, no distinct cell borders are present as in epithelial tumors (Stirtzinger, 1988). Eosinophilic osteoid matrix may be present in the background as homogenous matrix or as large, irregular, aggregated clumps (Stirtzinger, 1988). Islands of osteoid surrounded by osteoblasts may be seen (Mahaffey, 1999). Benign osteoblasts and osteoclasts may be intermixed with the malignant population.

The accuracy for correct diagnosis of bone lesions using aspiration cytology is frequently debated. In one study of 39 clinically and radiographically affected dogs, cytology was superior to histopathology. The study compared aspiration biopsy and core biopsy of the center zone and transition zone of affected dogs (Michels, 1997). Tumors were divided into osteosarcoma, sarcoma, carcinoma, and no neoplasia (Michels, 1997). The cytological diagnosis corresponded with the histopathological diagnosis in 29 of 39 biopsies from dogs (Michels, 1997). Cytology yielded a more specific diagnosis in 9 of 39 dogs, and histopathology was more specific in 1 of 39 dogs (Michels, 1997). Additional prospective studies are required to evaluate and compare the reliability of cytological versus histological diagnosis.

Chondrosarcoma (Figs. 11-17 to 11-20)

CLINICAL DIAGNOSIS

Cartilaginous matrix produced by neoplastic cells leads to the classification of chondrosarcoma. Chondrosarcomas are more commonly found in mature, large-breed dogs in the ribs, nose, sternum, and pelvis (Palmer, 1993). Chondrosarcomas account for 10% to 13% of all bone tumors in the dog (Davidson, 1995). Osteosarcomas are rare in the cat, accounting for 3 of 24 cases of primary bone tumors (Davidson, 1995; Liu, 1974). Clinical signs vary depending on the site of origin of the tumor. Chondrosarcomas are locally invasive with a reported metastatic rate of 20% (Davidson, 1995). The frequency of metastasis for sinonasal neoplasms is reduced compared with those in other sites (Patnaik, 1984).

CYTOLOGICAL DIAGNOSIS

Cell harvest in chondrosarcoma, as in osteosarcoma, can be variable. Low-power examination of chondrosarcomas often immediately reveals a very useful cytological feature: large lakes of bright pink metachromatic matrix may cover the slide. Single chondroblasts are interspersed in this matrix. This "chondroid" is the intercellular matrix of cartilage and suggests a cartilaginous origin to the tumor. However,

it is not always present in chondrosarcoma and can be seen in other bony lesions or tumors if a cartilaginous area is aspirated. The usual criteria of malignancy apply to chondroblasts. However, the extreme variations seen in osteosarcoma are often not seen in chondrosarcoma. Increased N:C ratio, hyperchromasia, and anisokaryosis may be subtle. Nucleoli, if present, are usually single, small, and regular (Evans, 1996; Stirtzinger, 1988). Binucleation and mitosis are supportive of a malignant diagnosis. Differentiation of a benign chondroma from chondrosarcoma can be difficult, if not impossible.

Rhabdosarcomas/Rhabdomyomas (Figs. 11-21 to 11-24)

CLINICAL DIAGNOSIS

Rhabdosarcomas are rare tumors of striated muscle that most often affect animals less than 2 years of age (Fallin, 1993; Palmer, 1993). These tumors are locally invasive and frequently metastasize to multiple sites (Fallin, 1993).

CYTOLOGICAL DIAGNOSIS

One report of a rhabdosarcoma in a feline subcutaneous mass described a pleomorphic population of stromal cells with large, unusual multinucleate forms (Perman, 1979). Rhabdosarcoma was reported in a 12-month-old Labrador retriever with multiple soft-tissue masses containing cells with high N:C ratio and marked anisocytosis and anisokaryosis (Fallin, 1993). These large cells were assumed to be rhabdomyoblasts (Fallin, 1993). Multinucleated cells and mitosis were seen. Nuclei were organized in rows or ribbonlike arrangements and nucleoli were prominent, multiple, and irregular (Fallin, 1993). A second population of small, round cells was reported and presumed to be lymphocytes (Fallin, 1993). The human literature reports a population of small, round cells with scant cytoplasm and one to two nucleoli (Ackerman, 1992; Fallin, 1993). Differentiation from lymphocytes may be difficult. The cytological appearance of a botryoid rhabdomyosarcoma in the bladder of a dog was described (Alleman, 1991). Low numbers of spindle- to ribbon-shaped cells with abundant pale blue cytoplasm were present (Alleman, 1991). Occasional cells had basophilic cross striations. These small cells had eosinophilic longitudinal striations (Alleman, 1991). Nuclei were oval with coarse, clumped chromatin (Alleman, 1991). In our limited experience with rhabdosarcomas, multinucleation and marked anisocytosis are prominent features. Slides should be carefully scanned for evidence of striations within the cytoplasm that confirms the skeletal muscle origin. Differentiation from the malignant histiocytic diseases may be difficult. Although benign muscle tumors would be expected to lack the salient features of malignancy, a cytological diagnosis of rhabdomyoma is not documented.

Leiomyosarcoma (Fig. 11-25)

Clinical and Cytological Diagnoses

Tumors of smooth muscle are uncommon in both dogs and cats, with leiomyomas more frequent than leiomyosarcomas. Cigar-shaped nuclei with finely granular chromatin are typical of smooth-muscle tumors. Differentiation of leiomyomas and leiomyosarcomas may be impossible cytologically.

Giant Cell Tumor of Bone (Figs. 11-26 and 11-27)

Clinical and Cytological Diagnoses

Giant cell tumors of bone are rare neoplasms in the dog and cat, occurring primarily as osteocyte masses in the long bones (Palmer, 1993). These tumors are locally aggressive and rarely metastasize. Like most stromal masses, these tumors consist of single stromal cells with varying degrees of differentiation. Many of these stromal cells are typical osteoblast-like cells with multinucleation, uniform regular nuclei, and single regular nucleoli.

Synovial Sarcoma (Figs. 11-28 and 11-29)

Clinical Diagnosis

Synovial tumors are uncommon and can arise from bursae, joint capsules, and tendon sheaths (Lipowitz, 1979; Silva-Krott, 1993). In dogs the stifle and elbow are most commonly affected (Palmer, 1993). Synovial sarcomas destroy and cross the joint (Lowseth, 1984; Palmer, 1993). They can be difficult to remove and frequently recur (Palmer, 1993). Late-stage metastasis, especially to lung, is possible (Palmer, 1993). In the cat, local recurrence at the site has been reported, but the potential for metastasis is unknown (Silva-Krott, 1993). Differentiation of synovial sarcoma from histiocytic sarcoma (see Chapter 4) may be difficult.

Cytological Diagnosis

Synovial cell sarcoma is characterized by the presence of two cellular components: a spindlelike element intermixed with an epithelioid or synovioblastic element (Vail, 1992). The synovioblastic cells are round to polygonal (Silva-Krott, 1993) with variation in proportion (Vail, 1992). Large, pleomorphic mesenchymal cells resembling osteoclasts were observed in synovial fluid from a cat with forelimb lameness (Silva-Krott, 1993).

Synovial sarcoma was reported from the stifle joint of a dog (Lowseth, 1984). The synovial fluid contained many nonlytic neutrophils. Large, pleomorphic, spindle to polygonal cells were arranged singly or in groups. The cells had scant to abundant basophilic cytoplasm; eccentric nuclei; and prominent, angular nucleoli (Lowseth, 1984). Anisokaryosis was marked. Synovial sarcoma must be differentiated from metastatic carcinoma (Meinkoth, 1997).

References

Ackerman, M., Orell, S.R., Sterett, G.F., et al. Supporting tissues. In *Manual and Atlas of Fine Needle Aspiration Cytology*. ed 2. Churchill Livingstone, New York, 1992.

Alleman, A.R., Raskin, R.E., and Uhi, E.W. What is your diagnosis? *Vet Clin Pathol* 20:49-50, 1991.

Bitetto, W.V., Patnaik, A.K., Schrader, S.C., et al. Osteosarcoma in cats: 22 cases (1974-1984). *J Am Vet Med Assoc* 190:91-93, 1987.

Davidson, J.R. Canine and feline chondrosarcoma. *Compend Cont Ed Pract* 17:1109-1112, 1995.

Evans, E.W., Dubielzig, R.R., Carr, A.P., et al. What is your diagnosis? *Vet Clin Pathol* 25:37,57, 1996.

Fallin, C.W., Papendick, R.E., and Christopher, M.M. What is your diagnosis? *Vet Clin Pathol* 24:80,101, 1993.

LaRue, S.M., Withrow, S.J., and Wrigley, R.H. Radiographic bone surveys in the evaluation of primary bone tumors in dogs. *J Am Vet Med Assoc* 188:514-516, 1986.

Lipowitz, A.J., Fetter, A.W., and Walker, M.A. Synovial sarcoma of the dog. *J Am Vet Med Assoc* 174:76-81, 1979.

Liu, S., Dorfman, H., and Patnaik, A.K. Primary and secondary bone tumors in the cat. *J Small Anim Pract* 15: 141-156, 1974.

Lowseth, L.A., Herbert, R.A., Muggenburg, B.A., et al. What is your diagnosis? *Vet Clin Pathol* 18:5,74, 1984.

Mahaffey, E.A. Cytology of the musculoskeletal system. In *Diagnostic Cytology of the Dog and Cat*. R.L. Cowell, R.D. Tyler, J.H. Meinkoth (eds). Mosby, St Louis, 1999.

Meinkoth, J.H., Rochat, M.C., and Cowell, R.L. Metastatic carcinoma presenting as hind-limb lameness: diagnosis by synovial fluid cytology. *J Am Anim Hosp Assoc* 33:325-328, 1997.

Michels, G.M., DeNicola, D.B., and Waters, D.J. A prospective comparison of cytologic with histopathologic evaluation of neoplastic appendicular skeletal lesions in dogs. *Vet Pathol* 34:477, 1997 (abstract).

Palmer, N. Bones and joints. In *Pathology of Domestic Animals*. K.V.F. Jubb, P.C. Kennedy, and N. Palmer (eds). Academic Press, San Diego, 1993.

Patnaik, A.K., Lieberman, P.H., Erlandson, R.A., et al. Canine sinonasal skeletal neoplasms: chondrosarcomas and osteosarcomas. *Vet Pathol* 21:475-482, 1984.

Perman, V., Alasker, R.D., and Riis, R.C. *Cytology of the Dog and Cat*. American Animal Hospital Association, Lakewood, Colo, 1979.

Probst, C.W. and Ackerman, N. Malignant neoplasia of the canine appendicular skeleton. *Compend Cont Ed Pract* 4: 260-270, 1982.

Silva-Krott, U., Tucker, R.L., and Meeks, J.C. Synovial sarcoma in a cat. *J Am Vet Med Assoc* 203:1430-1431, 1993.

Stirtzinger, T. The cytologic diagnosis of mesenchymal tumors. *Semin Vet Med Surg (Small Anim)* 3:157-166, 1988.

Straw, R.C. and Withrow, S.J. Treatment of canine osteosarcoma. In *Current Veterinary Therapy XII, Small Animal Practice*. J.D. Bonagura (ed). WB Saunders, Philadelphia, 1995.

Vail, D.M., Powers, B.E., Getzy, D., et al. Prognostic importance of histological grade and cytochemical staining patterns for canine synovial cell sarcoma: preliminary results of a VCOG study. *Vet Cancer Soc* 17:1-4, 1992.

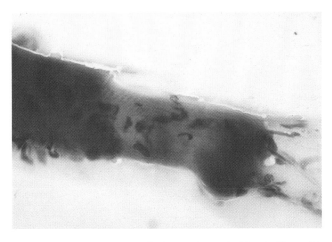

FIG. 11-1. Canine. Fine needle. Normal muscle. Muscle fiber with multiple small, elongate nuclei. (×100.)

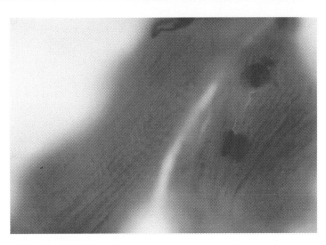

FIG. 11-2. Canine. Scraping. Normal muscle. Longitudinal and cross striations visible. Cigar-shaped nuclei. (×400.)

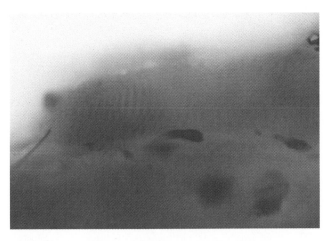

FIG. 11-3. Canine. Scraping. Normal muscle. Prominent striations and the typical green-blue tinctorial properties expected for Wright's-stained muscle fibers. (×400.)

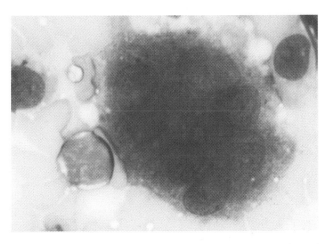

FIG. 11-4. Canine. Scraping. Normal bone. Large, multinucleated osteoclast. Note size compared with lymphocyte. (×500.)

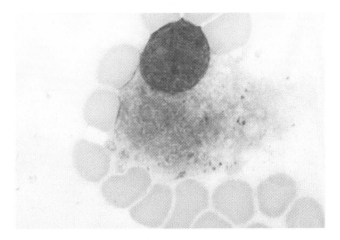

FIG. 11-5. Canine. Fine needle. Fracture callus. Osteoblast with small, azurophilic, cytoplasmic granules. (×630.)

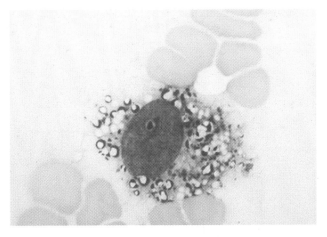

FIG. 11-6. Canine. Fine needle. Fracture callus. Stromal cell. The intracytoplasmic clear spaces outlined by metachromatic material suggest chondroblastic differentiation. (×630.)

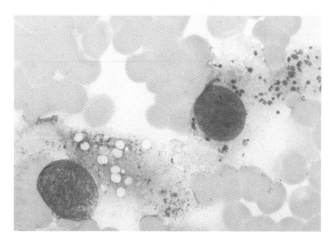

FIG. 11-7. Canine. Fine needle. Fracture callus. Stromal cells with elongate cytoplasm and indistinct boundaries, prominent metachromatic granulation, occasional vacuoles, low N:C ratio, and oval to elongate nucleus with indistinct nuclear chromatin. (×630.)

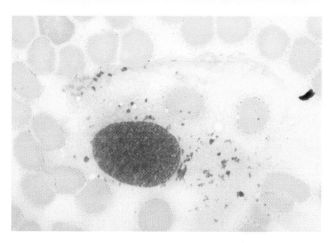

FIG. 11-8. Canine. Fine needle. Fracture callus. Similar cell to Fig. 11-7 at higher magnification. Nuclei are the diameter of two to three erythrocytes. Cytoplasmic metachromatic granules vary in size and are not specific for any one type of mesenchymal cell. (×500.)

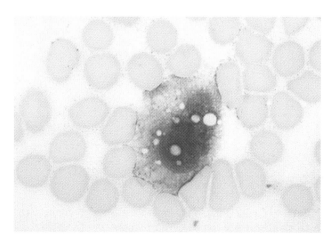

FIG. 11-9. Canine. Fine needle. Reactive bone. Single stromal cell with cytoplasmic accumulation of metachromatic material; consistent with early production of chondroid matrix. (×500.)

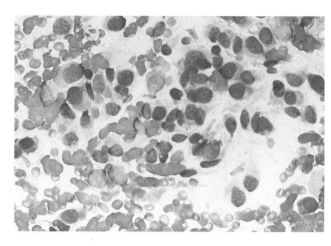

FIG. 11-10. Canine. Fine needle. Maxillary mass. Osteosarcoma. Low-powered view of numerous round to spindle-shaped cells with moderate anisokaryosis. (×100.)

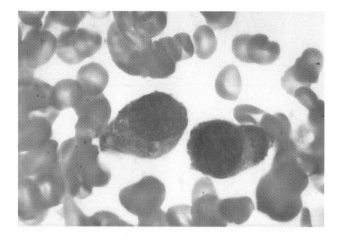

FIG. 11-11. Canine. Fine needle. Maxillary mass. Osteosarcoma. Two small, spindle-shaped cells with hyperchromatic eccentric nuclei. These may be benign osteoblasts, which can be found in productive areas of the tumor. (×500.)

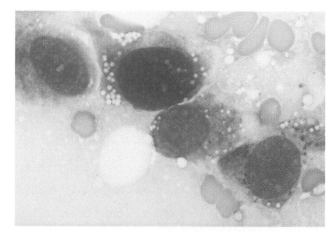

FIG. 11-12. Canine. Imprint. Hind-limb lameness. Osteosarcoma. Large cells with hyperchromatic nuclei, marked anisokaryosis, and prominent nucleoli consistent with malignant osteoblasts. Pink intracytoplasmic granules are not specific but may be precursor of osteoid matrix. (×400.)

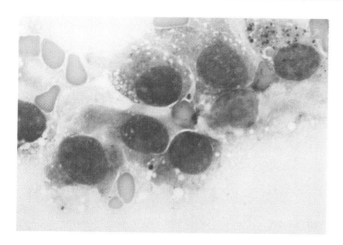

FIG. 11-13. Canine. Imprint. Hind-limb swelling. Osteosarcoma. (Same case as Fig. 11-12.) A cluster of round to spindle cells with eccentric large nuclei and increased N:C ratio consistent with malignant osteoblasts. (×400.)

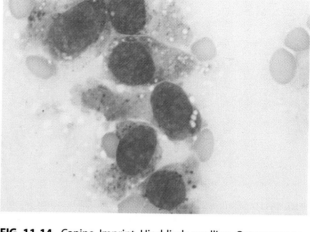

FIG. 11-14. Canine. Imprint. Hind-limb swelling. Osteosarcoma. (Same case as Fig. 11-12.) Spindle-shaped cells with indistinct basophilic cytoplasm containing numerous azurophilic cytoplasmic granules. (×400.)

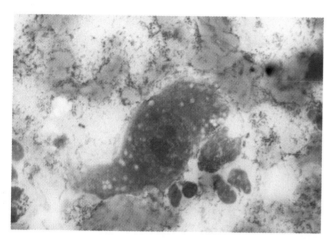

FIG. 11-15. Canine. Scraping. Leg mass. Osteosarcoma with osteomyelitis. Large, spindle-shaped cell surrounded by degenerate neutrophils and debris and free and phagocytized bacteria. The nuclear characteristics of malignancy can vary from mild to extreme in osteosarcoma. (×400.)

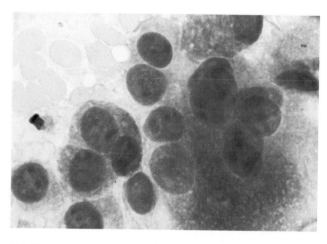

FIG. 11-16. Canine. Scraping. Leg mass. Osteosarcoma. A poorly preserved, large, multinucleated cell consistent with an osteoclast surrounded by smaller osteoblasts. Osteoclasts can be present with bone production and destruction. (×400.)

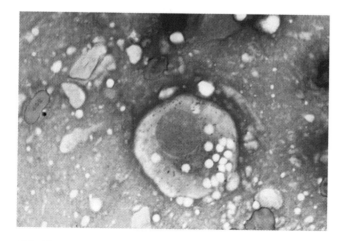

FIG. 11-17. Canine. Imprint. Mass in scapula. Chondrosarcoma. Abundant pink extracellular matrix surrounds a single cell with a large nucleus. The abundant bright pink amorphous to fibrillar extracellular matrix is consistent with chondroid matrix. (×400.)

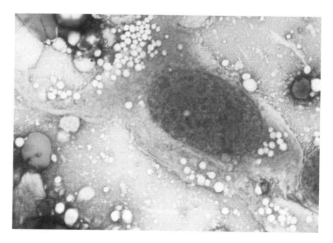

FIG. 11-18. Canine. Scraping. Scapular mass. Chondrosarcoma. (Same case as Fig. 11-17.) Spindle-shaped cell with a large nucleus, prominent heterochromatin, multiple nucleoli, and a high N:C ratio. (×400.)

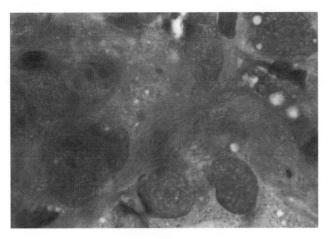

FIG. 11-19. Canine. Fine needle. Chest mass. Chondrosarcoma. Spindle-shaped cells with high N:C ratio; marked anisokaryosis; and prominent, variably sized nucleoli. There is abundant pink extracellular material that is typically observed in chondroid tumors. (×400.)

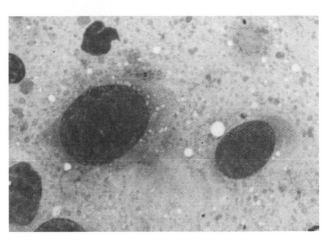

FIG. 11-20. Canine. Fine needle. Chest mass. Chondrosarcoma. Stromal cells with large, hyperchromatic nuclei and marked anisokaryosis. The limited background material is insufficient for differentiation but indicates the need to examine for additional evidence of matrix production. (×400.)

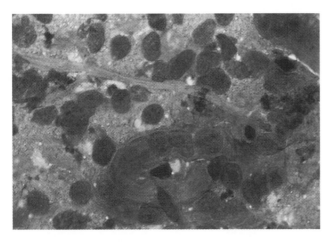

FIG. 11-21. Canine. Imprint. Left foreleg mass. Rhabdomyosarcoma. Small, bare nuclei within a pink matrix. The blue ribbonlike structure represents a multinucleated muscle fiber. (×250.)

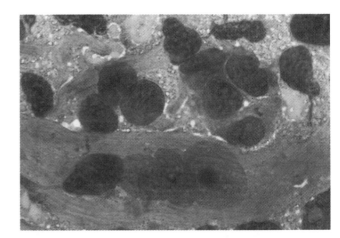

FIG 11-22. Canine. Imprint. Left foreleg mass. Rhabdomyosarcoma. (Same case as Fig. 11-21.) The multiple linearly arranged, variable-sized nuclei within a single muscle fiber; the small, bare nuclei; and the matrix are consistent with a tumor of skeletal muscle. Cytoplasmic striations indicate muscle fiber differentiation. (×400.)

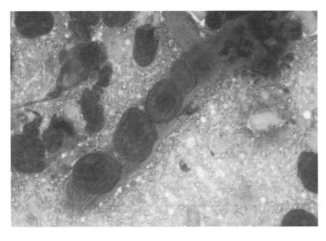

FIG. 11-23. Canine. Imprint. Left foreleg mass. Rhabdomyosarcoma. (Same case as Fig. 11-21.) Multinucleated cell with linearly arranged round nuclei and cytoplasmic striations. The nuclei display moderate anisokaryosis and prominent nucleoli. (×400.)

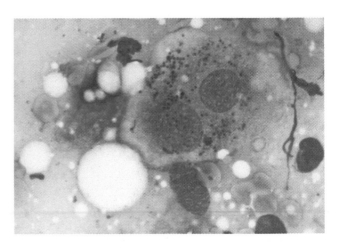

FIG. 11-24. Canine. Imprint. Mass on leg. Rhabdomyosarcoma. Large, binucleated stromal cell with prominent nonspecific cytoplasmic granulation. Multinucleation is a feature of rhabdomyosarcoma. (×400.)

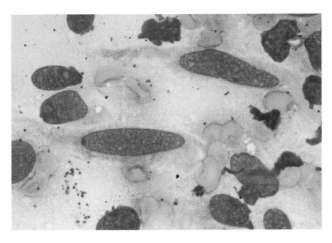

FIG. 11-25. Canine. Scraping. Vaginal mass. Leiomyosarcoma. The cigar-shaped nuclei with finely granular nuclear chromatin is typical of smooth-muscle tumors. Differentiation from other spindle cell tumors may be difficult. Differentiation between leiomyoma and leiomyosarcoma requires histological examination and special stains. (×400.)

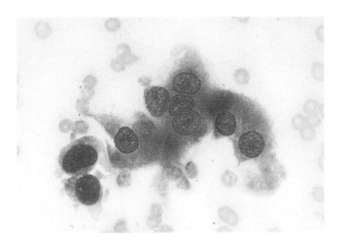

FIG. 11-26. Canine. Fine needle. Humerus. Giant cell tumor of bone. A multinucleated cell with uniform-sized round nuclei and lightly basophilic cytoplasm. Because of common association of giant cells and most stromal tumors, diagnosis is usually made by exclusion of other possibilities. (×250.)

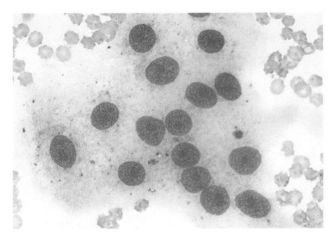

FIG. 11-27. Canine. Fine needle. Humerus. Giant cell tumor of bone. (Same case as Fig. 11-27.) Multinucleated cell with uniform nuclei, single nucleolus, and delicate cytoplasm. (×250.)

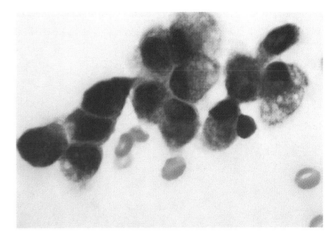

FIG. 11-28. Canine. Imprint. Mass in joint. Synovial sarcoma. Round to polygonal cells with hyperchromatic eccentric nuclei, low to high N:C ratio, and some cytoplasmic vacuolation. (×400.)

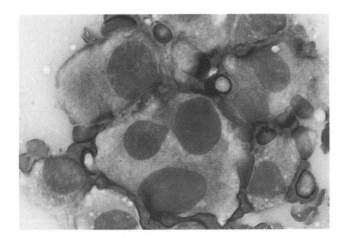

FIG. 11-29. Canine. Imprint. Synovial surface. Large, mononuclear cells with moderate anisokaryosis and abundant finely granular cytoplasm. The appearance of these cells contrasts sharply with Fig. 11-28. Recent developments suggest that some of these tumors may belong to the reactive histiocytosis. (×400.)

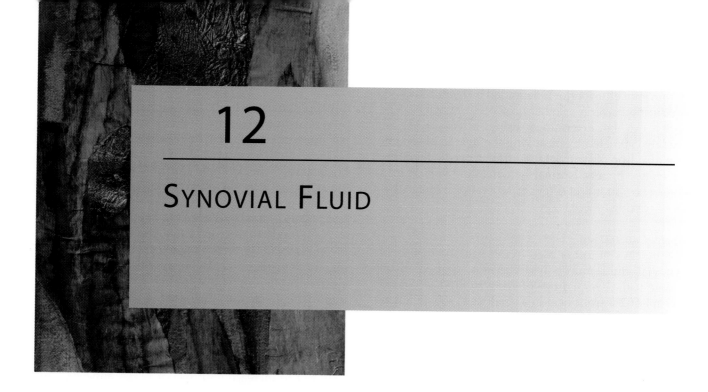

12

SYNOVIAL FLUID

Synovial fluid is frequently examined early in the investigation of suspect joint diseases. Radiology, microbiology, serology, histopathology of synovial biopsies, and tests for immune-mediated diseases may be required.

TECHNIQUE

ARTHROCENTESIS

During collection of synovial fluid, the animal must remain motionless to prevent iatrogenic trauma or blood contamination of the fluid. Sedation or anesthesia may or may not be required. The site is prepared as for a surgical approach. A 22-gauge needle is inserted into the flexed joint and fluid is gently aspirated into a 3-ml syringe. Preferred locations for arthrocentesis are described (Allen, 1991).

In small joints the aspirate volume may be minimal, allowing only immediate preparation of one or two air-dried smears. Slow movement of the spreader slide or use of the coverslip technique ensures a thin film that will enhance cell spreading and drying and improve detail of stained cells.

When there is adequate volume, fluid is placed in vials with and without EDTA. The anticoagulant is used to prevent clotting and aid cellular preservation. Normal synovial fluid does not clot but exhibits thixotropy and will return to the fluid state upon shaking. Clotting of the aliquot without anticoagulant indicates the entry of fibrinogen resulting from an inflammatory response or from the entry of blood before or during arthrocentesis. Heparin, if possible, is preferred as an anticoagulant for the mucin clot test because EDTA may cause minor depolymerization of the

hyaluronic acid and alter interpretation. A separate aliquot should be obtained for microbiological examination if an infectious cause is considered.

NORMAL SYNOVIAL FLUID (Figs. 12-1 to 12-12)

EXAMINATION

Synovial fluid is examined routinely in clinical diagnostical laboratories for volume, color, turbidity, viscosity, mucin clot formation, protein concentration, nucleated cell concentration, and morphology. Additional tests may be available on request.

VOLUME

Normal canine joints contain 0.1 to 1 ml of synovial fluid, with the greater volume found in the larger joints.

COLOR

Synovial fluid is clear and colorless. The fluid may be red-tinged because of hemarthrosis or iatrogenic blood contamination during arthrocentesis. Previous in vivo hemorrhage imparts a yellow-amber appearance to the fluid. Fresh hemorrhage may be indicated by the presence of platelets.

TURBIDITY

Turbidity indicates increased cellularity or the presence of flocculent material. Turbidity is not an indication of increased protein concentration.

VISCOSITY

The viscosity of synovial fluid is directly related to the concentration and quality of the hyaluronic acid. Viscosity is decreased when hyaluronic acid is diluted within joint effusions or if degraded by hyaluronidase-producing bacteria or other proteolytic enzymes. Viscosity can be determined using a viscometer or crudely estimated by observing the degree of separation of a drop of synovial fluid from a needle tip or between two fingers. Normal synovial fluid will create a connecting strand of a few to several centimeters before breaking.

MUCIN CLOT TEST

The mucin clot test is used to estimate the quality of synovial fluid mucopolysaccharides, that is, hyaluronic acid. Several drops of synovial fluid are added to 1 ml of 2% acetic acid in a small test tube. In a normal sample a white, ropelike clot is formed. Degradation of the hyaluronic acid produces a loose, friable clot. Dilution of the hyaluronic acid resulting from effusions affects viscosity to a greater degree than the mucin clot formation. In a synovial effusion that has a high cell count but a normal mucin clot test, the presence of adequate polymerized hyaluronic acid rules out the presence of hyaluronidase-producing bacteria and suggests the need to investigate further the reason for leukocytic chemotaxis.

TOTAL PROTEIN

Synovial fluid protein concentration can be determined using the biuret method or a refractometer. The synovial membrane is semipermeable to plasma proteins. Synovial fluid protein concentration increases when there is membrane disruption or in response to inflammatory mediators. Synovial fluid protein concentration and composition should be interpreted in parallel with serum or plasma proteins.

NUCLEATED CELL COUNT AND DIFFERENTIAL

Nucleated cells are counted using a Nebauer hemocytometer chamber or electronic particle cell counter. Acid diluents used for leukocyte counting precipitate mucin. A hypotonic saline solution is used as a diluent for synovial fluid and has the added advantage of lysing erythrocytes. The saline is simply substituted for the diluent in the WBC diluting pipette. Inadequate mixing of cells because of the thixotropic nature or small sample volume is a major contributor to variability in cell counts. Normal canine synovial fluid contains up to 3000×10^6/L (Duncan, 1994) but usually less than 500×10^6/L (Atilola, 1986; Fernandez, 1983). The larger joints in the dog, such as shoulder and stifle, have the higher cell counts (Fernandez, 1983). In a small study, the mean electronic cell count was slightly higher (1000×10^6/L) than the hemocytometer count (850×10^6/L) (Atilola, 1986). There is limited reference data available for feline synovial fluid, but it is assumed to be similar to values observed in dogs.

Cell Morphology

Cell morphology is best preserved if slides are prepared immediately on collection of fluid. Wet mount slides are recommended for crystal examination. Wright's-stained synovial fluid from a healthy joint cavity has a pink, finely granular background as a result of the presence of glycoproteins. Large crescents with increased staining intensity may be seen. With disease there may be dilution of background and increased granularity.

High fluid viscosity increases film thickness, reducing cell spreading, which together with slow-cell drying renders many cells indistinguishable. Mononuclear cells predominate in normal synovial fluid. It is impossible to classify each mononuclear cell because of the overlap in morphology. There may be low numbers of cells resembling lymphocytes and larger cells with cytoplasmic vacuolation resembling macrophages and synoviocytes. Cytoplasmic vacuolation is reported to increase with use of EDTA anticoagulant and with aging of fluid before slide preparation. Neutrophils and erythrocytes are rare in normal synovial fluid, unless there is iatrogenic contamination during arthrocentesis when platelets may be visible.

NONNEOPLASTIC DISEASE

Abnormalities of the canine joint have been classified according to several schemes. Examination of synovial fluid can classify joint abnormalities into traumatic, chronic degenerative, suppurative, and septic/nonseptic synovitis either independently or in conjunction with other clinical information. Further classification of the disease process requires culture and/or serology to rule out infectious agents and a range of tests to differentiate immune-mediated disorders. The following brief descriptions emphasize the salient features that have been reported in synovial fluid for the diseases described.

NONSUPPURATIVE INFLAMMATION

Trauma

CLINICAL DIAGNOSIS

Joint trauma usually presents clinically as an acute lameness restricted to one joint. A thorough history is essential for differentiating chronic degenerative joint problems.

CYTOLOGICAL DIAGNOSIS

Synovial fluid aspirated from an injured joint can be clear to yellow-tinged to bloody, has a normal mucin clot test, and usually has a mild increase in cellularity. Nucleated cell distribution may be normal. Degenerate to well-preserved red blood cells are present in the background. Erythrocytophagy may be present and supports a diagnosis of previous hemorrhage. Aspiration-related iatrogenic hemorrhage is indicated if there are platelets and well-preserved red cells on the slide.

Chronic Degenerative Joint Disease (Figs. 12-13 to 12-19)

CLINICAL DIAGNOSIS
Degenerative arthropathies usually result from previous trauma to the joint or from developmental abnormalities of the joints or articular surfaces. It is characterized by degenerative changes of the articular cartilage with secondary changes in the synovial membrane, bone, and cartilage (Pederson, 1983b).

CYTOLOGICAL DIAGNOSIS
This common joint abnormality of dogs presents with mild cytological changes. Nucleated cell counts may be normal or mildly increased, and cell distribution remains normal. Background staining may be slightly decreased as a result of dilution, but the mucin clot test often remains normal. Occasional to numerous single cells or clusters of synoviocytes are observed. The interpretation may be normal if few synoviocytes are present or a diagnosis of mild nonsuppurative synovitis compatible with degenerative disease may be possible.

In a study in which degenerative joint disease was created by unilateral severance of the anterior cruciate ligament, synovial fluid nucleated cell counts ranged from 1000 to 12,000 $\times$ 10^6/L with a mean of 3800 $\times$ 10^6/L (Lewis, 1987). In 7 of 10 dogs the percentage of neutrophils increased but never exceeded 34%. The mucin clot was considered poor in all 10 dogs (Lewis, 1987), although in our experience the mucin clot test is often normal.

Lymphocytic/Plasmacytic Polyarthritis

CLINICAL DIAGNOSIS
A bilateral inflammatory disease of the stifle joint reported in small- and medium-sized breeds of dogs is associated with joint laxity and instability, often leading to anterior cruciate damage. There is synovial hypertrophy and an intense lymphocytic plasmacytic synovial infiltrate (Bennett, 1995).

CYTOLOGICAL DIAGNOSIS
Synovial fluid nucleated cell counts ranged from 5000 to 20,000 $\times$ 10^6/L with 10% to 40% neutrophils and the remainder mononuclear cells (Hopper, 1989).

SUPPURATIVE INFLAMMATION

Infectious

Bacterial (Figs. 12-20 to 12-23)

CLINICAL DIAGNOSIS
A dog or cat with acute bacterial arthritis usually presents with systemic signs, including fever, inappe-

tence, and lethargy associated with enlargement of one or more joints. Leukocytosis is common.

CYTOLOGICAL DIAGNOSIS
The synovial fluid is usually turbid because of increased cells, has decreased viscosity, and may have a poor mucin clot depending on the bacterial hyaluronidase activity. Clotting is expected if fluid is collected without an anticoagulant. There is typically a marked increase in nucleated cells predominantly resulting from neutrophils. Bacteria may or may not be readily visible during slide examination. If bacteria are not visible, culture is necessary for confirmation of suspected bacterial synovitis, as well as for identification of the organism and determining antibiotic sensitivity. Synovial membrane culture may be more effective than synovial fluid culture in isolating the organism, especially if the volume of fluid does not allow concentration before culturing. Neutrophil nuclear degenerative changes, especially karyolysis, are often visible because of the presence of bacterial toxins. Nuclear morphology may be well preserved if the number of organisms is reduced as a result of antibiotic therapy or if the infectious agents are low toxin producers, as for many anaerobic bacteria. With the described features, the morphological interpretation would be septic suppurative synovitis.

In a study of 58 confirmed cases of bacterial arthritis, nucleated cell counts ranged from 4300 to 182,000 $\times$ 10^6/L. Polymorphonuclear cells predominated with a range of 43 to 99% and an average of 80% (Bennett, 1988b; Bennett, 1987f).

Mycoplasma

CLINICAL DIAGNOSIS
Arthritis caused by *Mycoplasma gatae* (Moise, 1983) and *Mycoplasma felis* (Hooper, 1985) have been reported in the cat. *Mycoplasma spumans* was cultured from a young greyhound dog with polyarthritis (Barton, 1985).

CYTOLOGICAL DIAGNOSIS
The synovial fluid from the greyhound was thin and cloudy (Barton, 1985). The neutrophils were increased and well preserved without the nuclear degenerative changes expected with bacterial synovitis (Bennett, 1995).

Viral

CLINICAL DIAGNOSIS
A systemic reaction was reported in cats with natural calicivirus infection and after administration of live calicivirus vaccine (Bennett, 1989; Levy, 1992). In kittens experimentally infected with two naturally occurring strains of calicivirus, a transient febrile illness developed with hyperesthesia and joints that were painful on manipulation (Pederson, 1983a).

CYTOLOGICAL DIAGNOSIS

Synovial fluid from a postvaccinal kitten contained $100,000 \times 10^6$/L cells with 80% small mononuclear cells, 14% neutrophils, and 6% large mononuclear cells. Calicivirus was isolated from the joint (Levy, 1992).

Borreliosis
CLINICAL DIAGNOSIS

The spirochete *Borrelia burgdorferi* causes a multisystem illness in humans and several domestic animals. It is transmitted by ticks of the *Ixodes* genus. In the dog, fever and acute lameness typically last several days but can recur cyclically. A positive diagnosis requires serological examination (Magnarelli, 1985). Recently, standardized criteria have been suggested for the diagnosis of *Borrelia* infection (Bennett, 1992).

CYTOLOGICAL DIAGNOSIS

Synovial fluid from nine affected dogs had a mean nucleated cell count of $46,300 \times 10^6$/L, of which 85% were nondegenerate neutrophils (Kornblatt, 1985). A cytological diagnosis of marked suppurative inflammation is appropriate. One dog with polyarthritis had a nucleated cell count of greater than $99,000 \times 10^6$/L (Moroff, 1990). The cells were primarily nonlytic neutrophils (Moroff, 1990).

Ehrlichiosis (Figs. 12-24 and 12-25)
CLINICAL DIAGNOSIS

A syndrome known as canine granulocytic ehrlichiosis has been reported in dogs (Stockham, 1992), which have clinical signs of acute lameness or muscular stiffness. Hematological abnormalities vary.

CYTOLOGICAL DIAGNOSIS

Analysis of synovial fluid from two affected dogs revealed a marked increase in cell count (30,000 to $50,000 \times 10^6$/L) with 60% to 80% nondegenerate neutrophils and 20% mononuclear cells (Cowell, 1988). The mucin clot test was normal. *Ehrlichia morula* were seen in approximately 1% of the synovial and blood neutrophils (Cowell, 1988; Stockham, 1992).

Additional agents that can cause synovitis include blastomycosis, leishmaniasis, and *Rickettsia rickettsii* (Rocky Mountain spotted fever), which are described in Chapter 3.

Noninfectious Erosive (Figs. 12-26 to 12-30)

Feline Periosteal Proliferative Polyarthritis
CLINICAL DIAGNOSIS

Feline periosteal proliferative polyarthritis (Bennett, 1988a) is also reported as feline chronic progressive polyarthritis (periosteal proliferative form) (Pederson, 1980; Peterson, 1983b). Cats present with fever, stiffness, lethargy, lymphadenopathy, and edema and erythema of the skin and subcutis overlying the affected joints (Pederson, 1980). This disease is similar to the rheumatoid syndrome and is characterized by extensive production of periosteal new bone. The carpus and hock are the primary joints involved. Severe destructive changes and enthesopathies can arise. An association with feline syncytium-forming virus and feline leukemia virus infection was suggested (Pederson, 1980).

CYTOLOGICAL DIAGNOSIS

In the synovial fluid of 17 affected cats, nucleated cell concentrations were 4000 to $70,000 \times 10^6$/L with 25% to 99% neutrophils (Pederson, 1980).

Rheumatoid Arthritis
CLINICAL DIAGNOSIS

Rheumatoid arthritis is an immunologically mediated arthropathy that causes a progressive destructive polyarthritis and polysynovitis in dogs and rarely in cats (Bennett, 1988b). In addition to lameness, dogs may present with inappetence, lethargy, fever, and lymphadenopathy (Bennett, 1987a). Chronic disease results in radiographic evidence of subchondral radiolucent foci and periarticular new bone formation. A relationship between canine distemper virus and rheumatoid arthritis in dogs has been postulated (Bell, 1991).

CYTOLOGICAL DIAGNOSIS

Synovial fluid in affected dogs has a moderate to marked increase in cellularity resulting predominantly from nondegenerate neutrophils. Synovial fluid analysis for 30 dogs with rheumatoid arthritis had nucleated cell counts ranging from 6200 to $87,200 \times 10^6$/L (mean $29,700 \times 10^6$/L) (Bennett, 1987a). The nucleated cells were predominantly neutrophils. Mucin clot tests were poor and friable (Bennett, 1987a). A rheumatoid factor (RF) titer of greater than or equal to 1/40 was observed in 73% of dogs in at least one sample (Bennett, 1987a). However, a negative titer was present in six of these positive dogs on one or more occasions (Bennett, 1987a). With chronicity, or with therapy, the cellular response frequently becomes mononuclear with increased lymphocytes and macrophages. Large numbers of synoviocytes, single, in large clusters, or in rafts, indicates associated synovial hyperplasia.

Greyhound Polyarthritis
CLINICAL DIAGNOSIS

An erosive polyarthritis of young greyhounds has been reported (Huxtable, 1976) in dogs that are rheumatoid factor and antinuclear antibody negative.

CYTOLOGICAL DIAGNOSIS

The synovial fluid from two affected dogs had nucleated cell counts from normal to $53,000 \times 6$/L with 80% neutrophils and 20% mononuclear cells (Huxtable, 1976; Woodward, 1991).

Noninfectious Nonerosive (Figs. 12-26 to 12-30)

Immune-mediated nonerosive arthritides are common in the dog. The causes are multiple and diverse but likely have similar immunopathogenic mechanisms. The causes include infectious diseases, immunological diseases, plasmacytic-lymphocytic synovitis, chronic hepatic disease, inflammatory bowel disease, allergic drug reactions, malignant neoplasms, and idiopathic diseases (Hopper, 1989). Most immune-mediated joint diseases present with similar clinical features of fever, anorexia, and lethargy accompanying the lameness. The clinical signs are usually cyclical, with the distal extremities most commonly affected (Hopper, 1989).

Systemic Lupus Erythematosus
CLINICAL DIAGNOSIS

Systemic lupus erythematosus (SLE) is a multisystem immunologically mediated condition that is characterized by circulating autoantibodies directed at nuclear antigens (Bennett, 1987b). A titer greater than 1 in 32 in the indirect immunofluorescence test, using rat liver as a substrate, is accepted as abnormal (Bennett, 1987b; Bennett, 1987e). Between 60% and 80% of dogs with SLE have polyarthritis (Scott, 1983). Skin disease was detected in 50% of affected dogs in one study (Bennett, 1987b). Also seen are muscular, neurological, vascular, and hematological abnormalities. Anemia was present in 35% of the cases and proteinuria in 50% (Hopper, 1989; Scott, 1983).

CYTOLOGICAL DIAGNOSIS

In dogs with SLE, the synovial fluid has a mild to marked increase in cellularity with the majority containing nonlytic neutrophils. There are low numbers of small lymphocytes, macrophages, and synoviocytes. The mucin clot test is often normal, which may help differentiate SLE from some bacterial arthritides. Rarely, LE cells can be seen in synovial fluid slides. LE cells are phagocytic cells, mainly neutrophils, with peripheralized nuclei and round, intracytoplasmic, homogenous, pink to purple dense material considered to be phagocytized partially degraded DNA. LE cells must not be confused with leukophagocytic macrophages.

Idiopathic Polyarthritis
CLINICAL DIAGNOSIS

Idiopathic polyarthritis is diagnosed by elimination and reported to be the most common polyarthritis in dogs. The clinical signs include pyrexia, lameness, inappetence, and lethargy (Bennett, 1987c). The pathogenesis is considered to be due to immune complex deposition in response to chronic antigenic stimulation from gastroenteritis, ulcerative colitis, parasites, respiratory or urinary tract infection, and neoplastic disease (Bennett, 1987c). Idiopathic polyarthritis has been sub-divided into four categories (Bennett, 1987c): uncomplicated idiopathic arthritis accounted for 51% of the reported cases, infections remote from the joint accounted for 26%, gastrointestinal disease accounted for 13%, and neoplasia 10% (Bennett, 1987c; Bennett, 1995).

CYTOLOGICAL DIAGNOSIS

In 67 cases of mixed etiology the joint fluid was generally turbid, watery, and increased in quantity, with a poor mucin clot. There was an increase in cellularity ranging from 3200 to 106,300 × 10^6/L (average 32,000 × 10^6/L) with 40% to 99.5% neutrophils (average 79%) (Bennett, 1987c).

Polyarthritis/Polymyositis
CLINICAL DIAGNOSIS

Idiopathic polymyositis/polyarthritis is an immune-based connective tissue disorder characterized by symmetrical polyarthritis, stiffness, joint swelling and pain, and muscle atrophy. Biopsies of muscle and synovium reveal a chronic active inflammatory process (Bennett, 1987d). These dogs are RF and ANA negative (Bennett, 1987d). Five of the six affected dogs were spaniels (Bennett, 1987d).

CYTOLOGICAL DIAGNOSIS

In six affected dogs, cell counts varied from 1900 to 81,000 × 10^6/L (mean = 25.3). Neutrophils accounted for 70% to 90% of the total cells. The mucin clot was generally poor (Bennett, 1987d).

Drug Hypersensitivity
CLINICAL DIAGNOSIS

A syndrome of nonseptic polyarthritis has been reported in dogs 1 to 3 weeks after commencement of therapy with trimethoprim/sulfonamide (Tribrissen) (Giger, 1985; Little, 1990; Werner, 1983). Large-breed dogs, particularly the Doberman, appear to be predisposed (Werner, 1983).

CYTOLOGICAL DIAGNOSIS

After challenge with Tribrissen, two affected Dobermans had synovial fluid cell counts of 20,000 to 44,000 × 10^6/L with 40% to 90% neutrophils and 11% to 50% large mononuclear cells (Werner, 1983). Recovery after cessation of therapy is reported. The syndrome has also been reported in a Pekinese (Little, 1990).

Juvenile-Onset Polyarthritis in Akitas
CLINICAL DIAGNOSIS

Eight Akitas less than 8 months of age presented with cyclic episodes of pain, high spiking fever, and nonseptic suppurative polyarthritis (Dougherty, 1991). An associated nonseptic meningitis was present in two dogs (Dougherty, 1991). Immunosuppressive therapy can be effective (Dougherty, 1991).

CYTOLOGICAL DIAGNOSIS

Synovial fluid nucleated cell counts ranged from 5000 to 62,000 $\times$ 10^6/L with a predominance of neutrophils in all samples (Dougherty, 1991).

Familial Renal Amyloidosis in Chinese Shar-Peis

CLINICAL DIAGNOSIS

A syndrome has been reported in shar-pei dogs that present with recurrent episodes of fever and swelling of one or both hocks. Involvement of other joints has been reported (Bennet, 1995; DiBartola, 1990; May, 1992). Some affected dogs develop renal amyloidosis, leading to renal failure and death (Bennett, 1995; May, 1992).

CYTOLOGICAL DIAGNOSIS

Synovial fluid examined from one dog with acute pyrexia had a nucleated cell count of 193,000 $\times$ 10^6/L, of which 90% were neutrophils (May, 1992).

NEOPLASTIC DISEASE

Synovial Sarcoma

Cytological characteristics of synovial sarcoma are described in Chapter 11. See Figs. 11-28 and 11-29.

References

Allen, D.G. Special techniques. In *Small Animal Medicine*. D.G. Allen (ed). JB Lippincott, Philadelphia, 1991.

Atilola, M.A.O., Lumsden, J.H., and Rooke, F.A. Comparison of manual and electronic counting for total nucleated cell counts on synovial fluid from canine stifle joints. *Can J Vet Res* 50:282-284, 1986.

Barton, M.D., Ireland, L., Kirschner, J.L., et al. Isolation of *Mycoplasma spumans* from polyarthritis in a greyhound. *Aust Vet J* 62:206, 1985.

Bell, S.C., Carter, S.D., and Bennett, D. Canine distemper viral antigens and antibodies in dogs with rheumatoid arthritis. *Res Vet Sci* 50:64-68, 1991.

Bennett, D. Immune-based erosive inflammatory joint disease of the dog: canine rheumatoid arthritis. *J Small Anim Pract* 28:779-819, 1987a.

Bennett, D. Immune based non-erosive inflammatory joint disease of the dog. 1. Canine systemic lupus erythematosus. *J Small Anim Pract* 28:871-889, 1987b.

Bennett, D., Gaskell, R.M., Mills, A., et al. Detection of feline calicivirus antigens in the joints of infected cats. *Vet Rec* 124:329-332, 1989.

Bennett, D. Immune-based non-erosive inflammatory joint disease of the dog. 3. Canine idiopathic polyarthritis. *J Small Anim Pract* 28:909-928, 1987c.

Bennett, D. and Kelly, D.F. Immune-based non-erosive inflammatory joint disease of the dog. 2. Polyarthritis/polymyositis syndrome *J Small Anim Pract* 28:891-908, 1987d.

Bennett, D. and Kirkham, D. The laboratory identification of serum antinuclear antibody in the dog. *J Comp Pathol* 97:523-539, 1987e.

Bennett, D. and May, C. Joint diseases of dogs and cats. In *Textbook of Veterinary Internal Medicine*. S.J. Ettinger and E.C. Feldman (eds). WB Saunders, Philadelphia, 1995.

Bennett, D., May, C., and Carter, S. Lyme disease. In *The Veterinary Annual 32 Issue*, M-R. Raw and T.J. Parkinson (eds). Blackwell Scientific Publications, London, 1992.

Bennett, D. and Nash, A.S. Feline immune-based polyarthritis: a study of thirty-one cases. *J Small Anim Pract* 29: 501-523, 1988a.

Bennett, D. and Taylor, D.J. Bacterial endocarditis and inflammatory joint disease in the dog. *J Small Anim Pract* 29:347-365, 1987f.

Bennett, D. and Taylor, D.J. Bacterial infective arthritis in the dog. *J Small Anim Pract* 29:207- 230, 1988b.

Cowell, R.L., Tyler, R.D., Clinkenbeard, K.D., et al. Ehrlichiosis and polyarthritis in three dogs. *J Am Vet Med Assoc* 192:1093-1095, 1988.

DiBartola, S.P., Tarr, M.J., Webb, D.M., et al. Familial renal amyloidosis in Chinese Shar Pei dogs. *J Am Vet Med Assoc* 197:483-487, 1990.

Dougherty, S.A, Center, S.A., Shaw, E.E., et al. Juvenile-onset polyarthritis syndrome in Akitas. *J Am Vet Med Assoc* 198:849-856, 1991.

Duncan, R.J., Prasse, K.W., and Mahaffey, E.A. Cytology. In *Veterinary Laboratory Medicine: Clinical Pathology*. ed 3. J.R. Duncan, K.W. Prasse, and E.A. Mahaffy (eds). Iowa State University Press, Ames, Iowa, 1994.

Fernandez, F.R., Grindem, C.B., Lipowitz, A.J., et al. Synovial fluid analysis: preparation of smears for cytologic examination of canine synovial fluid. *J Am Anim Hosp Assoc* 19:727-734, 1983.

Giger, H., Werner, L.L., Millichamp, N.J., et al. Sulfadiazine-induced allergy in six Doberman pinschers. *J Am Vet Med Assoc* 186:479-483, 1985.

Hooper, P.T., Ireland, L.A., and Carter, A. Mycoplasma polyarthritis in a cat with probable severe immune deficiency. *Aust Vet J* 62:352, 1985.

Hopper, P.E. Immune-mediated nonerosive arthritis in the dog. In *Current Veterinary Therapy X, Small Animal Practice*. R.W. Kirk and J.D. Bonagura (eds). WB Saunders, Philadelphia, 1989.

Huxtable, C.R. and Davis, P.E. The pathology of polyarthritis in young greyhounds. *J Comp Pathol* 86:11-21, 1976.

Kornblatt, A.N., Urband, P.H., and Steere, A.C. Arthritis caused by *Borrelia burgdorferi* in dogs. *J Am Vet Med Assoc* 186:960-963, 1985.

Levy, J, K. and Marsh, A. Isolation of calicivirus from the joint of a kitten with arthritis. *J Am Vet Med Assoc* 201: 753-755, 1992.

Lewis, D.D., Goring, R.L., Parker, R.B., et al. Comparison of diagnostic methods used in the evaluation of early degenerative joint disease in the dog. *J Am Anim Hosp Assoc* 23:305-315, 1987.

Little, D.J.L. and Carmichael, S. Trimethoprim sulphonamide hypersensitivity in dogs. *Vet Rec* 127:459-460, 1990.

Magnarelli, L.A., Anderson, J.F., Kaufman A.F., et al. Borreliosis in dogs from southern Connecticut. *J Am Vet Med Assoc* 186:955-959, 1985.

May, C., Hammill, J., and Bennett, D. Chinese Shar Pei fever syndrome: a preliminary report. *Vet Rec* 131:586-587, 1992.

Moise, N.S., Crissman, J.W., Fairbrother, J.F., et al. Mycoplasma gateae arthritis and tenosynovitis in cats: case report and experimental reproduction of the disease. *Am J Vet Res* 44:16-21, 1983.

Moroff, S. *Case 16.* ASVCP Annual Slide Review Session, Annual General Meeting, Phoenix, 1990.

Pederson, N.C., Laliberte, L., and Ekman, S. A transient febrile "limping" syndrome of kittens caused by two different strains of feline calicivirus. *Feline Practice* 13:26-35, 1983a.

Pederson, N.C., Pool, R.R., and Morgan, J.P. Joint diseases of dogs and cats. In *Textbook of Veterinary Internal Medicine.* S.J. Ettinger (ed). WB Saunders, Philadelphia, 1983b.

Pederson, N.C., Pool, R.R., and O'Brien, T. Feline chronic progressive polyarthritis. *Am J Vet Res* 41:522-535, 1980.

Scott, D.W, Walton, D.K., Manning, T.O, et al. Canine lupus erythematosus. 1. Systemic lupus erythematosus. *J Am Anim Hosp Assoc* 19:461-477, 1983.

Stockham, S.L., Schmidt, D.A., Curtis, K.S., et al. Evaluation of granulocytic ehrlichiosis in dogs of Missouri, including serologic status to *Ehrlichia canis, Ehrlichia equi,* and *Borrelia burgdorferi. Am J Vet Res* 53:63-68, 1992.

Werner, L.L. and Bright, J.M. Drug-induced immune hypersensitivity disorders in two dogs treated with trimethoprim sulfadiazine: case reports and drug challenge studies. *J Am Anim Hosp Assoc* 19:783-790, 1983.

Woodward, J.C., Riser, W.H., Bloomberg, M.S., et al. Erosive polyarthritis in two Greyhounds. *J Am Vet Med Assoc* 198:873-876, 1991.

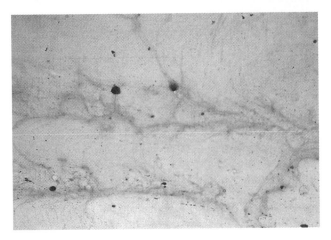

FIG. 12-1. Canine. Synovial fluid, direct smear. Low cellularity with lightly basophilic, lacy background typical for normal synovial fluid. (×50.)

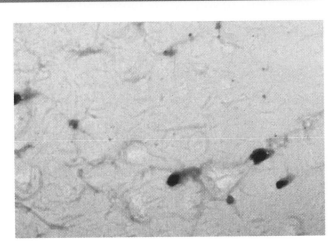

FIG. 12-2. Canine. Synovial fluid. Normal. Mononuclear cells predominate. The finely granular background and the dense crescents are artifactual and relate to the viscosity and mucopolysaccharide content. (×100.)

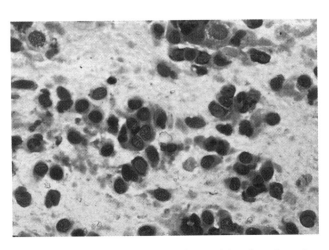

FIG. 12-3. Canine. Scraping. Normal synovial surface. Round to elongated synoviocytes with a pink, irregular, granular background. (×100.)

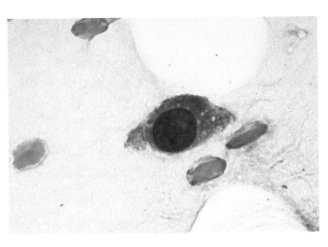

FIG. 12-4. Canine. Scraping. Normal synovial surface. The single synoviocyte has dense basophilic cytoplasm with mild vacuolation and a small, round nucleus. (×500.)

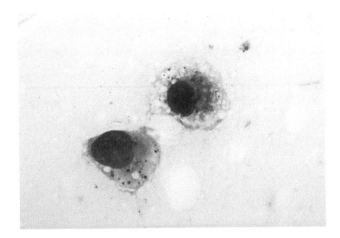

FIG. 12-5. Canine. Scraping. Normal synovial surface. Two synoviocytes with eccentric nuclei, low N:C ratio, and basophilic cytoplasm with vacuolation and metachromatic granules. Exfoliated synoviocytes with vacuolated cytoplasm can be very similar to macrophages. (×400.)

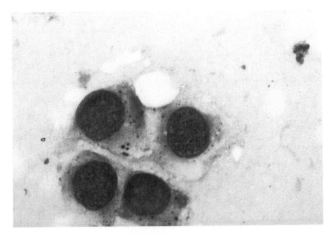

FIG. 12-6. Canine. Scraping. Normal synovial surface. Synoviocytes with dense to light basophilic cytoplasm; nonspecific metachromatic granulation; indistinct borders; small, round, dense, eccentric nuclei; and multiple small, indistinct nucleoli. (×500.)

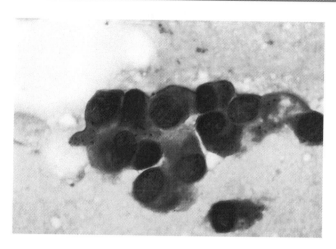

FIG. 12-7. Canine. Scraping. Normal synovial surface. Cluster of synoviocytes with eccentric nuclei and basophilic cytoplasm. (×400.)

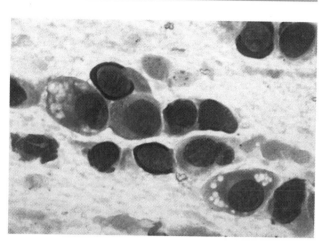

FIG. 12-8. Canine. Scraping. Normal synovial surface. Synoviocytes with variation in cytoplasmic vacuolation and basophilia. Prominent irregular granular background. (×400.)

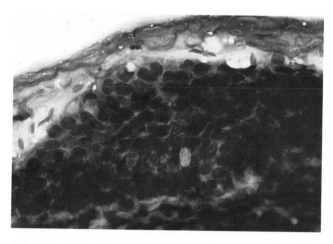

FIG. 12-9. Canine. Scraping. Normal synovial surface. Superficial layer of metachromatic material overlying a thick sheet of nucleated cells. The metachromatic material may be cartilaginous matrix or adherent glycosaminoglycans. (×160.)

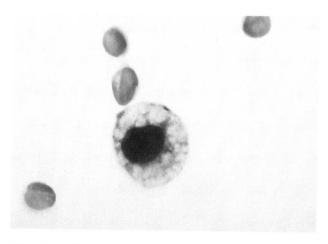

FIG. 12-10. Canine. Synovial fluid. Normal. A single vacuolated mononuclear cell that may be a degenerating synoviocyte or monocyte/macrophage. (×400.)

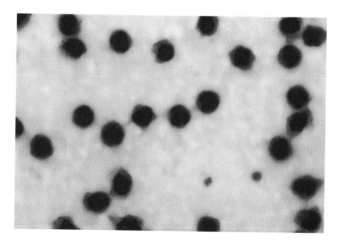

FIG. 12-11. Canine. Synovial fluid. Septic arthritis. Poor morphology because of slow drying. When cells are allowed to dry too slowly, especially neutrophils, condensation obscures nuclear details. Rapid air drying of cytological preparations is essential for preservation of cellular details. (×400.)

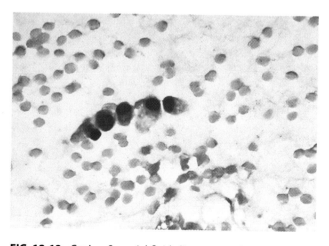

FIG. 12-12. Canine. Synovial fluid, direct smear. Iatrogenic hemorrhage created during sample collection. Streaming of erythrocytes and mononuclear cells is observed frequently in synovial fluid smears because of the viscosity. (×200.)

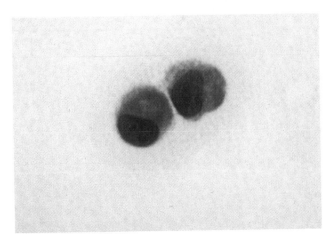

FIG. 12-13. Canine. Synovial fluid. Chronic degenerative joint disease. Nucleated cells 3000 × 10⁶/L. A slight to moderate increase in relatively normal synoviocytes may be the only cytological manifestation with chronic degenerative joint diseases. (×400.)

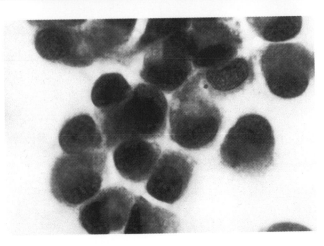

FIG. 12-14. Canine. Synovial fluid. Chronic degenerative joint disease. (Same case as Fig. 12-13.) The many cohesive synoviocytes are abnormal and indicate hyperplasia and exfoliation typical for chronic joint disorders. (×400.)

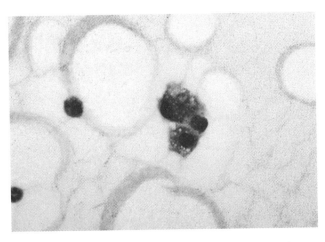

FIG. 12-15. Canine. Synovial fluid, direct smear. Chronic degenerative joint disease. Typical large crescents and foamy mononuclear cells. Cytoplasmic vacuolation develops within many cells in a fluid environment and has limited significance other than likely indicating degenerative changes within the cell. (×200.)

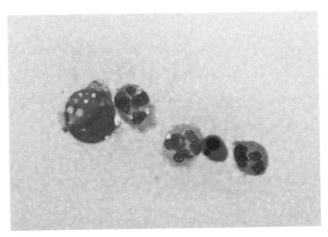

FIG. 12-16. Canine. Synovial fluid. Mixed inflammatory reaction. Degenerating neutrophils, one with karyopyknosis, and a macrophage consistent with mixed inflammatory response. With inflammation there may be loss of background density, possibly as a result of release of enzymes from phagocytic cells. (×400.)

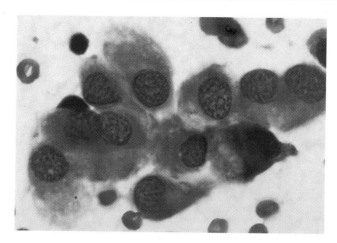

FIG. 12-17. Canine. Synovial fluid. Synovial cell hyperplasia. Clusters and sheets of basophilic synoviocytes with dark nuclei, prominent chromatin patterns, and visible nucleoli. Exfoliation of attached synoviocytes with this morphology is consistent with benign hyperplasia and usually indicates chronic irritation. (×400.)

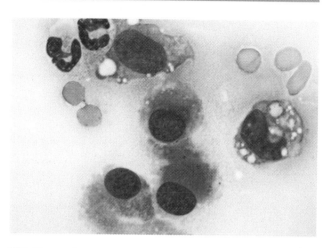

FIG. 12-18. Canine. Synovial fluid. Mixed inflammatory reaction. Chronic degenerative joint disease. Synoviocytes, neutrophils, and a macrophage. An increase in neutrophils may be indicative of a more severe underlying disorder. (×400.)

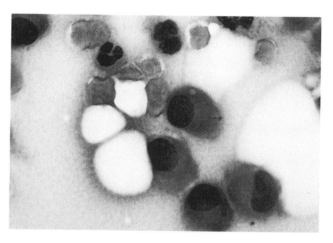

FIG. 12-19. Canine. Synovial fluid. Mixed inflammatory reaction. Chronic degenerative joint disease. A mixed cellular response, including synoviocytes and neutrophils. (×400.)

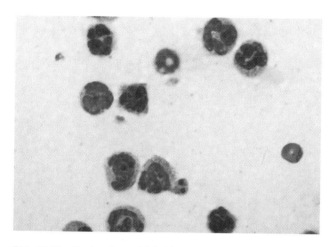

FIG. 12-20. Canine. Synovial fluid. Septic arthritis. Predominance of neutrophils with mild degeneration requires investigation of possible bacterial etiology, although bacteria are not visible in this field. (×400.)

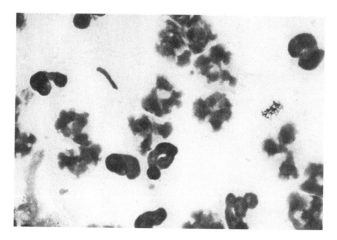

FIG. 12-21. Canine. Synovial fluid. Septic arthritis. Total cell count 89,000 × 10⁶/L. Marked neutrophil nuclear degeneration and extracellular large bacilli. (×400.)

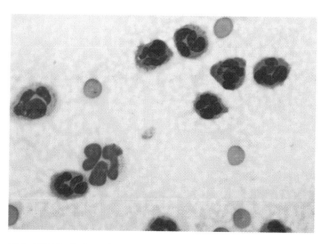

FIG. 12-22. Feline. Synovial fluid. Suppurative inflammation. Moderately well-preserved neutrophils and slight flocculation of background, suggesting changes in fluid viscosity. (×400.)

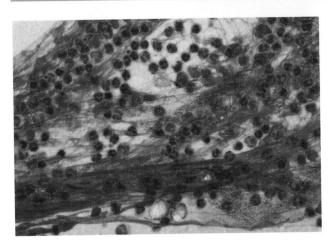

FIG. 12-23. Canine. Synovial fluid. Septic arthritis, direct smear. Marked suppurative inflammation with predominance of mildly degenerate neutrophils. The purple strands are consistent with nuclear debris released from ruptured nuclei. (×100.)

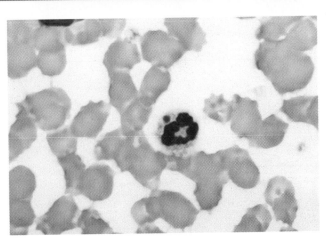

FIG. 12-24. Canine. Synovial fluid. Granulocytic ehrlichiosis. Small blue-gray inclusion consistent with morulae from *Ehrlichia* sp. is visible within the neutrophil cytoplasm. (×500.) (Courtesy A. Garma-Avina, 1985.)

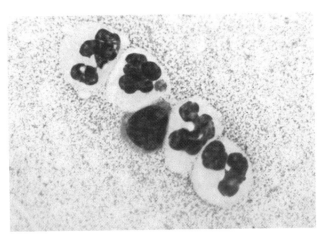

FIG. 12-25. Canine. Synovial fluid. Granulocytic ehrlichiosis. Nucleated cell count greater than 50,000 × 10⁶/L and included 90% nondegenerate neutrophils. The neutrophil contains a small, indistinct, blue-gray cytoplasmic inclusion compatible with *Ehrlichia* spp. (×400.) (Courtesy Rose Raskin, 1993.)

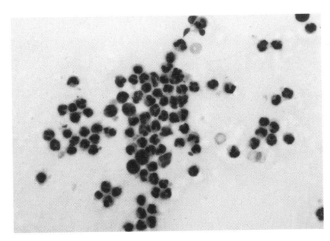

FIG. 12-26. Canine. Synovial fluid. Immune-mediated arthritis. Mixed inflammation with predominance of neutrophils is consistent with an immune-mediated cause. (×200.)

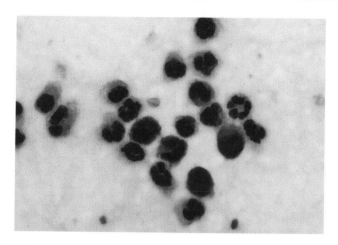

FIG. 12-27. Canine. Synovial fluid. Immune-mediated arthritis. Predominance of well-preserved neutrophils is consistent with an immune-mediated cause, although infectious agents must be ruled out. (×400.)

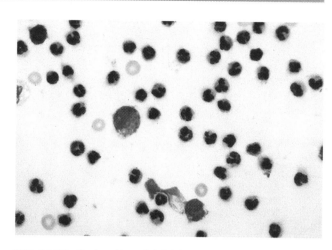

FIG. 12-28. Canine. Synovial fluid. Immune-mediated arthritis. Total cell count was 15,000 × 10⁶/L with predominance of neutrophils and a rare macrophage. Systemic lupus erythematosus and rheumatoid arthritis may present with similar inflammatory responses. The etiology behind joint disorders in many dogs with a neutrophilic response remains obscure. (×250.)

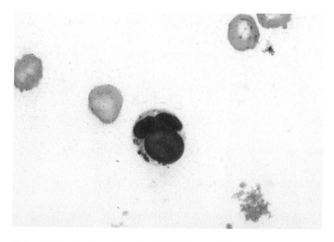

FIG. 12-29. Canine. Synovial fluid. Systemic lupus erythematosus. The neutrophil nucleus is encircling phagocytized depolymerized nucleic acids. Antinuclear antibodies initiate depolymerization and opsonization of nuclear material from ruptured cells. These cells are referred to as lupus erythematosus cells. Although the significance is high, the cells are rarely observed in suspect cases of SLE. (×400.)

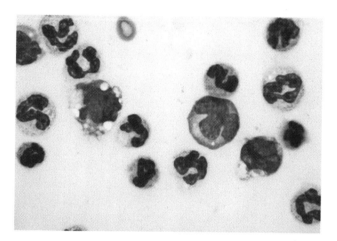

FIG. 12-30. Canine. Synovial fluid. Suppurative inflammation. Nondegenerate neutrophils with a few vacuolated mononuclear cells. No evidence of bacteria. Concurrent use of antibiotics can mask bacterial cause. Clinical history is important when differentiating immune-mediated disease from septic synovitis after therapy. (×400.)

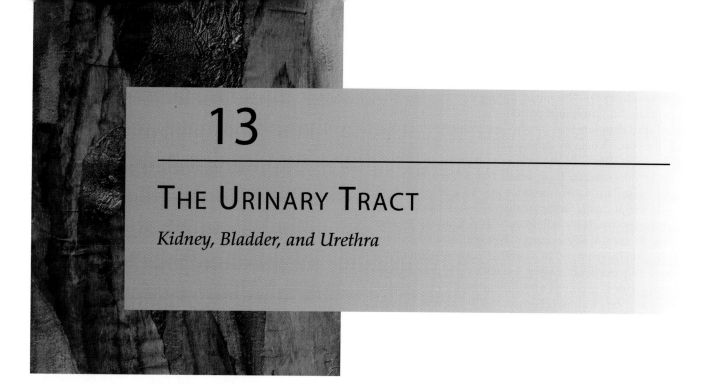

13

THE URINARY TRACT

Kidney, Bladder, and Urethra

Cytological examination of wet mount urine sediment is used routinely in most diagnostical laboratories. Additional techniques can be used to advantage. Reference is made to excellent photographs that illustrate the appearance of cells, casts, and crystals, as observed in wet mount preparations of urine sediment with and without use of staining (Osborne, 1981). The appearance of wet mount preparations is not described in this text. Cell fragility increases in a low protein environment in which morphology can be markedly influenced by urine pH, osmolality, and bacterial toxins. Such changes decrease the reliability of cytological details used to differentiate hyperplasia from suspect neoplastic changes.

When indicated, urine sediment examination should be used to obtain the most reliable cell morphology. The illustrations in this section demonstrate the appearance of air-dried Wright's-stained cells made from fine-needle or tissue imprints of biopsy samples and from fresh urine sediment.

TECHNIQUES

Urine

Increased or abnormal-appearing transitional epithelial cells are often initially identified during routine examination of wet mount urine sediment. Permanent slides should be prepared that allow use of additional stains and consultation as required. Slides for cytology examination should be made from freshly collected urine. Use of shorter centrifugation time and/or lower rpm than often recommended for routine urinalysis helps retain cell morphology. A drop of urine sediment is placed on a clean glass slide. Cells are spread using previously described techniques and rapidly air dried.

The appearance of transitional cells differs between wet mount preparations using aqueous stains and air-dried Romanowsky's-stained cells. Cells often imbibe fluid and appear larger and highly vacuolated. The nuclei appear degenerate and become small and pyknotic. Neutrophil nuclei lose lobulation and can resemble monocytes or macrophages. Neutrophils are typically about 1½ times the diameter of an erythrocyte and smaller than transitional epithelial cells. The appearance of the same source of cells may be different again when FNA or impression smears of the bladder are examined.

Solid Tissue

FNA is used if lesions can be palpated or, as increasingly described, where ultrasound-guided biopsies can be obtained. Surgical biopsy and postmortem specimens of the kidney or bladder can be used to make impression smears as previously described. FNA of the kidney has been effective in diagnosing lymphoma and FIP in the cat because the feline kidney is easily palpated and immobilized.

■ KIDNEY

NORMAL KIDNEY (Figs. 13-1 to 13-7)

FNA biopsy smears from the kidney contain a background of erythrocytes. The primary nucleated cells are of renal tubular origin. The cells are observed in sheets with prominent cell borders. Individual cells are approximately 3 to 5 times the diameter of a red blood cell and have a round central nucleus and a large amount of pale-blue granular cytoplasm (Meinkoth, 1999). The nuclei are regular in size with a fine granular chromatin pattern and one to two nucleoli. Lipid droplets may be present in the tubular cells of the cat. Nucleoli are usually small and round (Meinkoth, 1999). In the urine these cells can be difficult to differentiate from small transitional epithelial cells or inflammatory cells unless they are incorporated within casts. Occasionally cells may be observed in tubular structures where cellular details are unclear using Romanowsky's stains. Large spherical clumps of 20 to 25 cells arranged in a circular pattern without obvious cell borders, a very low N:C ratio, and cytoplasm with a granular appearance similar to hepatocytes may be observed (Barton, 1992). These structures appear to be a glomerular unit. Small capillary vessels may be seen within these structures (Barton, 1992). In the cat, renal tubule cells contain fat droplets and free fat may be present in the background from ruptured tubular cells (Barton, 1992).

NONNEOPLASTIC DISEASE

CLINICAL AND CYTOLOGICAL DIAGNOSES
Histopathology is usually necessary to confirm location of inflammatory lesions within the kidney. In cats, increased neutrophils and macrophages support suspect FIP, whereas a predominance of neutrophils, especially with nuclear lysis, and accompanying bacteria indicate acute bacterial pyelonephritis, especially if supported by radiography, urinalysis, and hematology. If pyelonephritis is suspected, aspiration biopsy should be considered only with extreme caution because of the risks associated with internal rupture.

NEOPLASTIC DISEASE

Renal Neoplasia (Figs. 13-8 and 13-9)

CLINICAL DIAGNOSIS
Primary renal tumors are rare. They comprise 0.5% of all feline neoplasms and 1% of all canine neoplasms (Maxie, 1993). In dogs, carcinomas account for 85% of primary renal neoplasms and almost all are malignant (Cuypers, 1997). The carcinomas occur in aged animals. Most dogs have metastasis at the time of presentation, probably resulting from delays in diagnosis (Maxie, 1993). Lymphoma is the most common renal neoplasm in the cat. Other primary renal tumors are rare (Cuypers, 1997).

CYTOLOGICAL DIAGNOSIS
Because the cytological descriptions for renal carcinoma are rare, we must be guided by the histological descriptions for renal carcinomas and the appearance of "clear cells" that have vacuolated cytoplasm and a basilar nucleus. Cellularity from renal carcinoma aspirates are often highly cellular, and cellular atypia may

be minimal (Meinkoth, 1999). With cytological examination, carcinoma may be the most definitive diagnosis possible.

Lymphosarcoma of the kidney can be diagnosed using FNA biopsy. The tumor may be an isolated nodule within one kidney or may diffusely affect both kidneys. A cytological description of lymphoma is included in Chapter 5.

■ BLADDER

NORMAL BLADDER (Figs. 13-10 to 13-15)

Urine sediment from healthy dogs and cats contains a few transitional epithelial cells, crystals, hyaline casts, fat droplets in cats, amorphous material, and contaminants. In voided samples, squamous epithelial cells from the distal urethra and vagina may be present. Similarly, hyperplastic and neoplastic transformation of bladder transitional cells can overlap in cellular appearance.

Impression smears made from the bladder of a clinically healthy dog contain many transitional epithelial cells. The cells may be arranged singly, in clusters, or in sheets of coherent cells. The cell size and appearance varies greatly depending on the depth of origin within the bladder mucosa. Nuclei are generally two to three red blood cells in diameter, regardless of site of origin. Most cells have 1 to 2 small regular nucleoli. The parabasal cells are two to four, whereas superficial cells are 5 to 10 red blood cells in diameter. The appearance of the cytoplasm can vary from smooth and amorphous to finely granular or reticulated, whereas the amount of cytoplasm varies with the depth of origin of the cell. In some cells, presumably of superficial origin, the cytoplasmic characteristics are suggestive of squamous differentiation with lighter-staining cytoplasm and angular borders.

Bladder washings were examined from 19 normal dogs (Rozengurt, 1985). The superficial epithelial cells were large, polygonal, and approximately 80 μ in diameter. They were present singly and in sheets, with one or two central nuclei. Occasionally a small central nucleolus was present. The bladder washings had fewer sheets of urothelial cells and less amorphous material than the comparable urine samples (Rozegurt, 1985).

NONNEOPLASTIC DISEASE

Cystitis (Figs. 13-16 to 13-20)

CLINICAL DIAGNOSIS
Urinary tract inflammation is most commonly caused by microbial infection of the urinary tract. Seven genera of aerobic bacteria, *Escherichia, Staphylococcus,*

Streptococcus, Proteus, Klebsiella, Pseudomonas, and *Enterobacter,* are the most common etiological agents (Lees, 1992). Care in collection and culture is required for reliable identification and to prevent contamination. *Candida albicans* is the most commonly reported fungal pathogen (Lulich, 1992).

CYTOLOGICAL DIAGNOSIS

Simple inflammation of the urinary tract can be identified by routine examination of midstream-collected urine sediment. In voided samples, vaginal or preputial contamination during initial or late stages of micturition can markedly influence cytological content. Sample collection techniques must be known by the microscopist for reliable interpretation of urine sediment. Hematuria and pyuria are the most common indicators of cystitis. Cells difficult to identify on wet mount preparations can frequently be classified using air-dried Romanowsky's-stained urine sediment smears. Because neutrophils and erythrocytes are not normally present in the urine of healthy dogs and cats, neutrophils, alone or in the presence of erythrocytes, are indicative of an inflammatory response. Localization to bladder origin, that is, cystitis, cannot be made on the basis of cytology alone. Neutrophils from urine sediment may retain lobulation or may be mononuclear with indistinct cytoplasmic margins. Bacteria are readily observed in urine sediment slides. Bacterial contamination must be considered when bacteria are present without accompanying inflammatory cells.

Chronic cystitis is observed frequently in the dog and is associated with profound hyperplastic changes in urothelial lining cells. Hyperplastic and dysplastic transitional cells can exfoliate in large numbers, often in cluster formation. Nuclear variability and an increase in N:C ratio are common, as is metaplastic squamous differentiation of the cytoplasm. If neoplastic cells are suspected in an animal with accompanying cystitis, confirmation of neoplasia should require directed biopsy or surgical exploration and biopsy.

NEOPLASTIC DISEASE

Bladder Carcinoma (Figs. 13-21 to 13-34)

CLINICAL DIAGNOSIS

In the dog, 1% of all neoplasms occur in the bladder (Osborne, 1968). Approximately 80% of lower urinary tract neoplasms are epithelial tumors (Maxie, 1993), the most common of which is the transitional cell carcinoma (Clemo, 1994). In one study of 115 dogs, transitional cell carcinoma accounted for 87% of all bladder and urethral tumors (Norris, 1992). Only three of the canine bladder tumors were benign (Norris, 1992). Transitional cell carcinomas metastasize approximately 50% of the time (Maxie, 1993). The metastasis can be variable and wide, but regional lymph nodes,

soft tissues, and bones of the hindquarters and lung seem predisposed (Maxie, 1993). Feline bladder cancer is considered rare, accounting for less than 0.8% of all tumors in cats (Brearley, 1986). Approximately 60% to 70% of the cases reported in the cat are epithelial in origin (Brearley, 1986; Schwarz, 1984; Walker, 1993). In one study, squamous carcinomas account for 4 of 27 reported cases (Schwarz, 1984).

CYTOLOGICAL DIAGNOSIS

Cytological examination of fresh urine is always the initial step for evaluation of the urinary tract. However, epithelial cells in urine are often greatly distorted because of variations in urine pH and tonicities. If a mass is suspected, FNA biopsy bypasses the cellular alterations that occur in urine. Obviously, a palpable mass must be present to succeed with FNA biopsy. One study reported 90% diagnostic accuracy using FNA biopsy in 22 dogs (Norris, 1992). The diagnostic accuracy of urine alone was reported at 30% (Norris, 1992). Although recent histological classification of canine transitional cell tumors relates prognosis to tumor grade and depth of invasion, correlation with cytological classification is not reported (Valli, 1995).

Transitional cells exfoliate readily when using impression smears or aspiration biopsy. Transitional cells are distinctly epithelial in morphology. They may be arranged in large clusters or sheets having discrete cell borders. As the name indicates, the cells vary markedly in size. Anisokaryosis is prominent, with large, angular, irregular nucleoli common. Nuclei may be multiple and irregular in shape with notches or angular sides. Cytoplasmic vacuolation is common and most often observed as small, discrete aggregates or less frequently as a single large, secretory type of vacuole. Mitosis may be present. Transitional epithelial cells may undergo a squamous type of transformation with light blue-gray cytoplasm and a more pyknotic nucleus. This is often prominent in cells from fresh urine.

Because bladder neoplasia is frequently accompanied by inflammation, the tumor cells are often intermixed with neutrophils and bacteria. Whenever there is significant inflammation, a hyperplastic response of the transitional epithelial cells is expected. In these cases, even with supporting clinical evidence, confirmation of neoplasia on the basis of cytological evidence must be made with considerable caution. Hyperchromasia, anisokaryosis, and an increase in N:C ratio are common to both hyperplasia and neoplasia. A definitive diagnosis of transitional cell carcinoma in the face of inflammation is one of the greatest challenges to the cytologist. In the presence of marked inflammation, a high cytological degree of suspicion for neoplasia should be interpreted by the clinician as an indication of the requirement for further confirmation using imaging studies and/or surgical exploration.

In one case study in a cat, pleomorphic epithelial cells with large, multiple nuclei were observed during cytological examination of a fine-needle biopsy of a posterior abdominal mass. Atypical squamous types of epithelial cells were observed on an impression smear 7 weeks later, emphasizing the squamous differentiation that frequently occurs in transitional cell tumors and that is reported in humans (Walker, 1993).

■ URETHRA

NORMAL URETHRA

The transitional epithelial cells in the proximal urethra are replaced with nonkeratinizing squamous epithelial cells at the urethral opening (Barton, 1992).

TECHNIQUE

If an obstructive urethral lesion is present, a flexible urethral catheter can be passed to the level of the urethral mass (Matthiesen, 1989). This may be guided by rectal palpation. From 5 to 10 ml of normal saline is infused from an attached syringe. Plugs of mucosa are aspirated into the tip of the catheter (Matthiesen, 1989). The cellular aspirate material is quickly and gently transferred to clean glass slides for fixation and staining.

NONNEOPLASTIC DISEASE

Urethritis

CLINICAL DIAGNOSIS

Granulomatous urethritis described in dogs is clinically indistinguishable from neoplasia (Matthiesen, 1989). It is characterized histologically by aggregates of lymphocytes and macrophages within the mucosa and submucosa of the urethra (Matthiesen, 1989). Aged female dogs appear to be predisposed. Treatment with antibiotics and antiinflammatory drugs is effective (Matthiesen, 1989). In one study of 41 cases of infiltrative urethral disease, granulomatous urethritis accounted for 10 cases (Moroff, 1991). Twenty-nine cases were due to epithelial neoplasia and two were leiomyoma (Moroff, 1991). In 11 of 15 cases, fine-needle biopsy correlated with the histological diagnosis (Moroff, 1991). In the four dogs with the discrepancy, one carcinoma was diagnosed cytologically as granulomatous urethritis, one epithelial neoplasia was diagnosed cytologically as urethritis, and one leiomyoma was diagnosed cytologically as an epithelial neoplasm (Moroff, 1991). The one remaining dog was diagnosed cytologically as epithelial neoplasia but urethritis histologically (Moroff, 1991). The dog had an epithelial neoplasm confirmed 1 month later (Moroff, 1991). Cytological diagnosis was accurate 80% of the time (Moroff, 1991).

CYTOLOGICAL DIAGNOSIS

Granulomatous urethritis is characterized cytologically by large numbers of macrophages and lymphocytes, intermixed with low numbers of neutrophils (Matthiesen, 1989). Epithelial cells may be normal to hyperplastic (Moroff, 1991).

NEOPLASTIC DISEASE

CLINICAL DIAGNOSIS

The most common urethral tumors are transitional cell carcinomas (Matthiesen, 1989). They may be an extension of a primary bladder tumor or originate within the prostate. Tumors of the urethra occur more frequently in older female dogs (Matthiesen, 1989) and are associated with a poor prognosis (Matthiesen, 1989).

CYTOLOGICAL DIAGNOSIS

The cytological appearance of transitional cell carcinomas is similar irrespective of origin. If located within the prostate, differentiation from primary carcinoma or adenocarcinoma may be difficult.

References

Barton, C.L. and Rogers, K.S. *Diagnostic cytology of the urogenital system.* Proceedings of the 10th ACVIM Forum, pp. 771-782, San Diego, 1992.

Brearley, M.J., Thatcher, C., and Cooper, J.E. Three cases of transitional cell carcinoma in the cat and a review of the literature. *Vet Rec* 118:91-94, 1986.

Clemo, F.A.S., DeNicola, D.B., Carlton, W.W., et al. Flow cytometric DNA ploidy analysis in canine transitional cell carcinoma of urinary bladders. *Vet Pathol* 31:207-215, 1994.

Cuypers, M.D., Grooters, A.M., Williams, J., et al. Renomegaly in dogs and cats. Part 1. Differential diagnosis *Compend Cont Ed Pract* 19:1019-1031,1997.

Lees, G.E. and Forrester, S.D. Update: Bacterial urinary tract infections. In *Current Veterinary Therapy XI, Small Animal Practice.* R.W. Kirk and J.D. Bonagura (eds). WB Saunders, Philadelphia, 1992.

Lulich, J.P. and Osborne, C.A. Fungal urinary tract infections. In *Current Veterinary Therapy XI, Small Animal Practice.* R.W. Kirk and J.D. Bonagura (eds). WB Saunders, Philadelphia, 1992.

Matthiesen, D.T. and Moroff, S.D. Infiltrative urethral diseases in the dog. In *Current Veterinary Therapy X, Small Animal Practice.* R.W. Kirk and J.D. Bonagura (eds). WB Saunders, Philadelphia, 1989.

Maxie, M.G. The urinary system. In *Pathology of Domestic Animals.* ed 4. K.V.F. Jubb, P.C. Kennedy, and N. Palmer (eds). Academic Press, San Diego, 1993.

Meinkoth, J.H., Cowell, R.L., and Tyler, RD. The renal parenchyma. In *Diagnostic Cytology of the Dog and Cat.* R.D. Cowell, R.D. Tyler, and J.H. Meinkoth (eds). Mosby, St Louis, 1999.

Moroff, S.D., Brown, B.A., Matthiesen, D.T., et al. Infiltrative urethral disease in female dogs: 41 cases (1980-1987). *J Am Vet Med Assoc* 199:247–251, 1991.

Norris, A.M., Laing, E.J., Valli, V.E., et al. Canine bladder and urethral tumors: a retrospective study of 115 cases (1980-1985). *J Vet Intern Med* 6:145–153, 1992.

Osborne, C.A., Low, D.G., Perman, V., et al. Neoplasms of the canine and feline urinary bladder: incidence, etiologic factors, occurrence and pathologic features. *Am J Vet Res* 29:2041-2053, 1968.

Osborne, C.A. and Stevens, J.B. *Handbook of Canine and Feline Urinalysis.* Ralston Purina Company, St Louis, 1981.

Rozengurt, N., Hyman, W.J., Berry, A., et al. Exfoliative cytology of the canine urinary bladder: a technique utilising Millipore filtration. *Vet Rec* 116:414-415, 1985.

Schwarz, P.D., Greene, R.W., and Patnaik, A.K. Urinary bladder tumors in the cat: a review of 27 cases. *J Am Anim Hosp Assoc* 21:237-245, 1984.

Valli, V.E., Norris, A., Jacobs, R.M., et al. Pathology of canine bladder and urethral cancer and correlation with tumour progression and survival. *J Comp Pathol* 113:113-130, 1995.

Walker, D.B., Cowell, R.L., Clinkenbeard, K.D., et al. Carcinoma in the urinary bladder of a cat: cytologic findings and a review of the literature. *Vet Clin Pathol* 22:103-108, 1993.

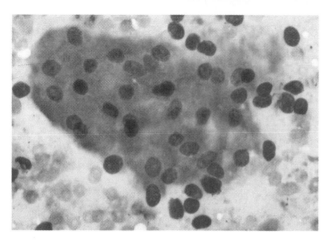

FIG. 13-1. Canine. Scraping. Normal kidney, cortical region. Large cluster of cells consistent with glomerulus. (×200.)

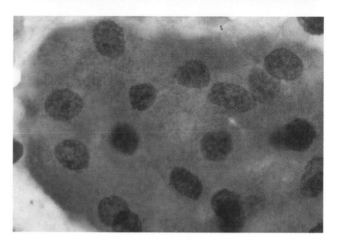

FIG. 13-2. Canine. Scraping. Normal kidney, cortical region. Higher magnification illustrating abundant, dense cytoplasm and round to oval nuclei. (×400.)

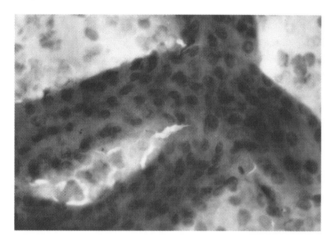

FIG. 13-3. Canine. Scraping. Normal kidney, cortical region. Arrangement of cells and cortical origin suggests that these are proximal tubular epithelial cells. (×100.)

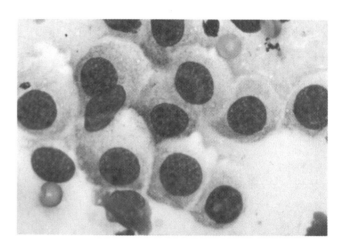

FIG. 13-4. Canine. Scraping. Normal kidney. Medium to large cells with irregular density of cytoplasm; round to oval nuclei with irregular chromatin pattern, and single large nucleolus consistent with tubular epithelial cells. (×630.)

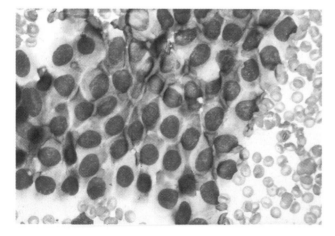

FIG. 13-5. Canine. Scraping. Normal kidney, cortical region. Sheet of medium to large cells with abundant, pale cytoplasm and round to slightly oval nuclei. Epithelial cells of unconfirmed type. (×200.)

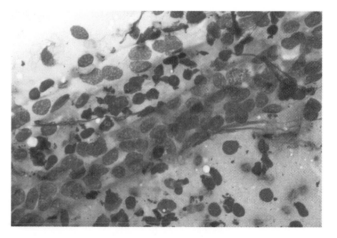

FIG. 13-6. Canine. Scraping. Normal kidney, medullary region. Many ruptured cells; arrangement of cells in the center of the slide suggests renal tubular origin. (×100.)

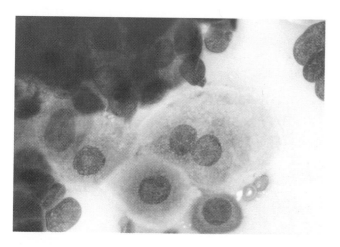

FIG. 13-7. Canine. Scraping. Normal kidney, medullary region. Round cells with distinct cytoplasmic borders; clear to lightly basophilic cytoplasm; large, round nuclei with irregular chromatin pattern and indistinct small nucleoli consistent with tubular epithelial cells, but cannot rule out transitional origin. (×400.)

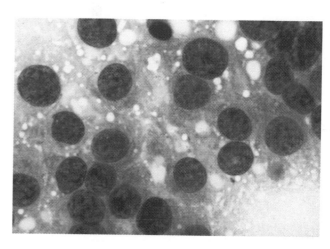

FIG. 13-8. Canine. Imprint. Abdominal mass. Renal tubular adenocarcinoma. Uniform population of cells with indistinct cytoplasmic borders; abundant, moderately granular cytoplasm with occasional vacuoles; and round to oval nuclei with fine to coarse chromatin and indistinct nucleoli. Cell arrangement consistent with acinar or tubular formation. (×500.) (Courtesy G.S. Elliott, 1991.)

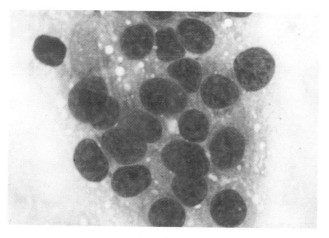

FIG. 13-9. Canine. Imprint. Abdominal mass. Renal tubular adenocarcinoma. (Same case as Fig. 13-8.) Epithelial cells with indistinct cell borders, moderate anisokaryosis and mild cytoplasmic vacuolation. (×400.) (Courtesy G.S. Elliott, 1991.)

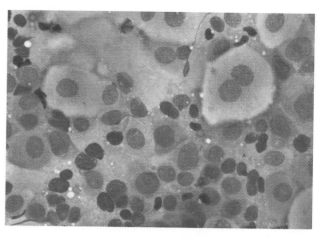

FIG. 13-10. Canine. Imprint. Normal bladder. Round to angular transitional cells with anisocytosis and low N:C ratio. Cytoplasm is lightly basophilic with variation in density. (×250.)

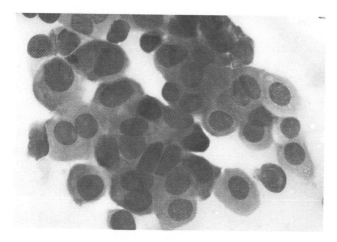

FIG. 13-11. Canine. Imprint. Normal bladder. Marked anisocytosis of cells with abundant cytoplasm typical of transitional epithelial cells. The size and N:C ratio have similarities to intermediate squamous epithelial cells. (×100.)

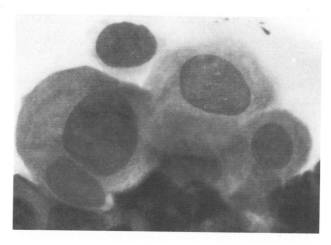

FIG. 13-12. Canine. Imprint. Normal bladder. Transitional epithelial cells illustrating the degree of anisocytosis, anisokaryosis, and hyperchromasia that can be expected within healthy benign cells. (×400.)

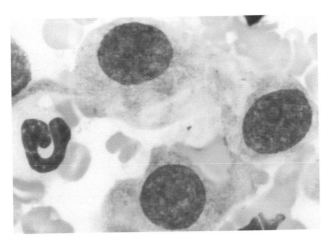

FIG. 13-13. Canine. Imprint. Normal bladder. Transitional epithelial cells illustrating anisocytosis and anisokaryosis. Note intracytoplasmic aggregation of azurophilic material present in cells. (×400.)

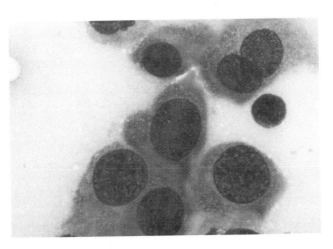

FIG. 13-14. Canine. Imprint. Normal bladder. Marked anisocytosis, anisokaryosis, and binucleation observed in normal transitional epithelial cells. Differentiation between normal, proplasia, and neoplasia based on cytological morphology must be conservative and incorporate all additional clinical information. (×400.)

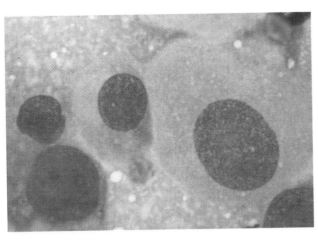

FIG. 13-15. Canine. Imprint. Normal bladder. Transitional epithelial cells illustrating marked anisokaryosis and a low N:C ratio. Note nuclear size relative to the erythrocyte. Nuclei have a fine chromatin pattern and small, multiple nucleoli. (×500.)

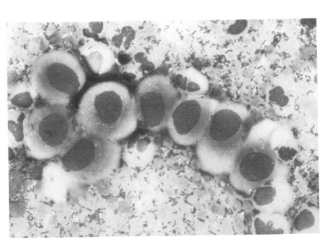

FIG. 13-16. Canine. Urine sediment. Cystitis. Background contains many bacteria, neutrophils, bare nuclei and uniform transitional epithelial cells. (×200.)

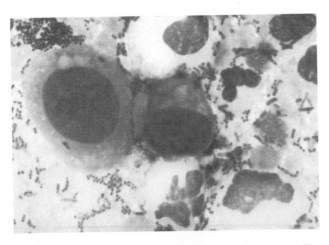

FIG. 13-17. Canine. Urine sediment. Cystitis. (Same case as Fig. 13-16.) Bacteria, degenerate neutrophils, and two transitional epithelial cells with moderate anisokaryosis and basophilic cytoplasm. Dysplasia is expected in association with inflammation. (×500.)

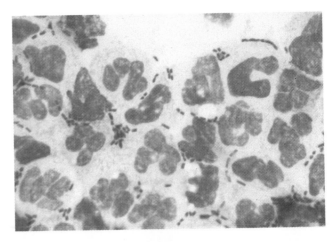

FIG. 13-18. Canine. Urine sediment. Cystitis. Degenerate neutrophils with many free and phagocytized bacteria. Neutrophil nuclear morphology can appear very different in air-dried and wet mount urine sediment. (×500.)

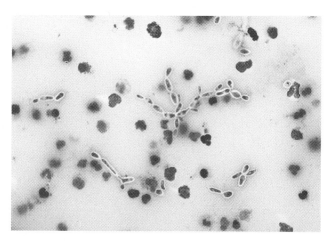

FIG. 13-19. Canine. Urine sediment. Fungal cystitis. Degenerate and ruptured neutrophils with numerous yeast organisms consistent with *Candida* sp. (×100.)

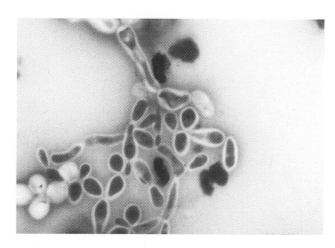

FIG. 13-20. Canine. Urine sediment. Fungal cystitis. Numerous drumstick yeastlike organisms consistent with *Candida* sp. (×400.)

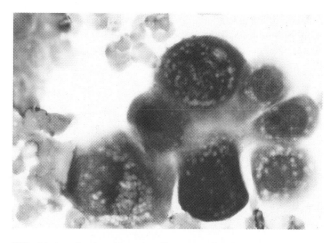

FIG. 13-21. Canine. Fine needle. Mass dorsal to penis. Transitional cell carcinoma. Moderately cohesive cluster of epithelial cells with basophilic vacuolated cytoplasm, marked anisokaryosis, and very high N:C ratio consistent with carcinoma. (×400.)

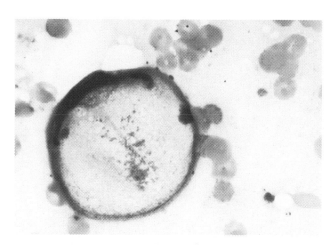

FIG. 13-22. Canine. Fine needle. Mass dorsal to penis. Transitional cell carcinoma. (Same case as Fig. 13-21.) A single, large cell with an eccentric, small nucleus and a large secretory vacuole. The light pink intracytoplasmic material is frequently observed within cells of a transitional cell carcinoma. (×400.)

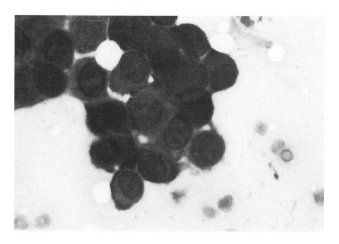

FIG. 13-23. Canine. Fine needle. Mass in tibia. Transitional cell carcinoma. A cohesive cluster of epithelial cells with high N:C ratio, hyperchromasia, and mild anisokaryosis. The cytoplasmic features are consistent with transitional cells. Morphology and location within bone both support a diagnosis of malignancy. (×250.)

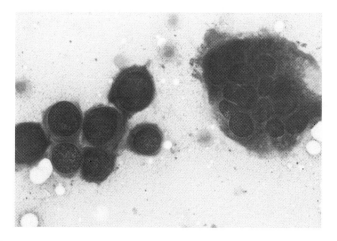

FIG. 13-24. Canine. Fine needle. Mass in tibia. Transitional cell carcinoma. (Same case as Fig. 13-23.) Cells with marked hyperchromasia, anisokaryosis, and high N:C ratio consistent with transitional epithelial cells, that is, malignant metastasis. Multinucleated cell is consistent with osteoclast for normal or reactive bone. (×250.)

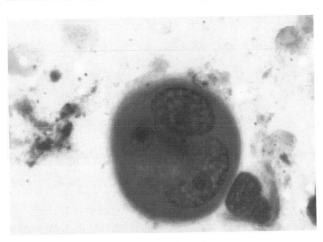

FIG. 13-25. Canine. Fine needle. Mass in tibia. Transitional cell carcinoma. (Same case as Fig. 13-23.) Anisokaryosis of trinucleated cell, prominent nucleoli, and poor cytoplasmic differentiation indicative of severity of anaplasia that may be observed in transitional cell carcinomas. (×500.)

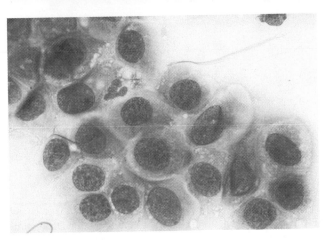

FIG. 13-26. Canine. Urine sediment. Transitional cell carcinoma. A sheet of transitional epithelial cells with few features of malignancy. Exfoliation of many cells, especially sheets or fronds, in the absence of inflammation or urolithiasis leads to increased suspicion for neoplasia. There is spectrum of mild to severe morphological change observed in transitional cell carcinomas. (×250.)

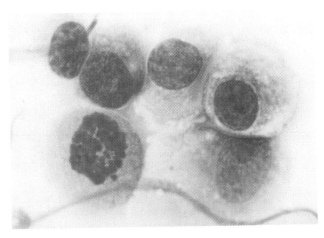

FIG. 13-27. Canine. Urine sediment. Transitional cell carcinoma. Mitosis is apparent within one nucleus. Access to the clinical information helps counterbalance the recognized need for conservative interpretation of cytological changes. (×400.)

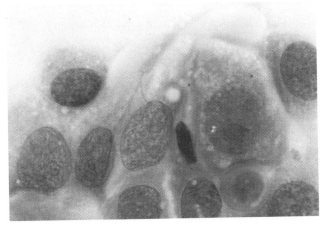

FIG. 13-28. Canine. Urine sediment. Transitional cell carcinoma. (Same case as Fig. 13-27.) Marked anisocytosis and anisokaryosis, multiple large nucleoli. (×400.)

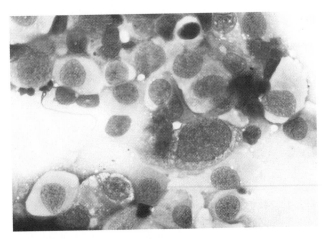

FIG. 13-29. Canine. Urine sediment. Transitional cell carcinoma. Single and cohesive cells; some with a marked increase in N:C ratio and hyperchromasia. (×200.)

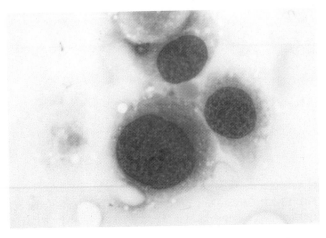

FIG. 13-30. Canine. Urine sediment. Transitional cell carcinoma. (Same case as Fig. 13-29.) Marked anisokaryosis consistent with transitional cell carcinoma. (×400.)

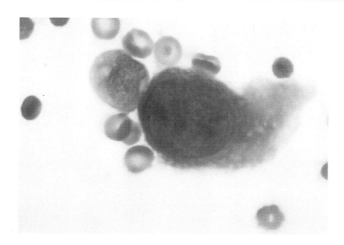

FIG. 13-31. Canine. Urine sediment. Transitional cell carcinoma. Marked anisokaryosis, hyperchromasia, high N:C ratio, and multiple nucleoli are consistent with transitional cell carcinoma. (×500.)

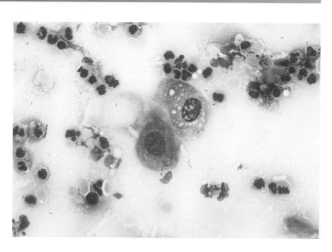

FIG. 13-32. Canine. Urine sediment. Cytological diagnosis: transitional cell carcinoma. Histological diagnosis: malacoplakia. Two large transitional cells surrounded by neutrophils. When inflammation is present, diagnosis of malignancy should be made very conservatively. (×100.)

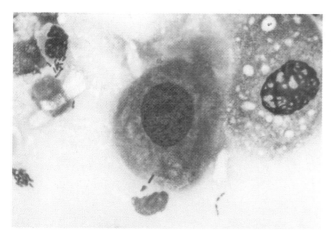

FIG. 13-33. Canine. Urine sediment. Malacoplakia. (Same case as Fig. 13-32.) Large transitional cells, one illustrating proplastic and one retroplastic changes likely resulting from the septic inflammation evident. (×400.)

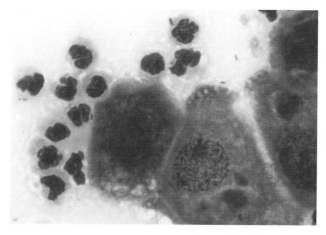

FIG. 13-34. Canine. Urine sediment. Malacoplakia. (Same case as Fig. 13-32.) Marked hyperchromasia, prominent chromatin pattern, and large nucleoli of transitional epithelial cells. Inflammation, bacteria, and low N:C ratio collectively require conservative interpretation of the cells illustrated. (×400.)

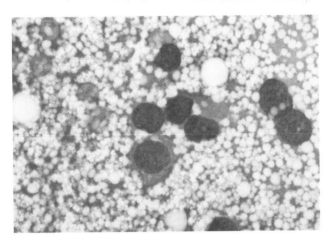

FIG. 13-35. Canine. Imprint. Normal adrenal. Finely vacuolated background indicative of lipid content. Individual small cells have basophilic amorphous cytoplasm and small, round nuclei with a fine chromatin pattern. (×400.)

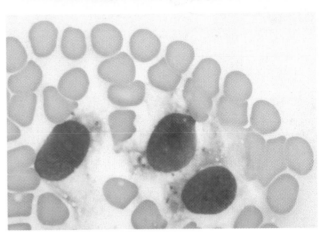

FIG. 13-36. Canine. Imprint. Normal adrenal. Cytoplasm has an indistinct outline and contains fine granulation. Nuclei are about two to three erythrocytes in diameter and contain multiple small nucleoli. (×500.)

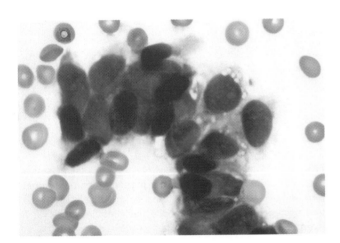

FIG. 13-37. Canine. Imprint. Normal adrenal. A heterogeneous cluster of cells with round to oval nuclei; indistinct small, multiple nucleoli; and poorly defined cytoplasmic boundaries. (×400.)

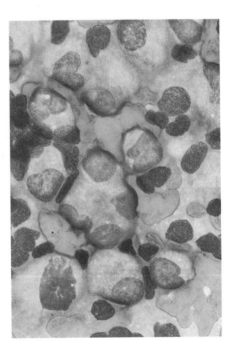

FIG. 13-38. Canine. Fine needle. Adrenal. Adrenal carcinoma. Round cells with pale cytoplasm, moderate N:C ratio and mild variation in nuclear size and shape. The arrangement of the small clusters of cells suggests an acinar origin. If the cells were known to originate from an adrenal mass, cytological diagnosis would be limited to "compatible with tumor of endocrine origin." (×400.)

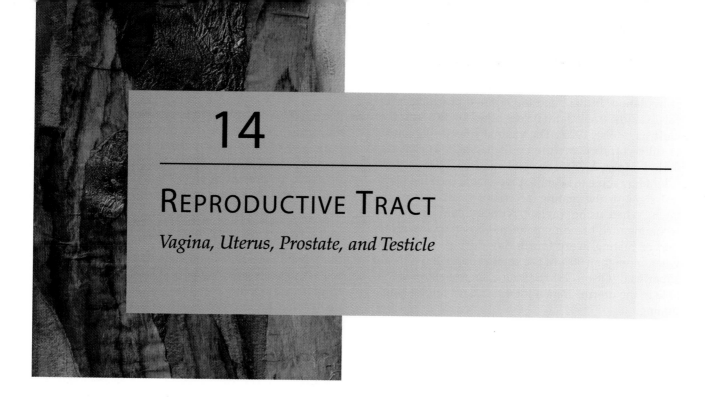

14

REPRODUCTIVE TRACT

Vagina, Uterus, Prostate, and Testicle

■ VAGINA

Assessment of the estrous cycle in the bitch, using vaginal cytology, is one of the earlier procedures describing exfoliative cytology in veterinary medicine (Roszel, 1975). Although observation of behavior is used for routine situations, vaginal cytology is still used for assessing individual problem cases, for evaluating mating status, and for assisting diagnosis of several reproductive disorders.

TECHNIQUE

Cells are obtained from the anterior vagina using a saline-moistened cotton swab. The swab is passed craniodorsally into the anterior vagina. Here the swab is brushed against the vaginal surface to harvest the cells present. The swab is removed and rolled gently over the surface of a clean glass slide. Sliding the swab along the glass surface can increase rupture of the cells. The swab should not touch the clitoral fossa or outer vaginal area. Superficial epithelial cells and leukocytes harvested from these areas can confound the interpretation (Thrall, 1999).

Another approach recommends the use of a medicine dropper containing 0.25 to 0.5 ml of physiological saline (Dahlgren, 1979). The medicine dropper is inserted into the vagina and the bulb is pressed and released several times, aspirating cells and saline into the dropper. A thin layer of the saline-cell mixture is spread onto a slide and then air dried (Dahlgren, 1979). Slides can be dipped into 95% methanol to prevent cellular deterioration (Olson, 1984).

A variety of stains have been described for examination of vaginal cytology. These include aqueous stains, such as toluidine blue and new methylene blue; Romanowsky's stains, including Wright's, Wright's Giemsa, and Diff-Quick; and trichrome stains, such as Papanicolaou's, Shorr's, Sano's modified, and H&E. Familiarity and convenience appear to dictate choice and use of staining. The various trichrome stains are less convenient for routine use but do assist in identification of the degree of keratin production within superficial epithelial cells. Keratin precursors are orange with many trichrome stains. Orangeophilia peaks during standing estrus (Olson, 1984). Experienced clinicians and theriogenologists are able to assess the effects of estrogen on the differentiation of superficial epithelial cells using a variety of morphological criteria and tend to use quick-staining procedures in conjunction with clinical history and examination.

NORMAL CANINE VAGINAL CYTOLOGY (Fig. 14-1)

Four types of epithelial cells characterize the vaginal epithelium at different stages of estrus. Starting from the basement membrane and moving superficially, these cells are basal, parabasal, intermediate, and superficial epithelial cells. Red blood cells and leukocytes are present at various stages of the estrous cycle, but their occurrence is not as reliable as the degree of differentiation, and thus appearance, of the epithelial cells.

When vaginal cytology is used to estimate optimal breeding time, examinations must be made every 1 or, at most, 2 days. The changing ovarian hormone concentrations are associated with characteristic changes in the appearance of the vaginal superficial epithelium. These changes in differentiation of the superficial epithelial cells can be used to assist identification of ovulation. In the bitch the optimal breeding interval extends from 3 to 10 days before the onset of diestrus (Holst, 1975). The vaginal smear will consist of fully cornified mature epithelial cells during this period (Holst, 1975). The cytological changes are considered by some to be more predictable than the physical signs or the mating/acceptance behavior of the bitch. When using vaginal cytology as a guide, the recommended breeding pattern is based on insemination or mating every fourth day during the interval when more than 90% of the vaginal epithelial cells are superficial (Olson, 1984). Canine spermatozoa are viable in the uterine lumen for 4 to 6 days after a single mating.

Basal Cells

The basal cells located next to the basement membrane are precursors for all vaginal epithelial cells. They are uniform small, round basophilic cells with scant cytoplasm. Because of their origin, they are rarely observed on vaginal smears made at any stage of the estrous cycle.

Parabasal Cells

Parabasal cells are the smallest epithelial cells seen on routine vaginal smears. They have a high N:C ratio and round nuclei and are very uniform in size. They are seen in low numbers and only when there is minimal differentiation of epithelial cells, as in diestrus, early proestrus, and anestrus (Holst, 1975). In prepubertal animals, parabasal cells can exfoliate in sheets that can be mistaken for neoplasia (Olson, 1984).

Intermediate Cells

Parabasal, intermediate, and superficial epithelial cells all have nuclei of similar size and shape. However, as the cell differentiates and cytoplasm diameter increases, the relative size of the nucleus, and thus N:C ratio, decreases. Intermediate cells have approximately twice the diameter of parabasal cells. The cytoplasm is abundant and pale blue to blue-green with Romanowsky's stains. As intermediate cells differentiate further, the cytoplasm becomes more irregular and folded. Large intermediate cells are sometimes referred to as *superficial intermediate cells* (Olson, 1984; Thrall, 1999).

Superficial Cells

These cells have the greatest diameter. Nuclei, when present, are faded or pyknotic, and cell borders are angulated and folded. The cytoplasm is abundant and blue-green.

Red Blood Cells

Red blood cells are frequently associated with early proestrus. However, neither the presence nor concentration of erythrocytes is a reliable indicator of the stage of estrus (Holst, 1975). They may be absent in proestrus or present in large numbers from proestrus to estrus through diestrus (Holst, 1975).

Metestrum Cells and Foam Cells

Metestrum cells and foam cells have been described. Metestrum cells are parabasal cells that contain a neutrophil in the cytoplasm and can be seen whenever neutrophils are present. Foam cells are parabasal cells that contain cytoplasmic vacuoles of unknown significance.

STAGING THE ESTROUS CYCLE (Figs. 14-2 to 14-11)

Proestrus

With increasing levels of estradiol associated with follicular maturation, the vaginal epithelium proliferates and red blood cells diapedese through uterine capillaries. In early proestrus the smear is characterized by neutrophils; red blood cells; and parabasal, intermediate, and superficial cells. The presence of erythrocytes can be unreliable in proestrus (Olson, 1984). The background has a dirty blue appearance caused by mucus. Bacteria are frequently observed. Toward the end of proestrus, neutrophils and red blood cells decrease in number, whereas intermediate and superficial cells predominate. Parabasal and small intermediate cells are absent toward the end of proestrus (Thrall, 1999).

Estrus

During estrus, neutrophils are absent and the background is clear (Roszel, 1977). Red blood cells are usually absent but can be observed throughout estrus and diestrus (Olson, 1984). Superficial epithelial cells account for 90% of the cells seen during estrus (Olson, 1984). Parabasal cells and intermediate cells account for less than 5% of the total nucleated cells (Olson, 1984). Bacteria may or may not be numerous and adhere to the surface of the superficial epithelial cells. They are not accompanied by leukocytes unless inflammation coexists.

Diestrus

With the onset of diestrus the number of superficial epithelial cells decreases, whereas the parabasal cells and intermediate cells increase up to 50% of the total

(Olson, 1984). The onset of diestrus is defined as (1) a decrease in the percentage of superficial cells by 20% or more, and (2) an increase in small intermediate cells from less than 5% to greater than 10% (Holst, 1975). Usually the changes are more dramatic than this minimum requirement (Holst, 1975). It has been observed that vaginal cytology correlates more closely with the hormonal events than behavioral patterns (i.e., refusal to accept mating). Neutrophils frequently reappear in association with parabasal and intermediate cells. Red blood cells may also be seen, and thus early diestrus and proestrus may be difficult to differentiate with one vaginal smear (Olson, 1984). Behavior patterns and vulvar examination aid in this differentiation.

Anestrus

In anestrus, parabasal cells and intermediate cells are the predominant cell types, but their ratio fluctuates (Roszel, 1977). A constant feature is the absence of orange (with trichrome stains) or blue (with Wright's or Giemsa stains) superficial cells (Roszel, 1977). Neutrophils and bacteria may or may not be present (Olson, 1984).

FELINE ESTROUS VAGINAL CYTOLOGY

Vaginal epithelial changes during estrus in the cat are similar to those in the dog. Superficial cells are greater than 70% of the epithelial cells. However, no erythrocytes are seen in proestrus or estrus. Also, changes associated with diestrus do not occur unless the cat is bred (Barton, 1992; Herron, 1977).

NONNEOPLASTIC DISEASE

Vaginitis

CLINICAL AND CYTOLOGICAL DIAGNOSES
Large numbers of neutrophils characterize vaginal smears from bitches with acute vaginitis. If there is a bacterial component, the neutrophils may be degenerate and contain phagocytized bacteria (Olson, 1984). Neutrophils are normally present during diestrus but decrease dramatically by 1 week postestrus, unlike the neutrophils present in dogs with vaginitis (Olson, 1984). The neutrophil concentration during anestrus and proestrus is much lower than with vaginitis.

NEOPLASTIC DISEASE

Vaginal Tumors

CLINICAL DIAGNOSES
Vaginal tumors are uncommon and tend to occur in older dogs (Olson, 1984). Tumors of the female tubular genital tract account for 3% of all canine tumors (Kang, 1983). Mesenchymal tumors, leiomyomas, and fibromas are the most common (Kang, 1983). Leiomyomas of the canine reproductive tract account for 2.4% of all canine neoplasms, and 85% of these occur in the vagina and vulva (Kang, 1983). Leiomyomas are the most common neoplasm of the uterus and vagina in the queen, as well (Johnson, 1989).

CYTOLOGICAL DIAGNOSIS
Mesenchymal tumors and transmissible venereal tumors can be diagnosed from vaginal smears. Urethral transitional cell carcinomas, which invade the vagina, have also been identified with vaginal smears (Olson, 1984b). One impression smear of a vaginal leiomyoma revealed only stromal cells (Kang, 1983).

■ *UTERUS*

NORMAL UTERUS (Figs. 14-12 to 14-14)

Limited experience with normal uterine cytology suggests a uniform population of round to cuboidal epithelial cells. These epithelial cells have distinct cell borders; mild cytoplasmic vacuolation; and bland, round to oval nuclei. Further examination of the normal canine and feline uterus in the gravid and nongravid states is required.

NONNEOPLASTIC DISEASE

Pyometra and Metritis

CLINICAL DIAGNOSIS
Escherichia coli, Staphylococcus aureus, Streptococcus, Pseudomonas, and *Proteus* spp. are the most common organisms isolated from pyometra in the dog (Gilbert, 1992; Olson, 1984b). In the bitch the condition most commonly affects older unbred animals who are presented several weeks after the onset of estrus (Kennedy, 1993). Depression, anorexia, and polyuria or polydipsia are common presenting signs (Kennedy, 1993). Pyometra in the cat is reported but is less common than in the dog, presumably because cats are induced ovulators, limiting the exposure to progesterone in the nongravid uterus (Gilbert, 1992; Kennedy, 1993). Pyometra usually occurs in cats 2 to 5 weeks after spontaneous ovulation (Kennedy, 1993).

Metritis in the bitch usually follows parturition. Dogs are systemically ill and have a noxious uterine discharge (Olson, 1984).

CYTOLOGICAL DIAGNOSIS
In open pyometra the vaginal smear contains many degenerate neutrophils. Vacuolated endometrial cells

may be present but can be difficult to differentiate from macrophages (Olson, 1984b).

Subinvolution of Placental Sites

CLINICAL DIAGNOSIS
Retained tags of placental tissue, which continue to bleed after whelping, can occur in young bitches, usually after the first whelping (Olson, 1984). A bloody vulvar discharge can persist for weeks but usually resolves (Olson, 1984).

CLINICAL DIAGNOSIS
Vaginal smears demonstrate large numbers of red blood cells. Large syncytia of cells, possibly trophoblastic in origin, are reported (Olson, 1984).

NEOPLASTIC DISEASE

Uterine Tumors

CLINICAL DIAGNOSIS
Uterine tumors account for less than 0.5% of all canine tumors, and the most commonly reported are smooth muscle in origin (Baldwin, 1992). Smooth-muscle tumors can be benign or malignant and occur predominately in older bitches (Baldwin, 1992). Uterine carcinomas are rare and carry a poor prognosis because metastatic disease is usually present at the time of diagnosis (Baldwin, 1992).

CYTOLOGICAL DIAGNOSIS
Vaginal smears from a dog with uterine carcinoma contained erythrocytes and large numbers of neutrophils, consistent with inflammatory disease (Baldwin, 1992). Bleeding is described as a clinical sign of uterine cancer and should always be investigated.

■ PROSTATE

Canine prostatic diseases are divided broadly into infectious and noninfectious categories. The infectious categories include acute and chronic bacterial prostatitis and prostatic abscess. The noninfectious categories include benign prostatic hyperplasia, prostatic and paraprostatic cysts, and prostatic neoplasia. Infection may coexist with noninfectious diseases.

Suspicion of prostatic disease is based on history, clinical signs, and physical examination (Barsanti, 1995). The four primary presenting signs of prostatic disease are hemorrhagic urethral discharge (urinary tract signs), systemic febrile illness, and defecation and locomotion abnormalities (Hornbuckle, 1978). Differential diagnoses are developed from information obtained from urinalysis, microbiological, radiographic, and ultrasonographic studies. Confirmation may require cytology, microbiology, and/or histopathology. With adequate sampling techniques, cytological examination of prostatic fluid or FNA biopsy will lead to prostatic disease differentiation in many dogs. The inflammatory response is readily observed by cytological examination of prostatic fluid collected from urethral discharge, by catheterization or ejaculation. Culture and sensitivity of prostatic fluid is necessary for confirmation of bacterial prostatitis (Barsanti, 1995). Anaerobic bacterial, mycoplasmal, and fungal culture may be indicated in some cases. Cysts are aspirated to differentiate a walled abscess before core biopsy. Localization of origin of cells and cell details are optimized with urethral brush biopsy or FNA biopsy.

TECHNIQUES

Urethral Discharge Sampling

The simplest but least effective technique for examination of prostatic disorders is examination of the urethral discharge. The prepuce is retracted and the glans is cleaned. The discharge is collected into a vial or onto a glass slide for microscopic examination, or into a sterile container for culture and colony counts. Comparison with catheterized urine is necessary to differentiate normal lower urethral bacterial flora, bladder infection, or contamination. Large concentrations of bacteria ($>10^5$/ml) and the presence of inflammatory cells support prostatic infection.

Ejaculate Fluid

An ejaculate can be obtained from many intact dogs using manual manipulation (Barsanti, 1995). The initial clear fraction and the cloudy concentrated sperm fraction can be separated from the third clear prostatic fluid fraction using a collection funnel. If cloudy throughout, the total sample should be examined (Barsanti, 1995). Between 0.5 and 1.0 ml of the clear prostatic fluid is collected for cytological and microbiological examination. The aliquot for cytological examination should be placed into a vial containing EDTA if inflammation is suspected. A separate aliquot is collected into a sterile tube for quantitative bacterial culture and sensitivity. A distal urethral swab should be collected before ejaculation for comparative purposes.

Collection of ejaculate can be difficult in dogs affected with painful prostatic disorders. The collection of ejaculate was successful in 69% of dogs with prostatic hyperplasia, 50% with squamous metaplasia, 33% with bacterial prostatitis, 29% with nonbacterial prostatitis, and 0% with prostatic neoplasia (Kay, 1989).

Ejaculate fluid culture was accurate in the diagnosis of prostatic infection approximately 80% of the time where ejaculate fluid colony counts were 2 $\log_{10}$ greater than the distal urethral swab (Ling, 1990; Ling, 1983). Interpretation of distal urethral swabs has led to some confusion (Barsanti, 1995). Determination of the unique distal urethral flora of the individual dog is useful for comparison with the suspect infectious agent (Barsanti, 1995). Paired urethral swab and ejaculate sample cultures disagreed with prostatic tissue or cyst culture 20% of the time for diagnosis of prostatic infection (Ling, 1990).

Prostatic Massage

Prostatic fluid may be collected by combining catheterization and prostatic massage. This procedure is used if a dog is unable to ejaculate, when attempting to localize the source of infection, or if identification of abnormal cells is indicated (Cowan, 1991).

The simplest approach is to pass a urinary catheter, guided by rectal palpation, to the prostatic urethra. A syringe is attached to the catheter and aspirated while the prostate gland is massaged per rectum. A small amount of prostatic secretion is obtained using this technique. If unsuccessful, a few milliliters of sterile saline may be flushed into the catheter and aspirated while the prostatic gland is massaged (Olson, 1987).

An alternative method is described for use when urinary tract infection may accompany bacterial prostatitis. The bladder is emptied and flushed with sterile saline, and the fluid is aspirated and collected. The catheter is then withdrawn to the caudal pole of the prostate. Both sides of the prostate are massaged per rectum. While occluding the distal urethra, 5 ml of sterile saline is injected. The catheter is advanced into the bladder and the fluid is aspirated (Barsanti, 1980; Cowan, 1991). Bacterial colony counts and cell morphology are compared in the fluid taken before prostatic massage and after prostatic massage. Because urinary tract infection often accompanies bacterial prostatitis (Barsanti, 1983), if the postmassage bacterial colony count is 10^2/ml greater than the premassage sample, infection is more likely to originate in the prostate (Barsanti, 1983; Cowan, 1991). It has been suggested, however, that massage be reserved for dogs with suspect bacterial prostatitis and no urinary tract infection because culture results may not be interpretable in the presence of urinary tract infection (Barsanti, 1983). Cytological evidence of inflammation may help in making this distinction. If urinary infection is suspected, treatment with ampicillin is recommended one day before prostatic massage (Cowan, 1991) because ampicillin does not cross the lipid barrier and thus enters the urine but not the prostate (Barsanti, 1995). Low numbers of bacteria may be significant in the presence of antibiotics (Barsanti, 1995).

Urethral Brush Technique

An urethral brush technique is described for distal urethral and for prostatic urethral sampling. The glans penis is cleaned using a 1:1000 dilution of benzalkonium chloride. A sterile 90-cm microbiological specimen brush (Microinvasive Inc., Milford, Mass.) is advanced into the urethra (Kay, 1989). For prostatic urethral sampling, the tip of the catheter is inserted to the caudal pole of the prostate, guided via rectal palpation. The prostate gland is massaged per rectum. The inner catheter is advanced, dislodging the catheter plug. The brush is advanced and retracted five or six times within the urethra. The brush is withdrawn, cut off with sterile scissors, and dropped into a test tube containing 3 ml of sterile lactated Ringer's solution (Kay, 1989). Aliquots are cultured and examined for cells. Cytological observations from prostatic urethral brush biopsies have not been reported for normal dogs.

FNA Biopsy

FNA of the prostate is an effective means of localizing and diagnosing prostatic lesions, especially where cells are not obtained in prostatic ejaculate or wash (Thrall, 1985). A transabdominal approach may be used if the gland is large. Alternatively, perianal or transrectal approaches are described (Finco, 1974; Thrall, 1985). A 22-gauge needle is directed into the prostate gland. Cells and/or fluid are aspirated using a syringe. A drop of aspirate material or fluid sediment is spread on a slide for examination and then submitted for culture if possible.

Aspiration biopsy is useful for differentiating an abscess from prostatic cysts. If purulent fluid is observed, the fluid should be aspirated until all pressure is reduced to prevent leakage. Aspiration allows definition of the source of squamous epithelial cells for the diagnosis of squamous metaplasia. The origin and the excellent detail of cells provides greater confidence in diagnosing neoplasia. The main disadvantage of aspiration biopsy is that focal lesions may be missed (Barsanti, 1995; Thrall, 1985).

NORMAL TISSUE (Figs. 14-15 to 14-18)

Ejaculate Fluid

Prostatic ejaculate fluid from healthy dogs is clear; has a pH of 6.0 to 6.7; and may contain a few erythrocytes, leukocytes, and squamous epithelial cells (Barsanti, 1995; Dorfmann, 1995). In 12 of 18 normal dogs, the ejaculate fluid contained a small number of neutrophils (Barsanti, 1980). Dogs free of prostatic disease are reported to have less than 100 bacteria per ml of prostatic fluid (Olson, 1987). However, undetected urethral contamination may account for up to 10^5/ml bacteria, usually gram-positive, with no evidence of inflammation unless there is preputial contamination (Barsanti, 1995). Large numbers of gram-negative bacteria (>100,000/ml) and white blood cells usually indicate infection (Dorfmann, 1995).

Prostatic Massage

The samples taken before and after prostatic massage from 20 normal dogs were similar, but cells were more numerous in postmassage samples (Barsanti, 1980). The cells included spermatozoa, transitional epithelial cells, squamous epithelial cells, and erythrocytes (Barsanti, 1980). Prostatic epithelial cells were not observed in samples before or after prostatic massage from the normal dogs (Barsanti, 1980). Bacteria were not found in the urine or in the before- or after-massage samples in 19 of 20 dogs (Barsanti, 1980). Cultures from normal dogs are usually negative or have low numbers (<100/ml), suggestive of lower urethral contamination (Barsanti, 1995).

FNA Biopsy

An aspiration biopsy from a normal prostate contains clusters of cuboidal to low columnar prostatic epithelial cells. The epithelial cytoplasm is finely granular and basophilic and may be vacuolated. Nuclei are round to oval with a single, small, inconspicuous nucleoli (Thrall, 1985). Cells may exfoliate in sheets with a typical "honeycomb" appearance.

NONNEOPLASTIC DISEASE

Benign Prostatic Hyperplasia

CLINICAL DIAGNOSIS
Benign hypertrophy is the most common abnormality of the prostate gland in dogs, occurring only in intact males. During sexual development, increase in prostate size parallels testosterone production. The influence of hormone concentration on hyperplasia is less clear in the mature dog. Benign hypertrophy is evident in some dogs by 3 years, present in over 50% by 5 years, and over 90% by 8 years of age (Barsanti, 1995; Cowan, 1991). In one study, all beagles over 6 years had complex benign prostatic hyperplasia (Lowseth, 1990). There appears to be a greater risk for large-breed dogs (Kay, 1989). Benign hypertrophy is associated with an increase in gland size and weight (Lowseth, 1990). The increase in size is due primarily to an increase in interstitial tissue and gland lumens, leading to progressive symmetrical cystic dilation of the glands (Lowseth, 1990) or formation of intra-parenchymal cysts (Cowan, 1991).

Most dogs have no clinical signs associated with prostatic hypertrophy. The most common sign is a hemorrhagic nonsuppurative urethral discharge that can be localized to the prostatic urethra. Fecal tenesmus or dysuria may occur with marked hypertrophy. On palpation the gland is nonpainful and usually symmetrically enlarged. Castration is the most effective treatment. A marked reduction in size and hemorrhagic discharge occurs within a few weeks of surgery (Barsanti, 1995). Squamous metaplasia may develop in the presence of estrogen (Cowan, 1991).

CYTOLOGICAL DIAGNOSIS
Benign hyperplasia, diagnosed by histological examination, was identified in 7 of 11 dogs with prostatic urethral brush biopsies (Kay, 1989) and in 5 of 7 dogs with aspiration biopsies (Thrall, 1985). Hemorrhage was observed in semen and prostatic massage samples from 9 of 13 dogs with a histological diagnosis of benign hyperplasia (Barsanti, 1984). Histological examination may be required in those clinical cases requiring absolute confirmation (Barsanti, 1995).

Hyperplastic prostatic epithelial cells are similar in appearance to normal prostatic epithelial cells, but the cellularity of the massage sample may be increased. Epithelial fragments have a characteristic mosaic appearance with uniform cell size, abundant cytoplasm, and mature nuclei with a small, round nucleolus. There may be an increase in cell size and mild anisokaryosis, but N:C ratio is preserved. In general, the cells appear normal and hyperplasia is diagnosed when cells are seen in conjunction with a clinically enlarged prostate (Barton, 1992).

Squamous Metaplasia (Fig. 14-19)

CLINICAL DIAGNOSIS
Under the influence of estrogens, cuboidal to low columnar prostatic epithelial cells develop morphological and staining characteristics of squamous epithelial cells. Estrogen receptors are present on ductal, stromal, and about 10% of epithelial cells but can be induced in other epithelial cells (Barsanti, 1995). Sertoli's cell tumors are the most common endogenous source of estrogen. Squamous metaplasia induces ductal stasis, which can lead to cyst formation and possibly abscessation (Barsanti, 1995). The prostate gland will vary in size. It may be small in response to decreased testosterone production or large with development of cysts or abscessation (Barsanti, 1995). The primary clinical signs develop in response to hyperestrogenism. Removal of the estrogen source is the treatment.

CYTOLOGICAL DIAGNOSIS
Although biopsy confirmation is recommended (Barsanti, 1995), in one study, urethral brush biopsies were more sensitive than histology in identifying squamous metaplasia (Kay, 1989). Aspiration biopsy

identifies the origin of squamous cells but may have lower sensitivity than brush biopsies used in conjunction with prostatic massage.

On cytological examination of a prostatic urethral wash, or an aspiration biopsy, hyperplastic epithelial cells are arranged singly or in clusters intermixed with larger single epithelial cells, which have a low to moderate N:C ratio. The cytoplasm of these larger epithelial cells is blue-green with Romanowsky's stains and polyhedral or angular, typical of squamous differentiation. The nucleus may be open and vesiculated or small and pyknotic. The cells are often found at the feathered edge of the smear. If prostatic cysts are present, hemorrhagic debris and intact red blood cells may be observed.

Prostatic Cysts

CLINICAL DIAGNOSIS
Various types of intraprostatic cysts are reported. Cysts account for only 2% to 5% of prostatic abnormalities (Dorfmann, 1995). Multiple cysts can be associated with benign prostatic hypertrophy or with squamous metaplasia. Single intraprostatic and paraprostatic cysts are reported. Clinical signs are usually minimal unless the cysts impinge on the urethra or colon, or unless secondarily infected (Olson, 1987). There may be hemorrhagic urethral discharge unassociated with urination (Olson, 1987). Surgical removal of the cysts, or marsupialization of paraprostatic cysts, is the treatment of choice but is not without complications (Barsanti, 1995).

CYTOLOGICAL DIAGNOSIS
Urethral discharge or aspirate fluid from prostatic cysts is frequently bloody. Cytological examination of prostatic fluid can help differentiate prostatic cysts from abscesses that appear similar radiographically (Barsanti, 1995). Uninfected prostatic cysts contain a few to several milliliters of serosanguinous to brown fluid. On microscopic examination the fluid may be acellular with a dirty red to brown background or contain a few erythrocytes, leukocytes, or benign epithelial cells (Thrall, 1985).

Prostatitis (Figs. 14-20 to 14-23)

CLINICAL DIAGNOSIS
Bacteria are not normally present in the canine prostatic gland (Olson, 1987). Bacterial infection is implicated in 20% to 70% of dogs with clinical problems involving the prostate (Cowan, 1991). All dogs with lower urinary tract infection should be considered to have concurrent prostatic infection until proven negative (Barsanti, 1995). Ascending infection through the prostatic urethra is the usual route of infection. The most common organisms are *E. coli, Proteus, Staphylococcus,* and *Streptococcus* spp. (Cowan, 1991). Infection may occur as a result of altered prostatic architecture, resulting from either benign hypertrophy, squamous metaplasia, carcinoma, or cysts. This predisposes the gland to infection by providing a medium for bacterial growth or by interfering with normal defense mechanisms (Olson, 1987). Hematogenous infection may occur. Infection is not common with simple benign hyperplasia (Barsanti, 1995).

Acute and chronic bacterial prostatitis is differentiated on the basis of systemic and local signs. With acute prostatitis, systemic illness is common. Obtaining a prostatic sample may be extremely painful for the dog. In contrast, dogs with chronic bacterial prostatitis usually have a history of recurrent urinary tract infection or urethral discharge without systemic signs (Cowan, 1991). If local areas of septic prostatitis coalesce, or if prostatic cysts become infected, an abscess may develop. In one report, 51.2% of dogs with abscesses died or were euthanized because of the disease (Hornbuckle, 1978).

CYTOLOGICAL DIAGNOSIS
Cytological preparations from bacterial prostatitis contain many degenerate neutrophils intermixed with benign epithelial cells. Intracellular and extracellular bacteria may be visible unless previously treated with antibiotics. The epithelial cells may appear normal to hyperplastic with hyperchromasia, increased N:C ratio, and mild anisokaryosis in response to the inflammation. Following a cardinal rule for cytological interpretation, a diagnosis of neoplasia should be avoided, or made very cautiously, in the presence of severe inflammation. In one study, the presence of macrophages correlated well with prostatic infection (Barsanti, 1983). Eight of 12 dogs with bacterial prostatitis had inflammatory cells and bacteria on urethral brush cytology slides (Kay, 1989). Cytological evidence of inflammation within the ejaculate may correlate better with histological evidence of prostatitis than bacterial culture of the prostate (Barsanti, 1983).

NEOPLASTIC DISEASE

Prostatic Carcinoma (Figs. 14-24 to 14-28)

CLINICAL DIAGNOSIS
Prostatic carcinoma is considered to be rare in dogs. A prevalence of 0.2% and 0.6% is reported from necropsy studies (Bell, 1991). In another study, 16% of the dogs with prostatic disease were reported to have prostatic adenocarcinoma (Olson, 1987). Transitional carcinoma frequently involves the prostatic urethra. Differentiation between prostatic carcinoma and transitional cell carcinomas may be difficult and requires careful concurrent histological examination of the bladder. Prostatic neoplasia is seen more frequently in older,

medium- to large-breed dogs (Cowan, 1991; Hargis, 1983). Prognosis is poor because widespread metastasis is common at the time of diagnosis (Bell, 1991; Hargis, 1983; Weaver, 1981). Most dogs are dead within 1 month of diagnosis (Hargis, 1983).

CYTOLOGICAL DIAGNOSIS

With fine-needle cytological examination, multiple, large clusters of prostatic epithelial cells are usually present. There is cellular disorientation and loss of the normal mosaic pattern. The N:C ratio is usually increased. There is mild to moderate anisokaryosis. Nucleoli are multiple and prominent (Barsanti, 1984). Occasional epithelial cells suggest secretory function, as indicated by the presence of large, round, eosinophilic granular areas. Some cell clusters may suggest acinar formation.

Of four dogs with prostatic carcinoma, two were diagnosed and one was suspected from urethral brush biopsies (Kay, 1989). Cytological biopsies were examined in 17 of 31 dogs with histological confirmation of prostatic carcinoma (Bell, 1991). From 19 biopsies, of which 14 were aspirations, the cytological interpretation agreed with the histological diagnosis in 14 dogs (Bell, 1991).

■ TESTICLE

Infrequently, cytological examination of the testicle is required. Examination of semen for fertility is not discussed in this atlas.

TECHNIQUE

FNA can be used to investigate palpable testicular lesions preoperatively, during surgery, or at postmortem. Because orchidectomy is the treatment of choice for palpable testicular masses, presurgical examination is seldom done. Fine-needle aspirates can be obtained readily; however, because of the increased fragility of testicular cells, greater care must be taken when preparing the cell monolayer. Gentle touch impression may be the most suitable method for preserving intact cells when tissue is available. Ruptured cells often predominate in the cell preparation even when using the gentlest techniques. If a biopsy is removed, cytological preparations should be made very soon because of the rapid rate of cell deterioration.

NORMAL TESTICLE (Figs. 14-29 to 14-33)

High cellularity with a predominance of ruptured nuclei is characteristic of testicular imprints. With rup-

ture of the nuclei, coarse nuclear chromatin and large, irregular nucleoli become prominent. Careful scanning may be required to locate intact well-preserved testicular cells. The cells are round, with coarse nuclear chromatin patterns and have a single, large, central nucleolus. N:C ratio is moderate. The cytoplasm is symmetrically arranged around the nucleus. Mitotic figures are numerous.

NONNEOPLASTIC DISEASE

Orchitis

CLINICAL AND CYTOLOGICAL DIAGNOSES

In the dog the two primary reasons for testicular enlargement are orchitis and neoplasia. Bacterial orchitis can be due to infection with *Brucella canis*, *Pseudomonas*, *E. coli*, or *Proteus* spp. (Ladds, 1993). When orchitis is due to distemper, intranuclear or intracytoplasmic inclusions may be observed (Ladds, 1993). The cellular inflammatory response is similar with orchitis as with other tissues. Occasionally the infectious agent may be visible on the cytological smears (Zinkl, 1999), but this is unusual, and culture is generally required.

NEOPLASTIC DISEASE

Testicular tumors account for 5% to 15% of all tumors in the male dog. They are extremely rare in the cat (O'Keefe, 1995).

Seminoma (Figs. 14-34 and 14-35)

CLINICAL DIAGNOSIS

Seminomas are common in dogs, accounting for 33% of all testicular tumors, especially in cryptorchids (Barton, 1992). Dogs are often asymptomatic, unless the seminoma is accompanied by a Sertoli's cell tumor. Seminomas are locally invasive, and although they tend not to metastasize, they do so more frequently than the other canine testicular tumors (Ladds, 1993). Tumors may be quite large at the time of consultation (Ladds, 1993).

CYTOLOGICAL DIAGNOSIS

Cytological distinction among the three canine testicular tumor types is not always possible. However, certain cellular characteristics are more suggestive of one type than another. Seminoma cells tend to be round, with one or two nuclei, each possessing one large nucleolus. The nuclear chromatin is uniformly finely reticular (Zinkl, 1999). Moderate anisokaryosis may be seen. The cytoplasm is faintly basophilic, and in some cells, N:C ratio may be high. Multinucleation and mitosis may be common (Barton, 1992).

Sertoli's Cell Tumor (Figs. 14-36 and 14-37)

CLINICAL DIAGNOSIS

Enlargement of the testicle is the main presenting clinical sign. Sertoli's cell tumors account for approximately 50% of all testicular tumors (Barton, 1992). The tumors are more common in cryptorchid dogs with undescended testes (Zinkl, 1999). A feminization syndrome is associated with the high estrogen content of the tumors. Excess endogenous estrogen may lead to bone marrow suppression and resulting thrombocytopenia, anemia, and granulocytopenia (Ladds, 1993).

CYTOLOGICAL DIAGNOSIS

Round cells with finely reticulated nuclear chromatin patterns are typical of Sertoli's cell tumors. Nuclei may exhibit large, multiple nucleoli. A unique feature of Sertoli's cell tumors is a pale-staining cytoplasm that contains prominent, variably sized vacuoles (Zinkl, 1999). Mitoses are common.

Interstitial Cell Tumors (Fig. 14-38)

CLINICAL DIAGNOSIS

Testicular enlargement is uncommon in interstitial cell tumors and as such these tumors are rarely aspirated for clinical purposes. Impression smears, for interest, may be made at necropsy when these tumors are found as an incidental finding. Interstitial cell tumors may secrete androgens, which explains their association with perianal gland neoplasia, tail-gland hyperplasia, and prostatic enlargement (Ladds, 1993).

CYTOLOGICAL DIAGNOSIS

With FNA there is a moderate harvest of small- to medium-sized cells with abundant cytoplasm (Zinkl, 1999). The N:C ratio is low and nucleoli are small and inconspicuous (Zinkl, 1999). Some cells may contain small vacuoles of uniform size (Barton, 1992; Zinkl, 1999).

References

Baldwin, C.J., Roszel, J.F., and Clark, T.P. Uterine adenocarcinoma in dogs. *Compend Cont Ed Pract* 14:31-737, 1992.

Barsanti, J.A. and Finco, D.R. Evaluation of techniques for diagnosis of canine prostatic diseases. *J Am Vet Med Assoc* 185:198-200, 1984.

Barsanti, J.A. and Finco, D.R. Prostatic diseases. In *Textbook of Veterinary Internal Medicine.* S.J. Ettinger and E.C. Feldman (eds). WB Saunders, Philadelphia, 1995.

Barsanti, J.A., Prasse, K.W., Crowell, W.A., et al. Evaluation of various techniques for diagnosis of chronic bacterial prostatitis in the dog. *J Am Vet Med Assoc* 183:219-224, 1983.

Barsanti, J.A., Shotts, E.B., Prasse, K., et al. Evaluation of diagnostic techniques for canine prostatic diseases. *J Am Vet Med Assoc* 177:160-163, 1980.

Barton, C.L. and Rogers, K.S. Diagnostic cytology of the urogenital system. *Proc 10th ACVIM Forum,* San Diego, pp 771-782, 1992.

Bell, F.W., Klausner, J.S., Hayden, D.W., et al. Clinical and pathologic features of prostatic adenocarcinoma in sexually intact and castrated dogs: 31 cases (1970-1987). *J Am Vet Med Assoc* 199:1623-1630, 1991.

Cowan, L.A. and Barsanti, J.A. Prostatic disease. In *Small Animal Medicine.* D.G. Allen, S.E. Kruth, and M.S. Garvey, (eds). JP Lippincott, Philadelphia, 1991.

Dahlgren, R.R. *Vaginal Cytology of the Dog.* Ralston Purina Company, GP 2738 A 7607, St Louis, 1979.

Dorfman, M. and Barsanti, J. Diseases of the canine prostate gland. *Compend Cont Ed Pract* 17:791-810, 1995.

Finco, D.R. Prostate gland biopsy. *Vet Clin North Am (Small Anim Pract)* 4:367-375, 1974.

Gilbert, R.O. Diagnosis and treatment of pyometra in bitches and queens. *Compend Cont Ed Pract* 6:777-783, 1992.

Hargis, A.M. and Miller, L.M. Prostatic carcinoma in dogs. *Compend Cont Ed Pract* 5:647-653, 1983.

Herron, M.A. Feline vaginal cytologic examination. *Feline Practice* 36-39, 1977.

Holst, P.A. and Phemister, R.D. Temporal sequence of events in the estrus cycle of the bitch. *Am J Vet Res* 36:705-706, 1975.

Hornbuckle, W.E., MacCoy, D.M., Allan, G.S., et al. Prostatic disease in the dog. *Cornell Vet* 68:284-298, 1978.

Johnson, C.A. Vulvar discharges. In *Current Veterinary Therapy X. Small Animal Practice.* R.W. Kirk and J.D. Bonagura (eds). WB Saunders, Philadelphia, 1989.

Kang, T.B. and Holmberg, D.L. Vaginal leiomyoma in a dog. *Can Vet J* 24:258-260, 1983.

Kay, N.D., Ling, G.V., and Johnson, D.L. A urethral brush technique for the diagnosis of canine bacterial prostatitis. *J Am Anim Hosp Assoc* 25:527-532, 1989.

Kay, N.D., Ling, G.V., Nyland, T.G., et al. Cytological diagnosis of canine prostatic disease using a urethral brush technique. *J Am Anim Hosp Assoc* 25:517-531, 1989.

Kennedy, P.C. and Miller, R.B. The female genital system. In *Pathology of Domestic Animals.* ed 4. K.V.F. Jubb, P.C. Kennedy and N. Palmer (eds). Academic Press, San Diego, 1993.

Ladds, P.W. The male genital system. In *Pathology of Domestic Animals. vol 3.* K.V.F. Jubb, P.C. Kennedy, and N. Palmer (eds). Academic Press, San Diego, 1993.

Ling, G.V., Branam, J.E., Ruby, A.L., et al. Canine prostatic fluid: techniques of collection, quantitative bacterial culture, and interpretation of results. *J Am Vet Med Assoc* 183:201-206, 1983.

Ling, G.V., Nyland, T.G., Kennedy, P.C., et al. Comparison of two sample collection methods for quantitative bacteriologic culture of canine prostatic fluid. *J Am Vet Med Assoc* 196:1479-1482, 1990.

Lowseth, L.A., Gerlach, R.F., Gillett, N.A., et al. Age-related changes in the prostate and testes of the beagle dog. *Vet Pathol* 27:347-353, 1990.

O'Keefe, D.A. Tumors of the genital system and mammary glands. In *Textbook of Veterinary Internal Medicine. Diseases of the Dog and Cat.* S.J. Ettinger and E.C. Feldman (eds). WB Saunders, Philadelphia, 1995.

Olson, P., Wrigley, R.H., Thrall, M.A., et al. Disorders of the canine prostate gland: pathogenesis, diagnosis, and medical therapy. *Compend Cont Ed Pract* 9:613-623, 1987.

Olson, P.N., Thrall, M.A., Wykes, P.M., et al. Vaginal cytology. Part 1. A useful tool for staging the canine estrous cycle. *Compend Cont Ed Pract* 6:288-296, 1984a.

Olson, P.N., Thrall, M.A., Wykes, P.M., et al. Vaginal cytology. Part 11. Its use in diagnosing canine reproductive disorders. *Compend Cont Ed Pract* 6:385-390, 1984b.

Roszel, J.F. Genital cytology of the bitch. *Vet Scope* 11:2, 1975.

Roszel, J.F. Normal canine vaginal cytology. *Vet Clin North Am (Small Anim)* 7:667-681, 1977.

Schutte, A.P. Canine vaginal cytology—I. Technique and cytological morphology. *J Small Anim Pract* 8:301-306, 1967.

Shorr, E. *Science* 91:321, 1940.

Thrall, M.A. and Olson, P.N. The vagina. In *Diagnostic Cytology of the Dog and Cat.* ed 2. R.L Cowell, R.D. Tyler, and J.H. Meinkoth (eds). Mosby, St Louis, 1999.

Thrall, M.A., Olson, P.N., and Freemyer, E.G. Cytologic diagnosis of canine prostatic disease. *J Am Anim Hosp Assoc* 21:94-102, 1985.

Weaver, A.D. Fifteen cases of prostatic carcinoma in the dog. *Vet Rec* 109:71-75, 1981.

Zinkl, J.G. and Feldman, B.F. The male reproductive tract: prostate, testes, semen. In *Diagnostic Cytology of the Dog and Cat.* ed 2. R.L. Cowell, R.D. Tyler, and J.H. Meinkoth (eds). Mosby, St Louis, 1999.

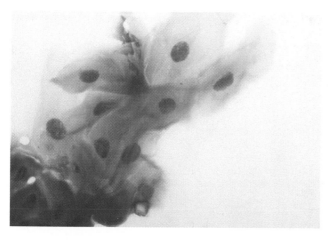

FIG. 14-1. Feline. Scraping. Normal vaginal wall. Intermediate squamous epithelial cells. (×100.)

FIG. 14-2. Canine. Swab. Vagina. Early estrus. Over 90% of cells are early superficial squamous epithelial cells; some have perinuclear clearing consistent with early keratin formation. Rare erythrocyte is still present. Many stains, especially trichrome stains, are preferable to Romanowsky's stains for demonstrating squamous differentiation and keratinization. When collated with clinical information, Romanowsky's stains are adequate. (×100.)

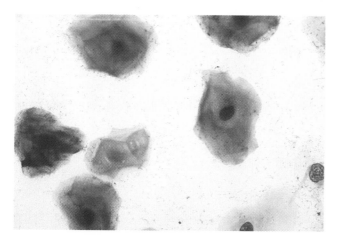

FIG. 14-3. Canine. Vaginal swab. Superficial squamous cells consistent with estrus. Leukostat stain. (×375.)

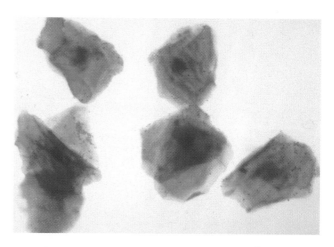

FIG. 14-4. Canine. Swab. Vagina. Estrus. Clear background and superficial squamous epithelial cells. Angularity of borders visible, but nuclei still present. (×100.)

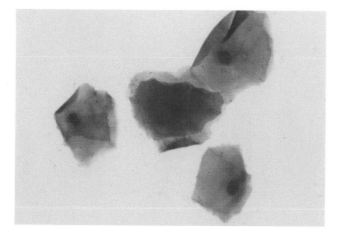

FIG. 14-5. Canine. Swab. Vagina. Estrus. Superficial squamous differentiation of epithelial cells typical of estrus. (×200.)

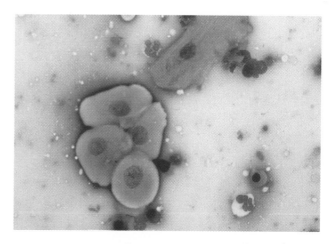

FIG. 14-6. Canine. Swab. Vagina. Proestrus. Abundant, pale cytoplasm that thins at the borders consistent with intermediate differentiation of epithelial cells. Occasional neutrophil is present. (×100.)

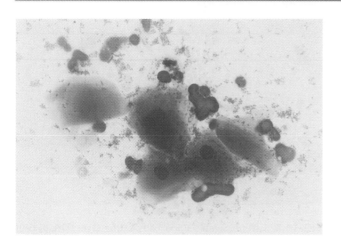

FIG. 14-7. Canine. Vaginal swab. Proestrus. Background of erythrocytes and intermediate to superficial squamous epithelial cells. Leukostat stain. (×200.)

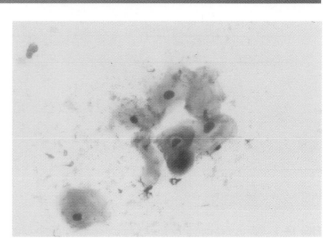

FIG. 14-8. Canine. Vaginal swab. Consistent with proestrus or diestrus. Background contains bacteria, erythrocytes, and cell debris. The epithelial cells are intermediate to superficial in differentiation. Clinical data and/or serial examinations are required for interpretation. (×125.)

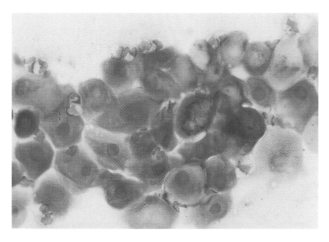

FIG. 14-9. Canine. Vaginal swab. Proestrus. Intermediate to superficial squamous epithelial cells. Note the cytoplasmic vacuolation within one degenerating cell and the few neutrophils. Leukostat stain. (×125.)

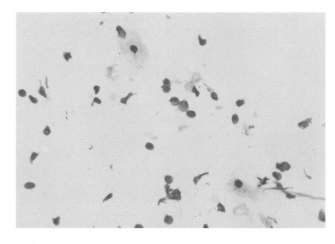

FIG. 14-10. Canine. Vaginal swab. Anestrus. Low cellularity consisting primarily of ruptured nuclei and a few intact intermediate epithelial cells. Leukostat stain. (×125.)

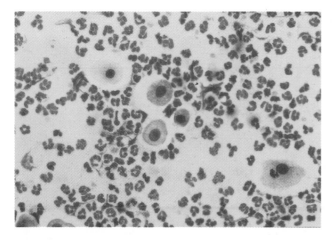

FIG. 14-11. Canine. Vaginal swab. Vaginitis. Parabasal to intermediate epithelial cells intermixed with neutrophils. (×125.)

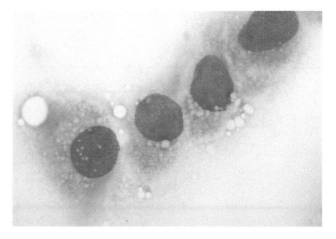

FIG. 14-12. Canine. Imprint. Normal uterus. Cuboidal epithelial cells with lightly staining basophilic cytoplasm; indistinct common borders; mild vacuolation; and bland, round to oval nuclei. (×400.)

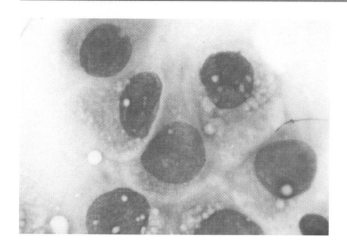

FIG. 14-13. Canine. Imprint. Normal uterus. (Same case as Fig. 14-12.) Round to cuboidal epithelial cells with occasional clear cytoplasmic vacuoles, common adjoining borders, indistinct chromatin, and small nucleoli. (×500.)

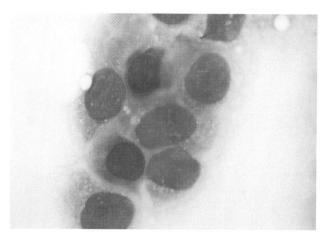

FIG. 14-14. Canine. Imprint. Normal uterus. (Same case as Fig. 14-12.) Epithelial cells with variation in nuclear size and density. (×400.)

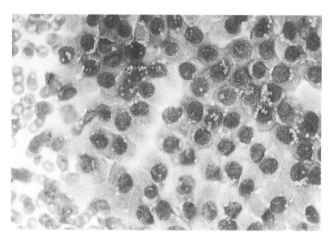

FIG. 14-15. Canine. Prostatic wash, normal. Sheet of benign prostatic epithelial cells demonstrating typical honeycomb mosaic, fine perinuclear vacuolation, and bland nuclear chromatin pattern. (×200.)

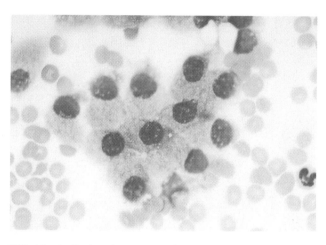

FIG. 14-16. Canine. Prostatic wash, normal. (Same case as Fig. 14-15.) Small sheet of prostatic cuboidal to columnar epithelial cells with eccentric nuclei and low N:C ratio. (×250.)

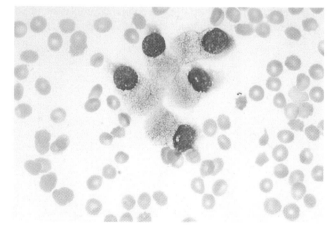

FIG. 14-17. Canine. Prostatic wash, normal. (Same case as Fig. 14-15.) Prostatic epithelial cells have a low N:C ratio, bland nuclear chromatin, and fine granular gray-blue cytoplasm. (×250.)

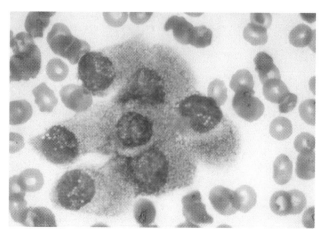

FIG. 14-18. Canine. Prostatic wash, normal. (Same case as Fig. 14-15.) Prostatic epithelial cells illustrating fine cytoplasmic granularity and vacuoles. The cytoplasmic characteristics resemble the appearance of hepatocytes and hepatoid perianal gland cells. The vacuoles obscure nuclear details. (×400.)

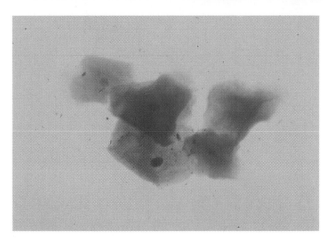

FIG. 14-19. Canine. Imprint. Prepuce. Squamous epithelial cells. This degree of differentiation is abnormal and indicates excessive estrogen production. This response is consistent with testicular tumor development within a bilateral cryptorchid dog. (×150.)

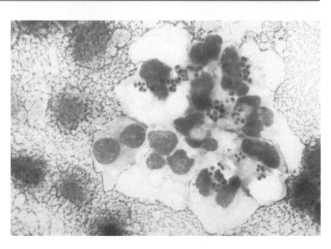

FIG. 14-20. Canine. Prostatic wash. Septic prostatitis. Cellular debris with degenerate neutrophils and large numbers of bacteria. (×400.)

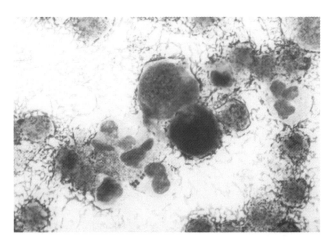

FIG. 14-21. Canine. Prostatic wash. Septic prostatitis. (Same case as Fig. 14-20.) Background contains bacteria and cell debris. There is an intact epithelial cell and degenerate neutrophils. (×400.)

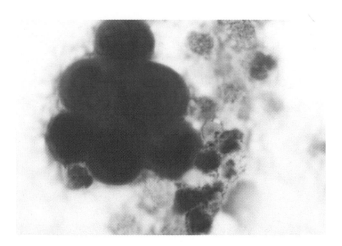

FIG. 14-22. Canine. Prostatic wash. Septic prostatitis. (Same case as Fig. 14-20.) Cluster of cells with high N:C ratio but limited detail resulting from marked hyperchromasia. There is nuclear debris, some degenerating neutrophils, and bacteria. Morphology of the epithelial cells illustrates the degree of proplasia and potential for misinterpretation when inflammation is present. (×500.)

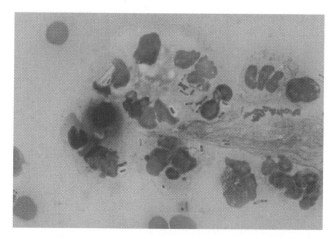

FIG. 14-23. Canine. Fine needle. Prostate. Prostatic abscess. Degenerating neutrophils with free and phagocytized bacteria. (×380.)

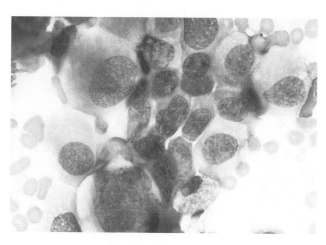

FIG. 14-24. Canine. Fine needle. Prostatic carcinoma. Epithelial cells with marked anisokaryosis. Note nuclear size compared with erythrocytes. Cytological differentiation of prostatic carcinoma and transitional cell carcinoma involving the prostate may not be possible. (×250.)

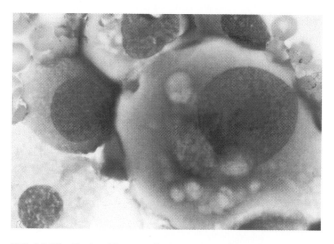

FIG. 14-25. Canine. Fine needle. Prostatic carcinoma. (Same case as Fig. 14-24.) Extreme variation in nuclear and cell size with large, irregular nucleolus. (×400.)

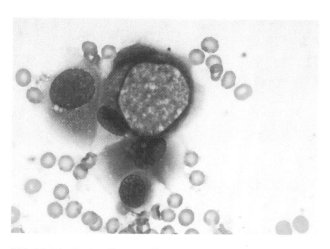

FIG. 14-26. Canine. Fine needle. Prostatic carcinoma. (Same case as Fig. 14-24.) Epithelial cells with anisokaryosis and hyperchromasia. The intracytoplasmic pink secretory product is a feature of many prostatic carcinomas but can be seen in transitional cell carcinomas. (×250.)

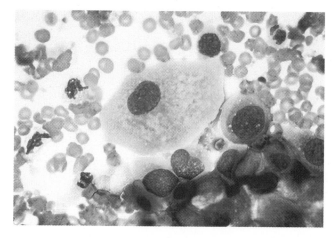

FIG. 14-27. Canine. Fine needle. Prostatic carcinoma. (Same case as Fig. 14-24.) Note the contrast between the large transitional cell and the smaller cells usually associated with prostatic origin. (×200.)

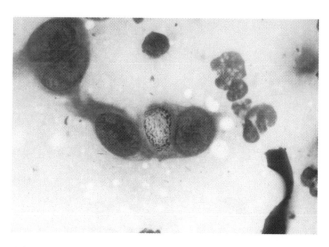

FIG. 14-28. Canine. Fine needle. Prostatic carcinoma. Anaplastic epithelial cells with high N:C ratio; hyperchromasia; large, irregular nucleoli; and, possibly, trinucleation. Metachromatic intracytoplasmic secretory product is present. (×400.)

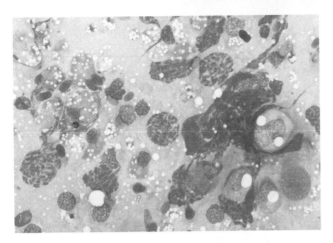

FIG. 14-29. Canine. Fine needle. Normal testicle. Few intact cells, many mitotic figures, and heterogeneous appearance of ruptured nuclei as commonly obtained from impressions or fine-needle aspirations of testicular tissue. (×200.)

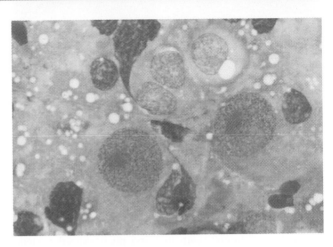

FIG. 14-30. Canine. Imprint. Normal testicle from a 4-month-old puppy. Heterogeneous population of round cells, dominated by large cells with prominent nuclei; distinct, fine chromatin pattern; central, large nucleoli; and lightly basophilic, indistinct cytoplasm. The large cells are consistent with seminiferous tubular cells. Because of fragility, rupture of many cells is expected, as indicated by the free nuclei present. (×400.)

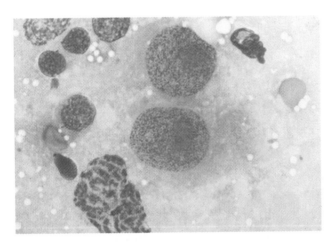

FIG. 14-31. Canine. Imprint. Normal testicle. Mitotic figure reflects cellular activity in normal testicular tissue. (×400.)

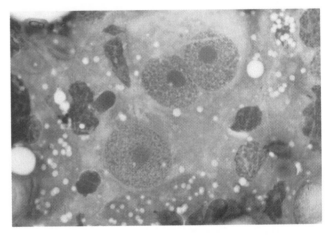

FIG. 14-32. Canine. Imprint. Normal testicle. Large, seminiferous tubule cells with moderate amount of blue-gray cytoplasm. Nuclei have a distinct chromatin pattern and prominent nucleoli. Clear vacuoles in background suggest lipid content. (×400.)

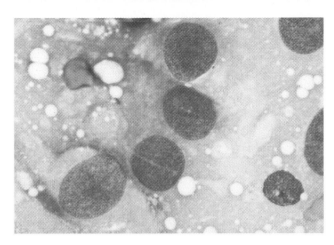

FIG. 14-33. Feline. Imprint. Normal testicle. Large cells with homogeneous, lightly basophilic cytoplasm and indistinct cytoplasmic borders. Note the anisokaryosis and occasional clear vacuoles in the intercellular space. (×400.)

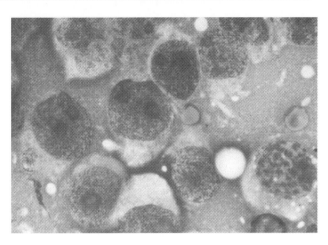

FIG. 14-34. Canine. Imprint. Seminoma. Large, round cells with large nuclei; fine to reticular chromatin pattern; one to two large nucleoli; and pale, mildly vacuolated cytoplasm. Testicular cells are extremely fragile and require gentle handling during slide preparation. (×400.)

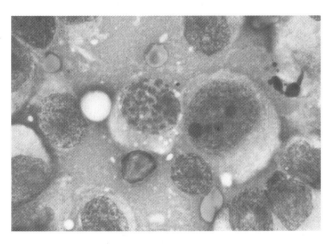

FIG. 14-35. Canine. Imprint. Seminoma. (Same case as Fig. 14-34.) The round cells have moderate anisokaryosis and include one mitotic figure. (×400.)

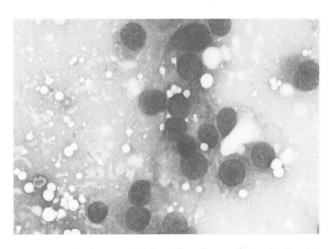

FIG. 14-36. Canine. Imprint. Sertoli's cell tumor. Round cells with pale-staining abundant cytoplasm and prominent, variably sized vacuoles characteristic of this tumor. (×250.)

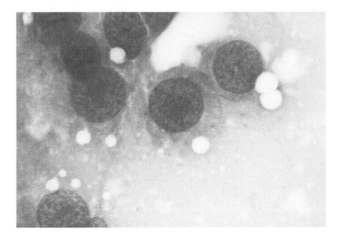

FIG. 14-37. Canine. Imprint. Sertoli's cell tumor. Large, round cells with reticulated nuclear chromatin; large, indistinct nucleoli; and discrete cytoplasmic vacuoles. (×500.)

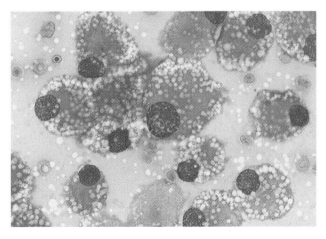

FIG. 14-38. Canine. Imprint. Interstitial cell tumor. Large, round cells with low N:C ratio and basophilic cytoplasm with diffuse, fine vacuolation. (×400.)

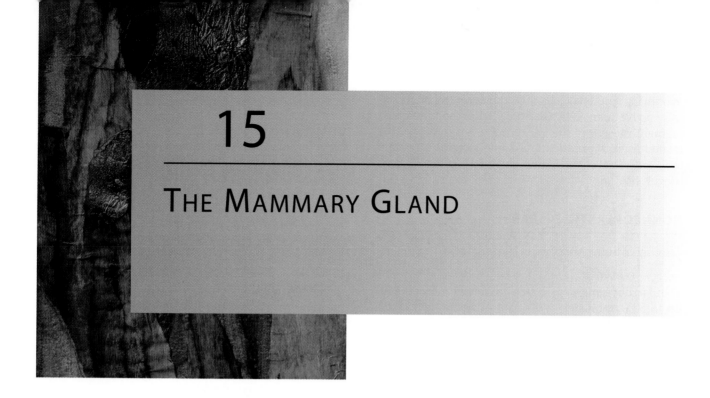

15

THE MAMMARY GLAND

Mammary lesions are common in bitches and queens. History and physical examination integrated with epidemiological data are used to establish differential diagnoses and possibly prognosis. Important observations include age of the patient, recent estrus, pregnancy or hormone therapy, whether intact or aged when ovariohysterectomy was performed, size and firmness of the lesion, rate of growth, attachment to skin or deeper tissues, and evidence for metastasis. Imaging and surgical biopsy, and more recently aspiration biopsy, are used for further investigation of tumors at early stages of development. Although the initial issue is to differentiate inflammation or hyperplasia from a tumor, the primary objective is to predict biological behavior, that is, prognosis.

Criteria for diagnosis and prognosis remains controversial for canine mammary tumors (Brodey, 1983; Gilbertson, 1983; Yager, 1993). The most reliable predictor of biological behavior is clinical or histological evidence of tumor infiltration or metastases (Yager, 1993). Other histological criteria or classifications for malignancy often correlate poorly with biological behavior. Comparisons between studies is not easy because of the different histological criteria used for malignancy and different criteria used for patient survival time and tumor recurrence endpoints.

Cytological examination appears to be useful in answering specific clinical questions relating to mammary lesions even though the few studies comparing cytology and histology report limited correlation. Optimal cytological interpretation depends on access to patient clinical information, a good understanding of the biology of these tumors in dogs and cats, examination of adequate representative cells, experience, and good communications with the clinician.

TECHNIQUES

FNA biopsies can be readily obtained from most mammary lesions. Because cell type and morphology vary within and between lesions, multiple aspirates are necessary to increase the probability of harvesting representative cells. Before-biopsy and after-biopsy aspirates and imprints are required to ensure similar origin of specimens when cytological and histological diagnoses are being compared. In general, fine-needle aspirates provide better cellular details than imprints.

NORMAL MAMMARY GLAND (Figs. 15-1 to 15-3)

FNAs from normal mammary gland tissue usually have low cellularity with fluid containing blood and/or adipocytes. The predominant cell is a large, vacuolated, foamy epithelial cell that resembles a macrophage (Maddux, 1999). Alcohol-fixed epithelial cells are round to oval, 6 to 8 μ in diameter, with nucleoli less than 2 μ (Allen, 1986). Ductular epithelial cells, which may be present in clusters or sheets, are basophilic with basilar nuclei and prominent intercellular borders.

NORMAL LACTATING MAMMARY GLAND (Figs. 15-4 to 15-8)

FNAs from lactating mammary glands have a higher cellularity than nonlactating glands. Clusters of cuboidal ductular epithelial cells, acinar cells with granular cytoplasm, and many pigment-laden epithelial cells are visible using Romanowsky's stains. These large, foamy cells may originate as histiocytes or as mammary epithelial cells that transform to phagocytically active foam cells (Barton, 1992). The blue-green pigment present in the background is assumed to be related to milk production. Nipple secretions contain lipid-laden cells and some ductular epithelial cells (Rozel, 1975).

NONNEOPLASTIC DISEASE

Canine Lobular and Cystic Hyperplasia

Clinical Diagnosis

Lobular hyperplasia is a benign change observed in up to 50% of bitches by 3 years of age (Yager, 1993). Lobular hyperplasia is suggested to be a preneoplastic lesion, because of the similar high prevalence of hyperplasia and mammary carcinomas within caudal mammary glands.

Cytological Diagnosis

In intact normal bitches, ductal and acinar epithelial cells and intralobular and interlobular connective tissue go through cycles of proliferation (Yager, 1993). With aging, hyperplastic and dysplastic cells become interspersed within the epithelium. Myoepithelial cells, which line the teat sinus and secretory acini, infiltrate the stroma and the connective tissue cores of papillary ductal growths in association with dysplastic and neoplastic changes (Yager, 1993). With time the connective tissue may condense to form collagen (Yager, 1993). The ground substance secreted by the myoepithelial cells can be converted to cartilage and may undergo secondary ossification to bone (Yager, 1993). In benign tumors this myoepithelial component may predominate. To confound the cellular picture, an inflammatory, cystic, or necrotic component may be superimposed within areas of hyperplasia, dysplasia, metaplasia, or neoplasia (Brodey, 1983).

With lobular hyperplasia, epithelial cells exhibit little pleomorphism. Papillary clusters with basophilic epithelium may be observed. A brown-green fluid with low cellularity may be aspirated from cystic cavitations. Foam cells laden with blue-green pigment may be present (Maddux, 1999).

Feline Mammary Fibroadenomatous Hyperplasia (Figs. 15-9 to 15-11)

Clinical Diagnosis

Feline fibroadenomatous hyperplasia is observed most frequently in young intact females or induced in older animals after the use of natural and synthetic progesterone compounds in male and female cats (Hayden, 1989; Yager, 1993). One or more glands become enlarged as a result of proliferation of stromal components and, to a lesser degree, ductal epithelium. The mammary enlargement is rapid and usually benign

(Hayden, 1989). Regression may occur spontaneously or after ovariohysterectomy.

Cytological Diagnosis

Mammary aspirates range from low to high cellularity and may include small clusters of epithelial cells with mild to moderate anisocytosis and low to high N:C ratio. Stromal cells are usually prominent and appear highly reactive with increased N:C ratio and prominent nucleoli. Pink intercellular substance is often prominent. One report described two distinct cell populations. The first was a uniform population of cuboidal epithelial cells in clusters. These epithelial cells had round nuclei, small nucleoli, and scant cytoplasm. The second mesenchymal population was embedded in a delicate pink extracellular matrix. These cells were spindle-shaped with oval nuclei and indistinct cytoplasmic boundaries (Mesher, 1997).

NEOPLASTIC DISEASE

Canine Mammary Tumors (Figs. 15-12 to 15-21)

Clinical Diagnosis

Mammary tumors account for about 50% of the neoplasms submitted from bitches for histological examination (Bostock, 1992; Gilbertson, 1983). About 95% of canine mammary tumors are now considered to be epithelial in origin, with less than 5% of mesenchymal origin (Brodey, 1983; Yager, 1993). About 20% of epithelial tumors are malignant based on histology, behavior, and survival times (Yager, 1993), in contrast to the 50% traditionally classified as malignant based only on histological classification (Brodey, 1983; O'Keefe, 1995). The primary mesenchymal tumors are predominantly osteosarcomas and fibrosarcomas and have a very poor prognosis (Yager, 1993).

The single most important criteria for predicting biological behavior is infiltration into surrounding tissue or vessels (Allen, 1986; Yager, 1993). Tumor size and degree of histological or nuclear differentiation provide additional predictive value (Allen, 1986; Gilbertson, 1983; Yager, 1993). Where invasion is evident clinically or histologically, 80% of bitches will be dead within 2 years, and most within the first year. In contrast, if no invasion is evident, 80% will remain alive after 2 years (Yager, 1993). This important criterion, invasion, is unavailable to the cytologist unless provided by the clinical evidence.

The progression from papillary to tubular to solid to anaplastic architecture is associated with decreasing median survival times (Gilbertson, 1983; Yager, 1993). The papillary/tubular tumors with well-differentiated epithelial cells and abundant myoepithelial stroma and cartilage or osseous metaplasia, but without invasiveness, account for approximately 80% of canine mammary tumors (Yager, 1993). These tumors, formerly classified as either benign or malignant mixed mammary tumors, may grow to a large size and become ulcerated but have a low expectation for invasion or metastasis (Yager, 1993). Classification of papillary and tubular tumors on the basis of histopathology, independent of infiltration or metastasis, can be challenging and appears to have limited prognostic value (Allen, 1986; Gilbertson, 1983). Nuclear differentiation and lymphocytic infiltration have some significance for predicting malignancy (Gilbertson, 1983).

CYTOLOGICAL DIAGNOSIS

Cytological examination of nipple secretion is useful for identification of inflammatory but seldom neoplastic pathology. The preferred technique, FNA biopsy, is readily obtained from mammary tumors.

A few studies examining cytological diagnosis of mammary tumors are available, but they use histopathology and not biological behavior as the standard (Allen, 1986; Griffiths, 1984; Hellman, 1989; Ménard, 1986). Some details of these studies are described. In one study using both Romanowsky's and Papanicolaou's stains, 8 of 19 mammary carcinomas were classified as malignant (Griffiths, 1984). Two tumors diagnosed cytologically as carcinomas were classified as histologically benign, that is, false positive. Biological behavior was not reported (Griffiths, 1984).

In the most detailed study, aspiration cytology with alcohol fixation and Papanicolaou's staining was used to examine 91 canine mammary masses (Allen, 1986). Adequate cytological and histological samples were obtained from 75 lesions in 33 dogs. A cytological grading system was established to assist as predictors of malignancy. On histological examination of these 75 masses, 36 were classified as malignant, 33 were benign tumors, and 6 were lobular hyperplasia. Because only five dogs had died within 1 year as a result of mammary cancer, a critical analysis of the prognostic significance for the cytological criteria could not be made. Ten of 20 cytological criteria correlated with the histological criteria of malignancy. Variation in nuclear size and macronuclei were significant criteria of malignancy, whereas absence was important in excluding malignancy. Nuclear molding and abnormal multinucleated cells did not differentiate malignant from benign lesions. The proposed grading scheme resulted in a cytological sensitivity for malignant tumors of 25% and 17% for the two cytopathologists (Allen, 1986). If the histological classification, as compared with biological activity, overestimated malignancy, these cytological observations are encouraging.

As part of a larger study, two of six mammary tumors were correctly diagnosed as malignant, three were suspicious, and no evaluation was possible for one (Ménard, 1986). The authors state that the results from fine-needle aspirates were poor because of specimen quality, including necrosis, contamination with blood and inflammatory cells, and dense cell clumps with little detail (Ménard, 1986).

In a study of DNA analysis in 84 tumors from 76 dogs, cytological diagnosis was compared with histological classification (Hellman, 1989). Cytology smears were prepared from surgically removed tumors. Staining methods were not described, and biological behavior after surgery was not reported. According to histological classification, 51 tumors were malignant and 33 were benign. On cytological examination, 21 tumors were malignant, 9 were suspicious, 45 were benign, and 9 were classified as being inadequate samples. Of 42 histologically classified carcinomas, on cytological examination, 23 were malignant, 14 were benign, and 5 had inadequate samples. Two histologically benign tumors were false positives on cytology, diagnosed as malignant and suspicious cytologically. The reliability of FNA biopsies was summarized as sensitivity 65%, specificity 94%, positive predictive value 93%, negative predictive value 67%, and accuracy 79% (Hellman, 1989).

The presentation of canine mammary tumors as a continuum from hyperplasia to adenoma to carcinoma makes differentiation difficult using aspiration cytology. Epithelial clusters and sheets can be observed from benign and malignant lesions (Allen, 1986). Poor intercellular cohesion did not help differentiate benign from malignant tumors, a useful criterion in human mammary lesion aspirates (Allen, 1986). The pink cartilaginous ground substance observed as small deposits or as a diffuse background may be present in both benign and malignant tumors. Cell morphology, primarily nuclear criteria, correlate poorly with the histological classification (Allen, 1986; Hellman, 1989). In contrast, anaplastic carcinomas, which are associated with a poor prognosis, should be identifiable if representative cells have been aspirated. As with most carcinomas, the primary criteria include clusters of epithelial cells that have marked anisokaryosis, hyperchromasia, and high N:C ratio. Occasional acinar arrangements and large secretory vacuoles may be visible. In mixed benign and malignant tumors, epithelial, fibrous, cartilaginous, osseous, and myoepithelial cells may be seen (Barton, 1992).

Because most histological classification systems have poor predictive value for biological behavior, the diagnostic value of cytology is still unproved. Prospective studies that include biological behavior are required to document the diagnostical and prognostic value of aspiration cytology for canine mammary tumors.

Malignant Mixed Mammary Tumor

CLINICAL AND CYTOLOGICAL DIAGNOSES

Carcinosarcomas, uncommon malignant mammary tumors of dogs, demonstrate the usual characteristics of malignancy in both the epithelial and stromal components (Brodey, 1983). Sarcomas are uncommon and may be difficult to differentiate from mixed tumors.

Most sarcomas are osteosarcomas or fibrosarcomas (Yager, 1993).

Feline Mammary Carcinoma (Figs. 15-22 to 15-25)

CLINICAL DIAGNOSIS

In cats, mammary tumors are common, with an incidence preceded only by skin tumors and lymphoma (Dorn, 1968; MacEwen, 1984a). Intact females have a higher risk of developing mammary cancer (Hayes, 1985). Mammary tumors have been reported in cats from 9 months to 19 years, with a median age of 10 years (Hayes, 1985). From 85% (Weijer, 1972) to over 90% (Yager, 1993) of feline mammary tumors are malignant, and most are adenocarcinomas (Weijer, 1972). Feline malignant mammary tumors tend to metastasize to local lymph nodes and lung (MacEwen, 1984). With surgery alone the median survival time is 10 to 12 months (Weijer, 1972), but cats with small tumors have enhanced survival time and a lower recurrence rate (MacEwen, 1984).

CYTOLOGICAL DIAGNOSIS

Differentiation from mammary fibroadenomatous hyperplasia must be considered in younger cats or if history includes progesterone therapy. Because reliability of cytological criteria differentiating hyperplasia from malignancy does not appear to have been reported, the criteria of malignancy as used for canine anaplastic carcinoma is recommended.

References

Allen, S.W., Prasse, K.W., and Mahaffey, E.A. Cytologic differentiation of benign from malignant canine mammary tumors. *Vet Pathol* 23:649-655, 1986.

Barton, C.L. Diagnostic cytology of the urogenital system. *Proc 10th ACVIM Forum*, San Diego, pp 770-782, 1992.

Bostock D.E., Moriarty, J., and Crocker, J. Correlation between histologic diagnosis mean nucleolar organizer region count and prognosis in canine mammary tumors. *Vet Pathol* 29:381-385, 1992.

Brodey, R.S., Goldschmidt, M.H., and Roszel, J.R. Canine mammary gland neoplasms. *J Am Anim Hosp Assoc* 19: 61-81, 1983.

Dorn, C.R., Taylor, D.O.N., Schneider, R., et al: Survey of animal neoplasms in Alameda and Contra Costa counties, California, II. Cancer morbidity in dogs and cats from Alameda county. *J Natl Cancer Inst* 40:307-318, 1968.

Gilbertson, S.R., Kurzman, I.D., Zachrau, R.E., et al. Canine mammary epithelial neoplasms: biologic implications of morphologic characteristics assessed in 232 dogs. *Vet Pathol* 20:127-142, 1983.

Griffiths, G.L., Lumsden, J.H., and Valli, V.E.O. Fine needle aspiration cytology and histologic correlation in canine tumours. *Vet Clin Pathol* 13:13-17, 1984.

Hayden, D.W., Barnes, D.M., and Johnson, K.H. Morphologic changes in the mammary gland of megestrol acetate-treated and untreated cats: a retrospective study. *Vet Pathol* 26:104-113, 1989.

Hayes, A.A. and Mooney, S. Feline mammary tumours. *Vet Clin North Am Small Anim Pract* 15:512-520, 1985.

Hellman, E. and Lingren, A. The accuracy of cytology in diagnosis and DNA analysis of canine mammary tumours. *J Comp Pathol* 101:443-449, 1989.

MacEwen, E.G., Hayes, A.A., Harvey, H.J., et al. Prognostic factors for feline mammary tumors. *J Am Vet Med Assoc* 185:201-204, 1984a.

MacEwen, E.G., Hayes, A.A., Mooney, S., et al. Evaluation of effect of levamisole on feline mammary cancer. *J Biol Response* 5:541-546, 1984b.

Maddux, J.M. and Shull, R.M. Subcutaneous glandular tissue: mammary, salivary, thyroid and parathyroid. In *Diagnostic Cytology of the Dog and Cat*. R.L Cowell, R.D. Tyler, and J.H. Meinkoth (eds). Mosby, St Louis, 1999.

Ménard, M., Fontaine, M., and Morin, M. Fine needle aspiration biopsy of malignant tumors in dogs and cats: a report of 102 cases. *Can Vet J* 27:504-510, 1986.

Mesher, C.I. What is your diagnosis? *Vet Clin Pathol* 26:4,13, 1997.

O'Keefe, D.A. Tumours of the genital system and mammary glands. In *Textbook of Veterinary Internal Medicine*. S.J. Ettinger and E.C. Feldman (eds). WB Saunders, Philadelphia, 1995.

Rozel, J.F. *Cells in canine mammary fluids associated with parturition, pseudocyesis, and tumor*. Doctoral dissertation, Oklahoma State University, Stillwater, Okla, 1975.

Weijer, K.O., Head, K.W., Misdorp, W., et al. Feline malignant mammary tumors. I. Morphology and biology: some comparisons with human and canine mammary carcinomas. *J Natl Cancer Inst* 49:1697–1704.

Yager, J.A., Scott, D.W., and Wilcock, B.P. The skin and appendages. In *Pathology of Domestic Animals*. ed 4. K.V.F. Jubb, P.C. Kennedy, and N. Palmer (eds). Academic Press, San Diego, 1993.

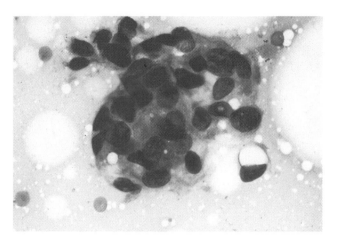

FIG. 15-1. Canine. Imprint. Normal nonlactating mammary gland. Epithelial cells with mild heterogeneity, anisokaryosis, and basophilic cytoplasm. These cells are most consistent with ductular origin. (×250.)

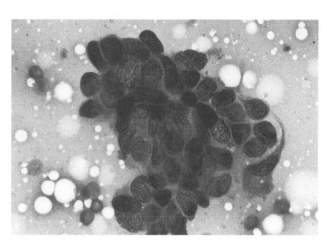

FIG. 15-2. Canine. Imprint. Normal mammary gland. Cluster of ductular epithelial cells illustrating mild variation in size, density, N:C ratio, and chromatin pattern for cells from noninflammatory healthy tissue. (×250.)

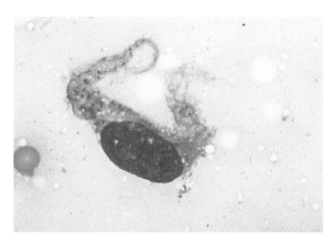

FIG. 15-3. Canine. Imprint. Normal mammary gland. Huge spindle-shaped cell with oval nucleus and granular cytoplasm likely of stromal origin. Myoepithelial cells are expected to have small, bipolar nuclei that can be observed within clusters of epithelial cells or as bare nuclei. (×500.)

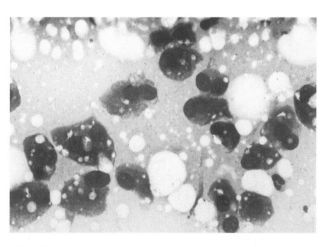

FIG. 15-4. Canine. Imprint. Normal lactating mammary gland. Disassociated epithelial cells with round nuclei, some binucleation, and basophilic vacuolated cytoplasm. The background density and large vacuoles are consistent with milk secretion. (×200.)

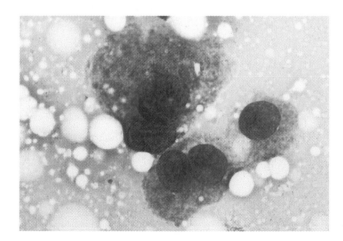

FIG. 15-5. Canine. Imprint. Normal lactating mammary gland. (Same case as Fig. 15-4.) Epithelial cells with round nuclei, indistinct chromatin patterns, large nucleoli, and basophilic granular cytoplasm. Large, extracellular, clear vacuoles suggest lipid accumulation. (×400.)

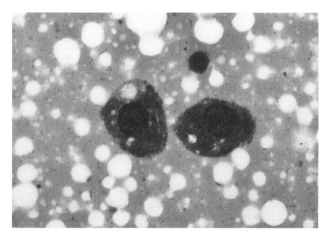

FIG. 15-6. Canine. Imprint. Normal lactating mammary gland. Epithelial cells with moderate N:C ratio, prominent nucleoli, and basophilic granular cytoplasm containing large vacuoles. The dense basophilic background with clear, round vacuoles is consistent with normal mammary secretion. (×400.)

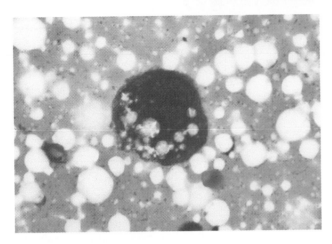

FIG. 15-7. Canine. Imprint. Normal lactating mammary gland. Large epithelial cell with binucleation; abundant vacuoles in cytoplasm and background indicative of secretory function. (×400.)

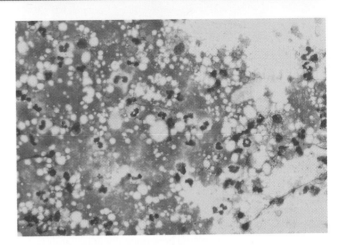

FIG. 15-8. Canine. Milk from a lactating healthy bitch. Note the amorphous to vacuolated dense background and the mixture of neutrophils and macrophages. Leukostat stain. (×125.)

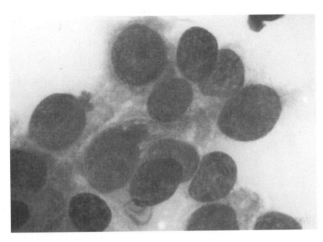

FIG. 15-9. Feline. Fine needle. Feline mammary fibroadenomatous hyperplasia. Cells with large, oval nuclei; moderate anisokaryosis; small, indistinct nucleoli; and gray-blue cytoplasm with indistinct boundaries. (×400.)

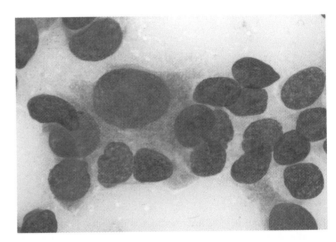

FIG. 15-10. Feline. Fine needle. Feline mammary fibroadenomatous hyperplasia. (Same case as Fig. 15-9.) Mildly cohesive epithelial cells, moderate anisokaryosis, and moderate to high N:C ratio. Although the extreme nuclear variation associated with carcinoma is not usually seen with this syndrome, clinical history is vital for correct interpretation. (×400.)

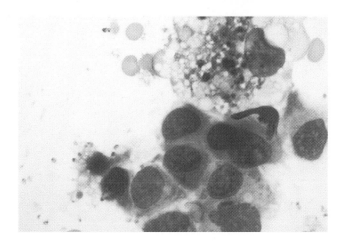

FIG. 15-11. Feline. Fine needle. Feline mammary fibroadenomatous hyperplasia. Cuboidal epithelial cells with moderate N:C ratio and bland nuclear chromatin. Blue-green pigment within macrophages is observed frequently in mammary cytological preparations. (×400.)

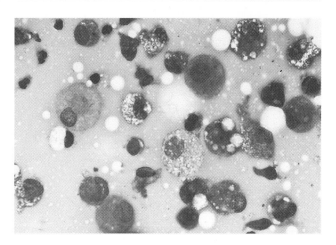

FIG. 15-12. Canine. Fine needle. Mammary tumor. High cellularity. Heterogeneous large, round epithelial cells with low N:C ratio, macrophages, small spindle cells, and a few neutrophils. Differentiation as to origin of the single round cells with prominent cytoplasmic vacuolation and occasional blue-green pigment may be difficult, for example, secretory cells or macrophages. (×200.)

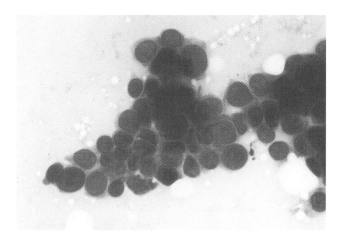

FIG. 15-13. Canine. Fine needle. Mammary carcinoma. Papillary arrangement of cells with marked anisokaryosis, hyperchromasia, high N:C ratio, and indistinct cytoplasmic borders. (×250.)

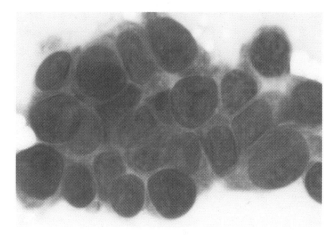

FIG. 15-14. Canine. Fine needle. Mammary carcinoma. (Same case as Fig. 15-13.) Round to oval epithelial cells with high N:C ratio; marked anisokaryosis; large, irregular nucleoli; and a few nuclei that appear to be in early prophase. (×500.)

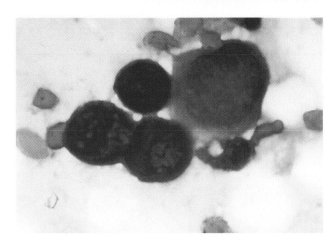

FIG. 15-15. Canine. Fine needle. Mammary carcinoma. Epithelial cells with marked anisokaryosis, hyperchromatic nuclei, and high N:C ratio. The discrete cytoplasmic vacuoles overlying the nuclei are consistent with secretory activity but are also similar to early squamous differentiation when using Romanowsky's stains. (×500.)

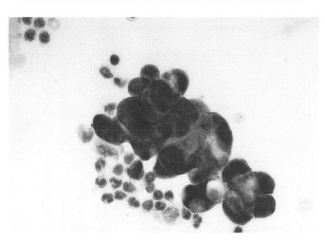

FIG. 15-16. Canine. Fine needle. Mammary carcinoma. Loosely cohesive epithelial cells with high N:C ratio, hyperchromasia, and acinar or papillary arrangement. Conservative interpretation is required because of the presence of neutrophils and the potential for epithelial proplasia (atypia) when inflammation is present. (×250.)

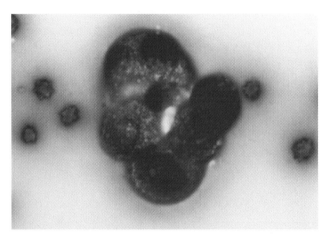

FIG. 15-17. Canine. Pleural fluid. Mammary carcinoma. Cluster of cells with hyperchromatic nuclei that vary from 1 to 3 erythrocytes in diameter and abundant cytoplasm with fine granular vacuolated cytoplasm. These cells are consistent with exfoliating (malignant) secretory epithelial cells, that is, adenocarcinoma, as opposed to hyperplastic mesothelial cells. (×400.)

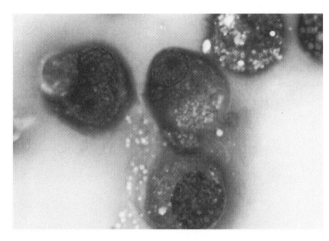

FIG. 15-18. Canine. Pleural fluid. Metastatic mammary carcinoma. (Same case as Fig. 15-17.) Single cells with prominent anisokaryosis; binucleation; large, irregular nucleoli; and basophilic cytoplasm with vacuolation consistent with malignancy of secretory origin epithelial cells. (×400.)

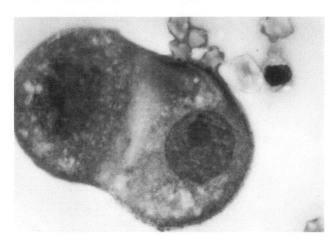

FIG. 15-19. Canine. Pleural fluid. Metastatic mammary carcinoma. Large epithelial cells with large nuclei, prominent heterochromatin and nucleoli, moderate anisokaryosis, and vacuolated cytoplasm consistent with secretory activity. (×500.)

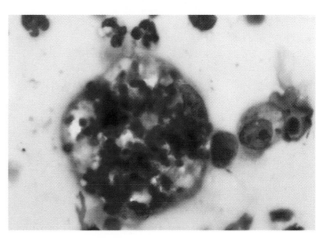

FIG. 15-20. Canine. Fine needle. Mammary carcinoma. Large cell distended with irregular round aggregates of blue-green pigment consistent with milk precursors. Necrosis and hemorrhage, often associated with mammary carcinoma, can lead to similar cytoplasmic pigmentation. (×400.)

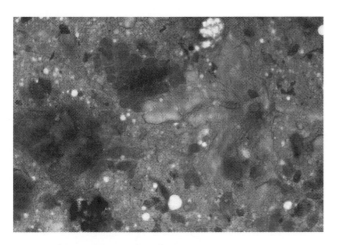

FIG. 15-21. Canine. Imprint. Mammary tumor. Prominent eosinophilic material, likely collagenous matrix, can be seen in any collagen-producing tumors. (×100.)

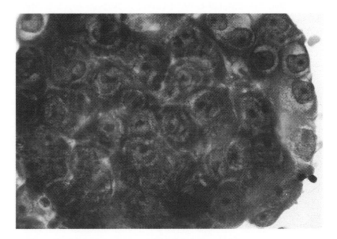

FIG. 15-22. Feline. Pleural fluid. Metastatic mammary carcinoma. Tightly associated cells with round nuclei; finely stippled chromatin; marked anisokaryosis; high N:C ratio; and large, irregular nucleoli. (×100.) (Courtesy Joyce S. Knoll, 1988.)

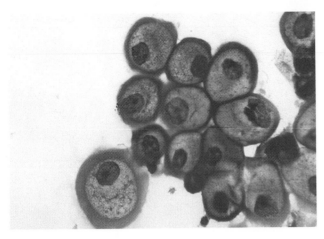

FIG. 15-23. Feline. Pleural fluid. Metastatic mammary carcinoma. (Same case as Fig. 15-22.) Individual cells exfoliating within the pleural fluid. Loosely cohesive large cells have pleomorphic nuclei and nucleoli and abundant basophilic cytoplasm with peripheral condensation. Original cytological interpretation was "degenerating carcinoma cells or an unusual manifestation of reactive mesothelial cells." (×200.) (Courtesy Joyce S. Knoll, 1988.)

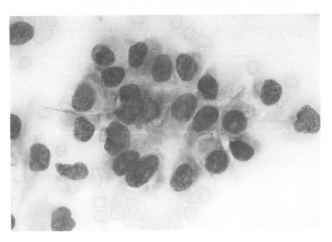

FIG. 15-24. Feline. Fine needle. Mammary carcinoma. Loosely cohesive cells with mild anisokaryosis, moderate N:C ratio, and inconspicuous nucleoli. Confirmation of malignancy can be difficult in well-differentiated carcinomas. (×250.)

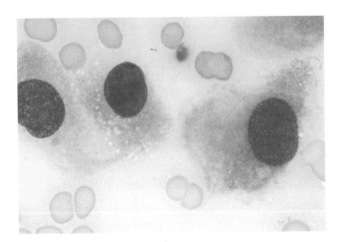

FIG. 15-25. Feline. Fine needle. Mammary carcinoma. (Same case as Fig. 15-24.) Increased magnification of similar cells illustrating moderately large nuclei, fine chromatin, prominent nucleoli, and abundant basophilic cytoplasm. Clinical details are essential when evaluating mammary cytological preparations. (×500.)

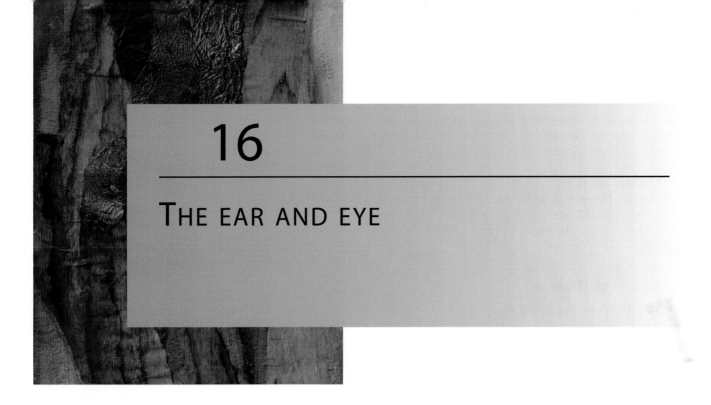

16

THE EAR AND EYE

■ *EAR*

INTRODUCTION

Diseases of the ear are very common in dogs and cats (Cowell, 1999; Scott, 1980). These disorders are often multifactorial and may involve the pinna alone or may be more extensive, involving the outer, middle, or inner ear canal (McKeever, 1997; Scott, 1980). The skin of the pinna may be involved in a variety of localized and generalized skin diseases. The external ear canal is readily accessible for diagnostical and therapeutic purposes and includes the vertical and horizontal canals terminating at the tympanic membrane.

TECHNIQUES

In the majority of cases a swab of the horizontal canal may be rolled onto a clean, dry glass slide. If the tympanic membrane is ruptured, swabs may be taken directly from the middle ear. Slides may be heat or alcohol fixed, or air dried, and stained by routine hematological stains. The swab may be obtained through the end of the otoscope or by visual placement. Gram's staining permits further microbial identification and may be supported by bacterial or fungal culture. In the case of suspected mite or fungal infection, slides may be examined unstained because some of the agents may be removed in the staining process.

FNA biopsy, scrapings, or imprints may be useful to diagnose exophytic masses identified on physical or otoscopic examination. Excess ear canal fluid may be collected by aspiration for cytocentrifugation or microbiological techniques. Scrapings of the skin of the earflaps may assist in the diagnosis of localized pinnal disease. Cytological examination facilitates identification of inflammatory cells, organisms, parasites, blood, cerumen, and/or atypical cells (Chickering, 1988; Cowell, 1999). Tissue biopsy has been reported to be the only technique available for the definitive diagnosis of otitis media (Little, 1991), and it may give a specific diagnosis in cases of polyps and in some autoimmune skin diseases (Rosser, 1988). Ancillary testing to rule out underlying dermatological or endocrine disease, or tympanic bullae involvement, may augment the cytological diagnosis.

PINNA

NONNEOPLASTIC DISEASE

Clinical signs in the animal with ear disease vary depending on the duration and severity of the disease, unilateral or bilateral involvement, therapeutics, and the extent and nature of any underlying disease. Typically the animal is presented with localizing signs, including heat, pain, pruritus, redness, swelling, and otorrhea (Pope, 1995).

Aural Hematoma

CLINICAL DIAGNOSIS
Auricular hematomas are frequently encountered, although cytology is rarely necessary to confirm the diagnosis. They occur most frequently in dogs with pendulous pinnae (Angarano, 1988). Hematomas may arise with or without concurrent otitis externa or otitis media (Dubielzig, 1994). Although the etiology is not clear, traumatic and immune-mediated causes have

been suggested (Angarano, 1988; Dubielzig, 1984; Griffin, 1994; Kuwahara, 1986). In cats, aural hematoma is most commonly seen in younger patients, secondary to otodectic mange. There is no gender or breed predilection (Scott, 1980).

CYTOLOGICAL DIAGNOSIS

Cytological features include low cellularity predominated by red cells and macrophages. The latter cells may show fresh erythrocytophagy and/or hemosiderin.

Parasitic Pinnal Disease

CLINICAL AND CYTOLOGICAL DIAGNOSES

Parasitic disease may cause pruritus and exudation of the pinna. *Sarcoptes scabiei*, *Demodex canis*, and *Notoedres cati* may be identified on skin scrapings and may be accompanied by variable numbers of mixed inflammatory cells, including eosinophils and mast cells, keratinized debris, and scale. Neutrophils, lymphocytes, and plasma cells may be attracted as a result of self-inflicted skin trauma. Fly bite dermatitis is most often identified by history (seasonality, exposure to *Simuliidae* sp. or *Stomoxys calcitrans*), the typical target skin lesions, and focal eosinophilic infiltration of the affected sites.

Infectious Diseases of the Pinna

CLINICAL AND CYTOLOGICAL DIAGNOSES

Infectious diseases of the pinna include localized bacterial or fungal infections. *Staphylococcus intermedius* is the most common bacterial isolate recovered (Berg, 1984). Cytology may reveal abundant neutrophils, crusts and debris, and intracellular cocci. Dermatophytes are frequently diagnosed in feline pinnal disease (Angarano, 1988). Microscopic examination of the hair may be helpful in confirming fungal dermatitis.

Immune-Mediated Pinnal Disease

CLINICAL DIAGNOSIS

Immune-mediated diseases often underlie disorders of the pinna. Canine atopy; food hypersensitivity; and autoimmune dermatoses, such as pemphigus foliaceous, pemphigus erythematosus, systemic lupus erythematosus, and discoid lupus erythematosus, may affect the skin of the pinna (Roth, 1988). Lesions of dermatomyositis often involve the skin of the pinna. The cause is unknown, and it is reported in collies and collie types of dogs.

CYTOLOGICAL DIAGNOSIS

Skin scrapings or imprints of blistered areas may reveal variable desquamation, crusting, and a prominent neutrophilic and/or eosinophilic infiltrate without evidence of sepsis or neutrophil toxicity. Acantholytic keratinocytes may be identified as large, round, basophilic single cells with pyknotic nuclei and are one of the hallmark findings in autoimmune dermatoses (Angarano, 1988; Chickering, 1988).

NEOPLASTIC DISEASE

CLINICAL DIAGNOSIS

The ears are not a common site for cutaneous tumors. The two most common tumors of the pinna are squamous cell carcinoma and histiocytoma (Angarano, 1988). Squamous cell carcinoma is a common sequela of chronic solar-induced actinic keratosis in white-haired cats. In one study of 61 cases of feline squamous cell carcinoma, 18 cats (30%) had lesions on the pinnae, and 13 (21%) had bilateral ear involvement. In this same study, five cats (8%) had both pinnal and nasal planum involvement. Of the cats with tumors, 95% were white or partially white animals (Lana, 1997). Ages of reported cases ranged from 5 to 17 years.

Histiocytomas are often found in young dogs, under the age of 4 years and often less than 2 years of age. These tumors may be ulcerated or crusted. They are benign and often spontaneously regress within weeks (Angarano, 1988).

CYTOLOGICAL DIAGNOSIS

The cytological appearance of squamous cell carcinoma cells varies with the degree of differentiation, as described in Chapter 4. It may be difficult to differentiate between epithelial dysplasia and neoplasia, especially with well-differentiated carcinomas.

The cytological features of histiocytoma are described in Chapter 4. Other tumors that are known to involve the pinna less frequently include papillomas, basal cell tumors, sebaceous gland tumors, fibromas/fibrosarcomas, and melanomas (Scott, 1980). The cytological appearance of tumors in this location are similar to the morphology observed in other body sites (Chapter 4).

EAR CANAL

NORMAL EAR CANAL (Figs. 16-1 to 16-2)

CYTOLOGICAL DIAGNOSIS

Cytological examination of the normal ear canal may reveal variable numbers of keratinized epithelial cells and small amounts of pale yellow ceruminous debris. Cerumen is a combination of desquamated cornified squamous epithelial cells and the oily secretion of the sebaceous and ceruminous glands (Chickering, 1988). Bacteria are absent or rarely found, and inflammatory cells are not present (Chickering, 1988; Cowell, 1999;

Dickson, 1983). *Malassezia canis* (formerly known *Pityrosporum pachydermatitis*) may be found in low numbers in normal ears and has been reported in 49% of normal dogs and 23% of normal cats (Baxter, 1976).

NONNEOPLASTIC DISEASE

Otitis Externa (Fig. 16-3)

CLINICAL DIAGNOSIS

Otitis externa is a very common disorder of the ear canal of dogs and cats (August, 1986). The prevalence of otitis externa has been reported to range from 5% to 20% in dogs and 2% to 10% in cats (August, 1986; Dickson, 1983; Scott, 1980). Otitis externa most frequently affects middle-aged dogs (Cowell, 1999). Otitis externa is less common in cats compared with dogs, although it is the most common ear disease in young cats 1 to 2 years of age (range 2 months to 16 years) (Scott, 1980).

CYTOLOGICAL DIAGNOSIS

Cytological evaluation of otic exudate has been reported as the most valuable technique for diagnosing etiological agents in the patient with otitis externa (Rosser, 1988). Smears of otic secretions reveal variable amounts of keratinaceous debris, red blood cells (in cases with ulceration of the skin of the canal), neutrophils, epithelial cells, and bacteria. Bacterial cocci can often be identified and are usually *Staphylococcus* or *Streptococcus* spp. Rod bacteria may be noted in patients with *Pseudomonas aeruginosa* or *Proteus mirabilis*. Infrequently isolates have been identified as *Klebsiella, Providencia,* and *Enterobacter* (Kowalski, 1988). Mixed infections involving two or more organisms are reported in up to 30% of cases (Baba, 1981). In cats, primary bacterial otitis externa is uncommon (Scott, 1980). *Staphylococcus aureus,* β-hemolytic *Streptococcus, Pasteurella multocida, Pseudomonas aeruginosa, Proteus,* and *Escherichia coli* have been reported in this species (Scott, 1980).

The most common cause of fungal otitis externa in dogs and cats is *Malassezia canis* (Griffin, 1981). Although it is found in normal ears, *Malassezia* is found 3 times more frequently in otitic ears than in normal ears (Scott, 1980). It has been isolated in up to 80% of otitis externa cases in dogs (Logas, 1994). Mycotic otitis externa is supported by the identification of more than 10 organisms per 40× objective, or greater than 4 organisms per oil-immersion field (Cowell, 1999; Rausch, 1978). The yeast are characteristically small, dark, basophilic, broad-based budding structures that resemble the sole of a shoe. Mixed bacteria and yeast infections are not uncommon. Other fungi, such as *Candida, Aspergillus, Trichophyton, Sporothrix,* and *Mi-*

crosporum, are less frequently identified as causes of otitis (August, 1986).

The primary parasite found in otic exudate is *Otodectes cynotis* (Chickering, 1988). Otodectic mange has been identified in 5% to 10% of canine otitis externa and in up to 50% to 84% of all cases of feline otitis externa (Griffin, 1981; Scott, 1980). Less common isolates include *Demodex canis, Demodex cati, Notoedres cati, Sarcoptes scabiei, Eutrombicula alfreddugèsi,* and, in the southwestern United States, *Otobius megnini* (August, 1986). Cytological evaluation may reveal cerumen; epidermal cells; red blood cells; and variable numbers of leukocytes, including neutrophils, eosinophils, plasma cells, lymphocytes, and mast cells.

Inflammatory Polyps

CLINICAL DIAGNOSIS

Inflammatory, nonneoplastic polyps arising from the mucosa of the nasopharynx, auditory tube, or middle ear are the most common masses in the external ear canal of cats (Pope, 1995). They are most common in young cats, but affected cats have ranged in age from 3 months to 15 years, with a mean age of 3.8 years reported. There is no reported breed or gender predisposition. Although the etiology is unknown, congenital and viral (calicivirus) causes have been suggested.

CYTOLOGICAL DIAGNOSIS

Swabs of inflammatory polyps are unlikely to establish a definitive diagnosis. FNA biopsy may yield variable numbers of mixed inflammatory cells (neutrophils, macrophages, lymphocytes, and plasma cells). Ciliated columnar respiratory epithelial cells with basal vesicular nuclei and/or benign squamous epithelium may be aspirated with a variable cell harvest.

Otitis Media/Interna

CLINICAL DIAGNOSIS

Otitis media is less common than otitis externa, although the exact prevalence is not known (McKeever, 1997). Most cases of otitis media are due to extension of otitis externa in dogs (Spreull, 1976). One report found otitis media in 16% of early cases of otitis externa and in up to 50% of chronic cases (Spreull, 1976). However, because perforations in the tympanic membrane were rarely found, the question of whether perforation must precede direct extension remains unanswered (Little, 1991). Clinical signs associated with otitis media are similar to those found with otitis externa. The prognosis is good if otitis media is diagnosed early and responds to therapy. However, the prognosis is guarded in cases with osteomyelitis of the tympanic bulla.

Otitis interna is suspected to be an extension of otitis media (Chrisman, 1979). It was reported in almost half of 83 cases of peripheral vestibular syndrome in dogs (Schunk, 1983). The prognosis is good in early cases that are treated appropriately. In cases with ascending brain stem infection or meningitis, or in some rapidly progressive central vestibular infections, the prognosis is poor (Shell, 1988). Clinical signs, such as nystagmus, limb ataxia, disorientation, circling, and difficult ambulation, may be noted with otitis interna.

CYTOLOGICAL DIAGNOSIS

The cytological findings in otitis media are similar to those of otitis externa and allow for the identification of etiological agents, inflammatory and epithelial cells. Cole et al (1998) concluded that the three most common organisms isolated from the horizontal and middle ear are *Staphylococcus intermedius,* yeast, and *Pseudomonas* spp.

In a recent study of 23 dogs with chronic bilateral otitis externa, cytological examination assisted in the diagnosis of otitis media in 38 of 46 (82.6%) of ears evaluated (Cole, 1998). However, when compared with bacterial culture results, cytological evaluation of middle ear exudate had a low rate of detection, identifying cocci and rods successfully in 25% and 26.3% of cases, respectively.

NEOPLASTIC DISEASE

CLINICAL DIAGNOSIS

Ear canal tumors are more common in the dog than in the cat (Cowell, 1999). They are found more frequently in the older dog and can arise from either the skin or adnexal structures. Neoplasm of the feline ear canal is uncommon (Scott, 1980). The cytological diagnosis of ear canal tumors is difficult by swab alone because cell exfoliation may be poor or the tumor may be masked by an associated inflammation. FNA biopsy may yield a higher harvest of cells for diagnosis. The clinical presentation of the animal with an ear canal tumor may be identical to that of the patient with chronic otitis externa.

Ceruminous Gland Tumors (Fig. 16-4)

CLINICAL DIAGNOSIS

Ceruminous gland tumors originate from the modified apocrine sweat glands found in the external ear canal. Although they are infrequent in both species, they are the most common tumor in the external ear canal in dogs and cats. Chronic inflammation and the products of cerumen decomposition have been suggested to be carcinogenic, possibly predisposing dysplastic glands to progress to neoplasia (Scott, 1980). Ceruminous gland tumors are usually unilateral but may be bilateral (Theon, 1994). It has been reported in cats that approximately half of these tumors are malignant (Van der Gaag, 1986), whereas in dogs, most

are benign (Pulley, 1990). In a study of 124 ceruminous gland tumors from dogs and cats, ceruminous gland adenocarcinomas were reportedly more prevalent than adenomas in both species and were more common in older animals (Moisan, 1996). The frequency of ceruminous gland tumors of any type was reported as 0.17% and 1.15% for canine and feline tumors diagnosed, respectively (Moisan, 1996). They have been reported to account for 1% to 2% of all feline tumors (Legendre, 1981). Ceruminous gland tumors are locally aggressive, invading the parotid region and the walls of the external ear canal. Recurrence is common. Distant metastasis to regional lymphatics, lungs, and distant viscera has been reported (Rogers, 1988). Ceruminous gland adenocarcinomas are very radiation-responsive tumors. The tumor-free survival time was estimated to be 39 months in a study of five dogs and six cats treated with either radiation alone or with a combination of surgery and radiation therapy (Theon, 1994).

CYTOLOGICAL DIAGNOSIS

In some cases, it may be difficult to distinguish between hyperplasia, benign disease, and malignant disease of the ceruminous glands. There is usually a good cell yield from these tumors, and cells are arranged in sheets and acinar structures. Cells from ceruminous adenomas display little atypia and are arranged in cohesive sheets with no evidence of acinar formation. Cells are large and pale-staining, with moderate to high N:C ratios, round to oval nuclei with vesicular or fine chromatin, and pale gray cytoplasm. Ceruminous adenocarcinomas show more cytological atypia with prominent hyperchromasia, anisocytosis, and anisokaryosis. The mitotic rate may be quite high.

Miscellaneous Tumors

Sebaceous gland adenoma and adenocarcinoma, basal cell carcinoma, mast cell tumor, chondroma, chondrosarcoma, trichoepithelioma, apocrine gland adenocarcinoma, histiocytoma, fibroma, fibrosarcoma, and papillomas are other neoplasms that have been reported in the ear (McKeever, 1988). Their appearance in this location resembles the morphology described in Chapter 4.

■ EYE

INTRODUCTION

Feline and canine eyes are subject to a variety of inflammatory, infectious, neoplastic, traumatic, degenerative, and anomalous conditions that may affect one or more ocular structures. It is not surprising that veterinary patients are commonly presented with ocular disease that may be a result of a very localized event or widespread systemic disorder.

TECHNIQUES

Exfoliative cytological examination of the eyelids, conjunctiva, cornea, aqueous or vitreous humor, and retrobulbar masses may aid in the diagnosis of canine and feline ocular disease. Lesions of the eyelids may be aspirated, imprinted, scraped, or swabbed in a manner similar to that used for other skin diseases. Care must be taken to remove superficial exudate. Slides are prepared and air dried or wet fixed in the standard manner for routine staining and cytology examination. Special stains, such as periodic acid–Schiff or Gomori's methenamine silver, may be requested where fungal involvement is suspected.

Cytology of conjunctival scrapings may confirm inflammatory, infectious, or neoplastic disease. Immunofluorescence testing of cytology specimens may definitively diagnose viral or chlamydial infection. Specimens for microbial culture or virus isolation should be collected before applying topical agents or manipulating ocular surface tissues. A topical anesthetic is placed in the conjunctival sac, and with gentle retropulsion of the globe, the lower eyelid and third eyelid should be exposed. A sterile Kimura platinum spatula (Spatula Platinum, Kimura, Storz Instrument Co., St. Louis) is used to scrape the palpebral surface of the third eyelid and adjacent conjunctiva (Murphy, 1988). The spatula should be scraped over the same area in one direction several times until a small droplet collects on the tip of the instrument (Lavach, 1977). The specimen is spread in a monolayer fashion on a glass slide for routine processing. Corneal lesions may be obtained in a similar manner, taking care in the patient with a deep ulcer to avoid excessive pressure, which may rupture the lesion. Multiple smears should be prepared so that different staining techniques, if preferred, may be used.

Intraocular sampling may include aspiration of iris lesions ("iris vacuuming") and aqueous and vitreous humors. In the case of iris lesions, with the patient anesthetized, the tip of a 25-gauge needle is advanced through the limbus and placed next to the lesion of interest. Capillary flow will allow collection of cells for examination. Vitreous humor sample is the most diagnostical but most traumatic to obtain and is only indicated in a blind eye with panuveitis. Aqueous humor samples may be helpful but are often nondiagnostical. Under general anesthesia, a 22- to 27-gauge needle is inserted 4 to 5 mm posterior to the corneal-scleral junction superorotemporally. The needle is directed towards the center of the eye and 0.5 to 1.0 ml of fluid is aspirated for cytology and microbiology. The cells in ocular fluids may be concentrated and preserved for cytological examination with use of a cytocentrifuge.

Orbital aspirates may be obtained with the animal anesthetized using a 1-inch, 22-gauge needle attached to a 12-ml syringe. Depending on the location of the lesion, an approach medial to the third eyelid or, alternatively, lateral and just posterior to the angle formed by the lateral orbital ligament and the zygomatic arch may be used.

EYELID

NORMAL EYELID

The eyelid is composed of thin layers of skin and palpebral conjunctiva (Prasse, 1999). The meibomian glands line the conjunctival surface of the eyelid margin, where they help prevent the evaporation of the precorneal tear film. Exfoliative cytology may reveal keratinized superficial, intermediate, or basilar squamous epithelium from the skin surface, or columnar, ciliated epithelium from the palpebral conjunctiva. A study of microbial isolates from the eyelid margin of each eye of 50 normal dogs and 50 normal cats revealed positive isolates from 94% of canine eyes and 54% of feline eyes. *Corynebacterium* spp. and *Staphylococcus* spp. were the most common isolates from the eyelids of dogs and cats, respectively (Gerding, 1990).

NONNEOPLASTIC DISEASE

CLINICAL DIAGNOSIS
Animals with eyelid disease or blepharitis may present clinically with hyperemia, chemosis, localized pain, squinting, or ocular discharge.

CYTOLOGICAL DIAGNOSIS
Bacterial blepharitis may feature many neutrophils with or without bacteria noted within and among the cells. There may be excessive debris and exudate associated with eyelid imprints and scrapings. Allergic blepharitis may be characterized by a mixed inflammatory cell infiltrate with variable numbers of neutrophils, macrophages, eosinophils, mast cells, lymphocytes, or plasma cells. Chalazion is a granuloma of the meibomian gland, whereas hordeolum is a localized abscess of the meibomian gland or eyelash. Because of the localized nature of the latter two lesions, cytology examination is rarely necessary to confirm the diagnosis.

NEOPLASTIC DISEASE

CLINICAL AND CYTOLOGICAL DIAGNOSES
The most common eyelid tumor in the dog is the meibomian gland adenoma (Kirschner, 1994). Other tumors encountered include papilloma, meibomian

gland adenocarcinoma, melanoma, histiocytoma, basal cell tumors, and squamous cell carcinoma. Squamous cell carcinoma (see Chapter 4) is one of the more frequent tumors diagnosed in feline eyelids and nictitans and is the most common feline adnexal tumor (Murphy, 1988; Williams, 1981). Melanoma, fibrosarcoma, neurofibroma, and basal cell tumor are other tumors that may involve the feline eyelid.

CONJUNCTIVA

NORMAL CONJUNCTIVA (Figs. 16-5 to 16-11)

Conjunctival mucosa covers the inner aspect of the eyelids (palpebral conjunctiva), the third eyelid, and reflects back upon the anterior sclera (bulbar conjunctiva). It extends from the lacrimal caruncle medially to the lateral canthus temporally. The palpebral layer is composed of pseudostratified columnar epithelial cells and goblet cells. The latter cells provide the preocular tear film and assist in the local immune response (Moore, 1994). Small numbers of keratinized cells have been reported from normal palpebral conjunctiva (Lavach, 1977). Goblet cells have a basilar nucleus and have variable amounts of globular, pale basophilic, intracytoplasmic mucus. These cells are most frequently recovered in the area near the fornix. The bulbar conjunctiva is a layer of noncornified squamous epithelium. Melanin granules are often detected in cells from this level. They appear as fine greenblack intracellular or extracellular granules. At the fornix, conjunctival lamina propria contains lymphoid tissue, which may be reflected in cytology specimens from this area by a mixed population of lymphocytes. Neutrophils are rare in conjunctival scrapings, and eosinophils and basophils are not found in cytological specimens from normal eyes. Occasional bacteria have been reported intracellularly or extracellularly from normal conjunctiva (Lavach, 1977; Murphy, 1988). Inclusions are not found in normal conjunctiva, but pseudoinclusions, such as ruptured nuclear debris or resulting from phagocytosed particles of recent topical therapy, may be identified (Lavach, 1977; Prasse, 1999).

NONNEOPLASTIC DISEASE

Bacterial Conjunctivitis (Figs. 16-12 to 16-18)

CLINICAL DIAGNOSIS
Conjunctivitis may be unilateral or bilateral and is usually manifested by variable hyperemia (red eye), pain, chemosis, epiphora, and lymphoid follicular hyperplasia. With chronic disease and secondary corneal involvement, blepharospasm and photophobia may be noted.

CYTOLOGICAL DIAGNOSIS
Increased numbers of neutrophils are noted in acute or chronic bacterial, fungal, and chlamydial infections of the conjunctiva. They may be well preserved or show degenerative changes, such as karyolysis. Bacteria may be noted within the cells or free in the background. Keratoconjunctivitis sicca is characterized by neutrophilic infiltration, with bacteria commonly detected on smears. Cytology specimens from "dry eye" cases may reveal numerous keratinized squamous epithelial cells with increased numbers of goblet cells and mucus. Chlamydial infections are characterized by a mixture of neutrophils, mononuclear cells, plasma cells, and multinucleated giant cells. Chlamydial inclusions may be found in the cytoplasm of epithelial cells or neutrophils, most commonly in the first 2 weeks of infection (Hoover, 1978; Murphy, 1988). These inclusions are discrete, large (3 to 5 μ) basophilic cytoplasmic bodies that often wrap around or form crescents adjacent to the nucleus. They may also be identified as aggregates of coccoid basophilic structures (elementary bodies), 0.5 to 1 μ in diameter (Prasse, 1999). Mycoplasma-induced conjunctivitis has been reported to be predominantly neutrophilic, with positive identification of clusters of pale-staining rodlike organisms on or within the epithelial cells (Campbell, 1973; Lavach, 1977; Murphy, 1988). Cytology was found to be highly sensitive in detecting mycoplasma bodies in 15 of 16 eyes scraped (Campbell, 1973).

Viral Conjunctivitis

CLINICAL AND CYTOLOGICAL DIAGNOSES
Herpes keratitis of cats is characterized by a neutrophilic conjunctivitis that is evident by day 3 of infection with FHV-1 (Murphy, 1988; Naisse, 1993). Epithelial giant cells have been reported inconsistently in association with FHV-1 infections (Bistner, 1971; Murphy, 1988). Inclusions are not seen in conjunctival smears of FHV infection (Bistner, 1971; Glaze, 1999), although intranuclear inclusions are reported to be easily detected in histological sections of affected tissue (Naisse, 1993). Based on this lack of detection of inclusions in cytology specimens and the nonspecific neutrophilic reaction, cytology has been reported to be of little value in the diagnosis of FHV-1 (Naisse, 1993). Canine distemper with secondary bacterial conjunctivitis may have an extensive neutrophilic infiltrate on conjunctival cytological examination. Basophilic to magenta inclusion bodies may be found in the cytoplasm of neutrophils and epithelial cells, although their identification lacks sensitivity in routine cases (Richardson, 1978). As the condition becomes chronic, lymphocytes and monocytes may comprise a larger proportion of the observed cellularity.

NEOPLASTIC DISEASE

CLINICAL AND CYTOLOGICAL DIAGNOSES

Tumors involving the conjunctiva may include papillomas, squamous cell carcinomas, melanomas, lipomas, hemangiomas, sarcomas, and mast cell neoplasia (Prasse, 1999; Williams, 1981). In one study of melanomas in 29 cats, there were 19 ocular tumors, of which 3 were palpebral. Metastasis occurred in all three cats with palpebral involvement (Williams, 1981). These tumors were characterized by large, heavily pigmented, anaplastic spindle and epithelioid cells arranged in groups. Neoplasms involving the nictitating membrane have been reported to include lymphomas, squamous cell carcinomas, and primary adenocarcinomas (Komaromy, 1997).

NASOLACRIMAL APPARATUS

CLINICAL AND CYTOLOGICAL DIAGNOSES

The most common lesions involving this area include inflammation of the lacrimal sac (dacryocystitis) and cystic lacrimal ducts (dacryops). Cytological specimens of dacryocystitis may be collected by flushing the upper or lower punctum and are characterized by neutrophils, macrophages, and occasionally bacteria. Dacryops often yields serosanguinous cystic fluid that has low cellularity composed of very few neutrophils, macrophages, and lymphocytes. The diagnosis of lacrimal duct cysts is usually based on cytological findings, location, and gross appearance of the lesion.

CORNEA

NORMAL CORNEA

The normal cornea is covered by noncornified stratified squamous epithelium covering a thick basal lamina (Descement's membrane). Staphylococci and streptococci are the most frequent isolates recovered from normal canine and feline eyes.

NONNEOPLASTIC DISEASE (Figs. 16-19 to 16-21)

CLINICAL AND CYTOLOGICAL DIAGNOSES

Although there are a variety of traumatic, degenerative, immune-based, nodular, ulcerative, and infectious causes of keratitis, cytology is most useful in the diagnosis of exudative and infectious corneal disorders. Cytological examination will aid in the characterization of the corneal exudate and confirmation of bacteria such as *Pseudomonas* spp. Keratomycosis is rare in dogs and cats compared with other species, such as the horse. However, *Aspergillus, Fusarium,* or

Candida may be positively identified on corneal scrapings and may require selective staining (periodic acid–Schiff or Gomori's methenamine silver) (Prasse, 1999). Although fungal lesions are rare in the cat, *Cladosporium* keratitis has been reported (Friedman, 1995). Feline eosinophilic keratitis is a disease of unknown etiology, readily identified on corneal scrapes by an abundance of eosinophils with fewer lymphocytes, plasma cells, neutrophils, and mast cells. Chronic superficial keratitis, or pannus, is characterized by a mixed inflammatory infiltrate including plasma cells. It is frequently diagnosed in German shepherds, and although the cause is unknown, an immune-mediated disorder, environmental factors, and a hereditary predisposition have been suggested (Dice, 1980). A proliferative corneal disease frequently identified in collies and collie crossbreeds known as nodular fasciitis may be examined using cytological methods and usually reveals an inflammatory component involving mixed lymphocytes, plasma cells, fibroblasts, macrophages, and neutrophils. These lesions involve the cornea at the limbus and extend into the cornea and sclera (Dice, 1980).

NEOPLASTIC DISEASE

CLINICAL AND CYTOLOGICAL DIAGNOSES

Primary corneal tumors are rare in dogs and cats. Viral papillomas are the most common primary corneal tumors in young dogs (Dice, 1980). Melanoma, hemangiosarcoma, fibrosarcoma, squamous cell carcinoma, and histiocytoma have been recognized in this site (Dice, 1980; Prasse, 1999) as described in Chapter 4.

ANTERIOR AND POSTERIOR CHAMBERS

NORMAL CYTOLOGY

Aqueous humor from normal dogs and cats has very low cellularity, with occasional mononuclear cells or melanocytes reported (Olin, 1977). Protein values were similar in both species, ranging from 0.11 to 0.55 g/L. In one study of aqueous humor from 12 healthy dogs and 15 healthy cats, cellularity was so low with such poor cell preservation that any intact cells in an aqueous humor were suggested to be abnormal (Hazel, 1985). Vitreous humor is normally acellular with rare red cells and melanin granules present (Prasse, 1999).

NONNEOPLASTIC DISEASE

CLINICAL AND CYTOLOGICAL DIAGNOSES

Aqueous centesis is an easy procedure but frequently fails to contribute to the diagnosis of intraocular diseases (Prasse, 1999; Wilke, 1994). Examination of aqueous humor was beneficial in only 3 of 37 (8%) cats and dogs examined with anterior uveitis (Olin, 1977). Two of these cases were diagnosed with lymphosarcoma. Aqueous cytology was found to be insufficiently specific to aid in the diagnosis of FIP (Olin, 1977). Infectious agents, such as bacteria, *Blastomyces dermatitidis*, and *Prototheca*, have been identified in both aqueous and vitreous humor. *Leishmania donovani* has been noted in aqueous aspirates (Prasse, 1999). Other fungi diagnosed in vitreous humor include *Cryptococcus neoformans* and *Histoplasma capsulatum*.

NEOPLASTIC DISEASE (Figs. 16-22 to 16-24)

CLINICAL AND CYTOLOGICAL DIAGNOSES

Most intraocular tumors are reported to be poorly exfoliative with the exception of lymphosarcoma (Prasse, 1999). Tumors found in the anterior uvea include ciliary body adenomas or adenocarcinomas, medulloepitheliomas, carcinomas, sarcomas, lymphosarcoma, melanomas, canine transmissible venereal tumors, and feline myeloproliferative tumors (Carlton, 1983, Prasse, 1999).

References

Angarano, D.W. Diseases of the pinna. *Vet Clin North Am Small Anim Pract* 18:869-884, 1988.

August, J.R. Diseases of the ear canal. In *The Complete Manual of Ear Care.* Veterinary Learning Systems, Lawrenceville, NJ, 1986.

Baba, E., and Fukata, T. Incidence of otitis externa in dogs and cats in Japan. *Vet Rec* 108:393-395, 1981.

Baxter, M. The association of Pityrosporum pachydermatis with the normal external ear canal of dogs and cats. *J Small Anim Pract* 17:231-234, 1976.

Berg, J.N., Wendell, D.E., Vegelweid, C., et al: Identification of the major coagulase-positive *Staphylococcus sp* of dogs as *Staphylococcus intermedius. Am J Vet Res* 45:1307, 1984.

Bistner, S.I., Carlson, J.H., Shively, J.H., et al. Ocular manifestations of feline herpes infection. *J Am Vet Med Assoc* 159:1223, 1971.

Campbell, L.H., Snyder, S.B., Reed, C.G., et al. Mycoplasma felis-associated conjunctivitis in cats. *J Am Vet Med Assoc* 163:991-995, 1973.

Carlton, W.W. Intraocular tumors. In *Comparative Ophthalmic Pathology.* R.L Peiffer (ed). Charles C Thomas, Springfield, Ill, 1983.

Chickering, W.R. Cytologic evaluation of otic exudates. *Vet Clin North Am Small Anim Pract* 18:773-782, 1988.

Chrisman, C.L. Disorders of the vestibular system. *Compend Cont Ed Pract Vet* 1:744-751, 1979.

Cole, L.K., Kwochka, K.W., Kowalski, J.J., et al. Microbial flora and antimicrobial susceptibility patterns of isolated pathogens from the horizontal ear canal and middle ear in dogs with otitis media. *J Am Vet Med Assoc* 212:534-538, 1998.

Cowell, R.L., Tyler, R.D., and Baldwin, C.J. The external ear canal. In *Diagnostic Cytology and Hematology of the Dog and Cat.* R.D. Tyler, R.L. Cowell, and J.H. Meinkoth (eds). Mosby, St Louis, 1999.

Dice, P.F. Primary corneal disease in the dog and cat. *Vet Clin North Am Small Anim Pract* 10:339-356, 1980.

Dickson, D.B. and Love, D.N. Bacteriology of the horizontal ear canal of dogs. *J Small Anim Pract* 24:413-421, 1983.

Dubielzig, R.R., Wilson, J.W., and Seireg, A.A. Pathogenesis of canine aural hematomas. *J Am Vet Med Assoc* 185: 873-875, 1984.

Friedman, D.S. Infectious feline keratoconjunctivitis. In *Current Veterinary Therapy XII.* J.D. Bonagura and R.W. Kirk (eds). WB Saunders, Philadelphia, 1995.

Gerding, P.A. and Kakoma, I. Microbiology of the canine and feline eye. *Vet Clin North Am Small Anim Pract* 20:615-625, 1990.

Glaze, M.B. and Gelatt, K.N. Feline ophthalmology. In *Veterinary Ophthalmology.* ed 3. K.N. Gelatt (ed). Williams & Wilkins, Philadelphia, 1999.

Griffin, C.E. Pinnal diseases. *Vet Clin North Am Small Anim Pract* 24:897-904, 1994.

Griffin, C.E. Otitis externa. *Comp Cont Ed Pract Vet* 3:741-749, 1981.

Hazel, S.J., Thrall, M.A., Severin, G.A., et al. Laboratory evaluation of aqueous humor in the healthy dog, cat, horse, and cow. *Am J Vet Res* 46:657-659, 1985.

Hoover, E.A., Kahn, D.E., and Langloss, J.M. Experimentally induced feline chlamydial infection (feline pneumonitis). *Am J Vet Res* 39:541-547, 1978.

Kirschner, S.E. Diseases of the eyelid. In *Saunders Manual of Small Animal Practice.* S.J. Birchard and R.G. Sherding (eds). WB Saunders, Philadelphia, 1994.

Komaromy, A.M., Ramsey, D.T., Render, J.A., et al. Primary adenocarcinoma of the gland of the nictitating membrane in a cat. *J Am Anim Hosp Assoc* 33:333-336, 1997.

Kowalski, J.J. The microbial environment of the ear canal in health and disease. *Vet Clin North Am Small Anim Pract* 18:743-754, 1988.

Kuwahara, J. Canine and feline aural hematoma: clinical, experimental, and clinicopathologic observations. *Am J Vet Res* 47:2300, 1986.

Lana, S.E., Ogilvie, G.K., Withrow, S.J., et al. Feline cutaneous squamous cell carcinoma of the nasal planum and the pinnae: 61 cases. *J Am Anim Hosp Assoc* 33:329-332, 1997.

Lavach, J.D., Thrall, M.A., Benjamin, M.M., et al. Cytology of normal and inflamed conjunctivas in dogs and cats. *J Am Vet Med Assoc* 170:722-727, 1977.

Legendre, A.M. and Krahwinkel, D.J. Feline ear tumors. *J Am Anim Hosp Assoc* 17:1035, 1981.

Little, C.J.L., Lane, J.G., and Pearson, G.R. Inflammatory middle ear disease of the dog: the pathology of otitis media. *Vet Rec* 128:293-296, 1991.

Logas, D.B. Diseases of the ear canal. *Vet Clin North Am Small Anim Pract* 24:905-919, 1994.

McKeever, P.J. and Jottes, S. Ear disease and its management. *Vet Clin North Am Small Anim Pract* 27:1523-1536, 1997.

McKeever, P.J. and Torres, S. Otitis externa, part 1: The ear and predisposing factors to otitis externa. *Comp Anim Pract* 2:7-14, 1988.

Moisan, P.G. and Watson, G.L. Ceruminous gland tumors in dogs and cats: a review of 124 cases. *J Am Anim Hosp Assoc* 32:449-453, 1996.

Moore, C.P. Conjunctiva. In *Saunders Manual of Small Animal Practice.* S.J. Birchard and R.G. Sherding (eds). WB Saunders, Philadelphia, 1994.

Murphy, J.M. Exfoliative cytologic examination as an aid in diagnosing ocular diseases in the dog and cat. *Semin Vet Med Surg (Small Anim)* 3:10-14, 1988.

Naisse, M.P., Guy, J.S., Stevens, J.B., et al. Clinical and laboratory findings in chronic conjunctivitis in cats: 91 cases (1983-1991). *J Am Vet Med Assoc* 203:834-837, 1993.

Olin, DD. Examination of the aqueous humor as a diagnostic aid in anterior uveitis. *J Am Vet Med Assoc* 171:557-559, 1977.

Pope, E.R. Feline inflammatory polyps. *Semin Vet Med Surg (Small Anim)* 10:87-93, 1995.

Prasse, K.W. and Winston, S.M. The eyes and associated structures. In *Diagnostic Cytology and Hematology of the Dog and Cat.* R.D. Tyler, R.L. Cowell, and J.H. Meinkoth (eds). Mosby, St Louis, 1999.

Pulley, L.T. and Stannard, A.A. Tumors of the skin and soft tissues. In *Tumors in Domestic Animals.* ed 3. J.E. Moulton (ed). University of California Press, Berkeley, Calif, 1990.

Rausch, F.D. and Skinner, G.W. Incidence and treatment of budding yeast in canine otitis externa. *Mod Vet Pract* 59:914-915, 1978.

Richardson, R.C. Diseases of the growing puppy. *Vet Clin North Am Small Anim Pract* 8:101, 1978.

Rogers, K.S. Tumors of the ear canal. *Vet Clin North Am Small Anim Pract* 18:859-868, 1988.

Rosser, E.J. Evaluation of the patient with otitis externa. *Vet Clin North Am Small Anim Pract* 18:765-773, 1988.

Roth, L. Pathologic changes in otitis externa. *Vet Clin North Am Small Anim Pract* 18:755-764, 1988.

Schunk, K.L. and Averill, D.R. Peripheral vestibular syndrome in the dog: a review of 83 cases. *J Am Vet Med Assoc* 182:1354-1357, 1983.

Scott, D.W. External ear disorders. *J Am Anim Hosp Assoc* 16:426-433, 1980.

Shell, L.G. Otitis media and otitis interna: etiology, diagnosis, and medical management. *Vet Clin North Am Small Anim Pract* 18:885-899, 1988.

Spreull, J.S.A. Otitis media in the dog. In *Current Veterinary Therapy V.* R.W. Kirk (ed). WB Saunders, Philadelphia, 1976.

Theon, A.P., Barthez, P.Y., Madewell, B.R., et al. Radiation therapy of ceruminous gland carcinomas in dogs and cats. *J Am Vet Med Assoc* 205:566-569, 1994.

Van der Gaag, I. The pathology of the external ear canal in dogs and cats. *Vet Q* 8:307-317, 1986.

Wilkie, D.A. Uvea. In *Saunders Manual of Small Animal Practice.* S.J. Birchard and R.G. Sherding (eds). WB Saunders, Philadelphia, 1994.

Williams, L.W., Gelatt, K.N., and Gwin, R.M. Opthalmic neoplasms in the cat. *J Am Anim Hosp Assoc* 17:999-1008, 1981.

Woog, J., Albert, D.M., Gonder, J.R., et al. Osteosarcoma in a phthisical feline eye. *Vet Pathol* 20:209-214, 1983.

FIG. 16-1. Canine. Scraping. Normal ear canal. Superficial squamous epithelial cells and debris. (×160.)

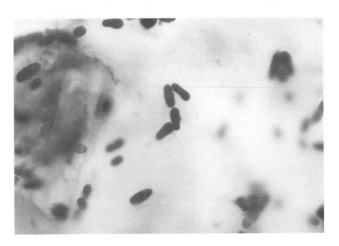

FIG. 16-2. Canine. Fine needle. Mass on eardrum. Malassezia. Several central organisms consistent with *Malassezia* sp., debris, and negative-staining cholesterol crystals. (×500.)

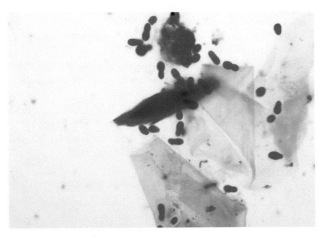

FIG. 16-3. Canine. Swab. Malassezia. Dumbbell-shaped organisms consistent with *Malassezia* sp. and superficial squamous epithelial cells. (×400.)

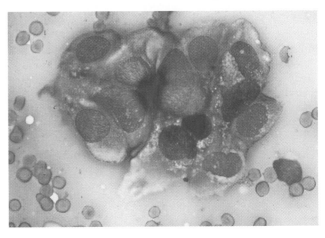

FIG. 16-4. Feline. Fine needle. Aural mass. Mixed ceruminous gland adenocarcinoma. Cohesive cluster of cells with cytological atypia. Coarse retiform nuclear chromatin, anisokaryosis, and nuclear hyperchromasia. (×312.)

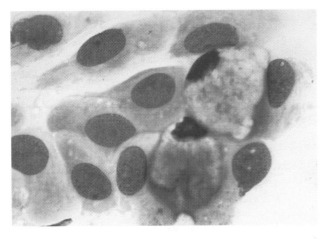

FIG. 16-5. Feline. Imprint. Normal nictitating membrane, inner surface. Uniform angular cells with amorphous nuclear chromatin and occasional large chromocenters. The cytoplasm is lightly basophilic with occasional vacuole. Two large cells have small, dense, eccentric nuclei and abundant, lightly basophilic and indistinctly vacuolated cytoplasm suggestive of mucus secretory activity. (×400.)

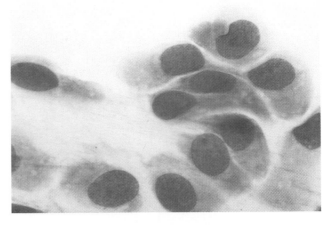

FIG. 16-6. Feline. Imprint. Normal nictitating membrane. Round to angular adjoining epithelial cells, with distinct cell borders and fine chromatin pattern. The cytoplasm is lightly basophilic. (×400.)

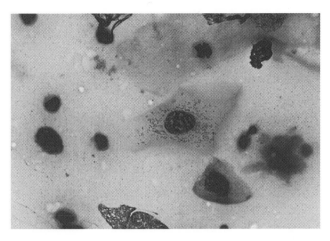

FIG. 16-7. Feline. Imprint. Conjunctiva. Normal melanin pigment within superficial epithelial cells. (×312.)

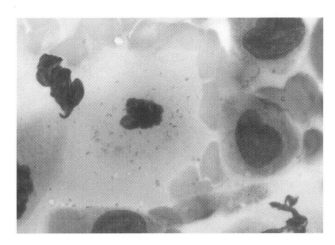

FIG 16-8. Feline. Scraping. Normal conjunctiva. Large, central, intermediate squamous epithelial cell contains moderate number of fine, elongated granules compatible with melanin pigment. Keratohyaline granules are less sharply outlined or pigmented with Wright's stain. (×500.)

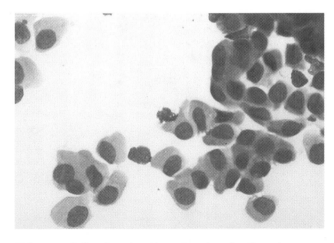

FIG. 16-9. Feline. Scraping. Normal conjunctiva. Round to angular epithelial cells, moderate uniform N:C ratio; abundant uniform cytoplasm. (×200.)

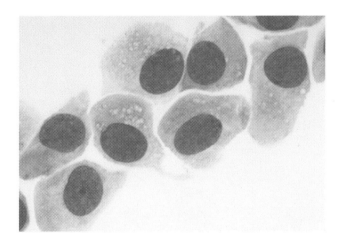

FIG. 16-10. Feline. Scraping. Normal conjunctiva. Conjunctival epithelial cells with round to oval nuclei, indistinct chromatin and nucleoli; abundant cytoplasm with uniform density and some small, indistinct, variably arranged vacuoles. (×400.)

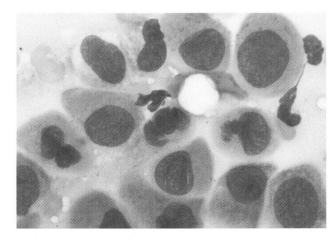

FIG. 16-11. Feline. Imprint. Normal conjunctiva. Individual round to angular epithelial cells with some variation in nuclear size, indistinct chromatin pattern and nucleoli; abundant, lightly basophilic amorphous cytoplasm containing indistinct blue-gray aggregates of RNA or precursors to keratohyaline granules. (×400.)

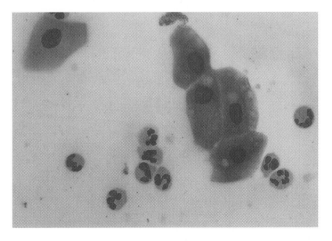

FIG. 16-12. Canine. Scraping. Suppurative nonseptic conjunctivitis. Nonlytic neutrophils and intermediate squamous epithelial cells. No evidence of etiological agents. (×200.)

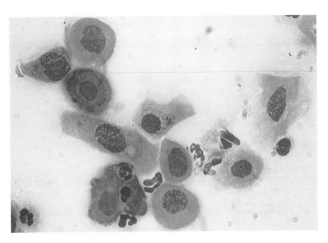

FIG. 16-13. Feline. Scraping. Suppurative nonseptic conjunctivitis. Neutrophils have mild karyolysis. A few superficial squamous epithelial cells with mild dysplasia are evident. (×312.)

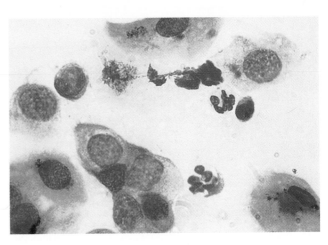

FIG. 16-14. Feline. Scraping. Conjunctiva. Melanin-laden squamous epithelial cells. There are two dense, basophilic cytoplasmic inclusions within one epithelial cell. These may represent residue from ophthalmic ointment. (×312.)

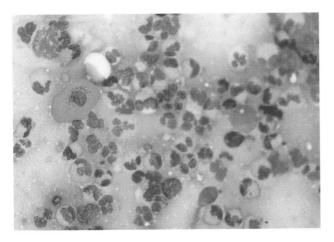

FIG. 16-15. Feline. Scraping. Eosinophilic conjunctivitis. Numerous eosinophils and a few mononuclear cells and neutrophils. A squamous epithelial cell is observed with light basophilic cytoplasm and a pyknotic nucleus. (×200.)

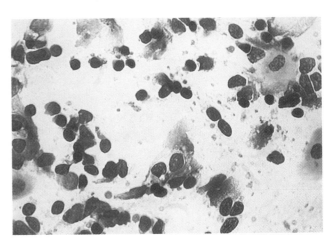

FIG. 16-16. Feline. Scraping. Lymphocytic conjunctivitis. Increased cellularity with many small, condensed, benign lymphocytes and few epithelial cells. (×250.)

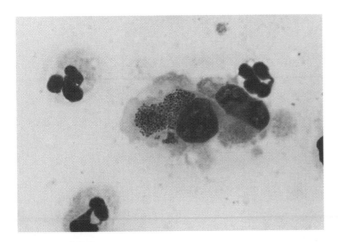

FIG. 16-17. Feline. Scraping. Chlamydial conjunctivitis. Few neutrophils surround squamous epithelial cells. The fine basophilic perinuclear inclusions in the cytoplasm of a squamous cell are the elementary bodies of *Chlamydia psittaci*. (×500.)

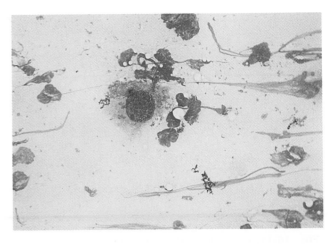

FIG. 16-18. Feline. Scraping. Mycoplasmal conjunctivitis. Squamous epithelial cell with many fine, lightly basophilic *Mycoplasma felis* organisms. Numerous lytic neutrophils in the background. (×500.)

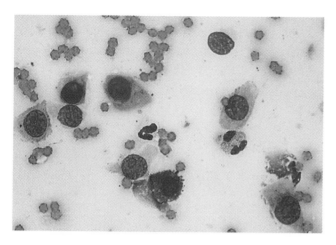

FIG. 16-19. Feline. Scraping. Eosinophilic and mast cell keratitis. Corneal epithelium, mast cells, and rare eosinophil. No etiological agents evident. (×250.)

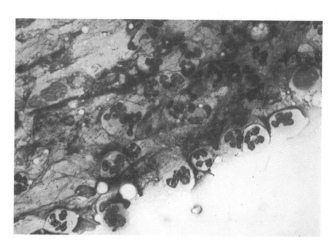

FIG. 16-20. Canine. Scraping. Suppurative bacterial keratitis. Abundant lytic cell debris in the background. Neutrophils show variable degrees of karyolysis or nuclear swelling. Rod bacteria are present intracellularly and extracellularly in large numbers. (×312.)

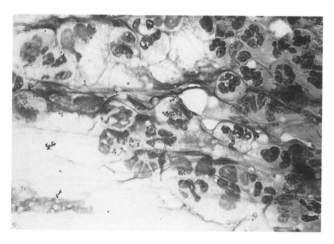

FIG. 16-21. Canine. Scraping. Suppurative bacterial keratitis. Neutrophils are present in high numbers with moderate to marked karyolysis with intracellular cocci. (×312.)

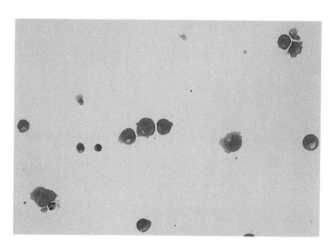

FIG. 16-22. Feline. Fine needle. Aqueous fluid. Ocular lymphoma. Increased cellularity with a population of large lymphocytes with moderate amounts of basophilic cytoplasm, and vesicular nuclei with single, pale nucleoli. Occasional small, benign lymphocytes are also present. (×50.)

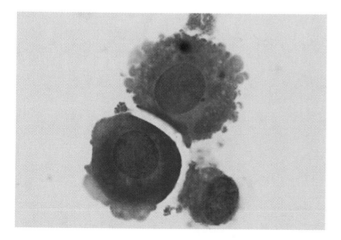

FIG. 16-23. Feline. Fine needle. Aqueous fluid. Iris melanoma. Large single cells with low N:C ratios; condensed, small central nuclei; and variable amounts of coarse intracytoplasmic pigment. Some anisokaryosis is evident. (×500.)

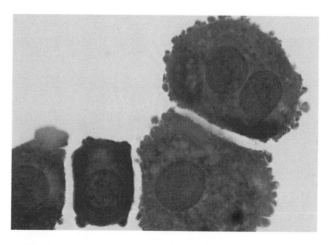

FIG. 16-24. Feline. Fine needle. Aqueous fluid. Iris melanoma. (Same case as Fig. 16-23.) Large, irregular cells with abundant intracytoplasmic pigment. (×500.)

INDEX